COPING WITH APHASIA

Coping with Aging Series

Series Editor
John C. Rosenbek, Ph.D.
Chief, Speech Pathology and Audiology Services
William S. Middleton Memorial Hospital
Madison, Wisconsin

Medical Editor
Molly Carnes, M.D.
Department of Medicine and Institute on Aging
University of Wisconsin
Madison, Wisconsin

Associate Director for
Clinical Services, Geriatric Research,
Education and Clinical Center
William S. Middleton Memorial Hospital
Madison, Wisconsin

COPING WITH APHASIA

Coping with Aging Series

Jon G. Lyon, Ph.D.

Living with Aphasia, Inc.
Mazomanie, Wisconsin

SINGULAR PUBLISHING GROUP, INC.
SAN DIEGO · LONDON

Singular Publishing Group
401 West "A" Street, Suite 325
San Diego, California 92101-7904

e-mail: singpub@singpub.com
Website: http://www.singpub.com

Typeset in 11/14 Times by So Cal Graphics
Printed in the United States of America by BookCrafters

Library of Congress Cataloging-in-Publication Data

Lyon, Jon G.
    Coping with Aphasia / Jon G. Lyon.
      p.   cm. — (Coping with aging series)
    Includes bibliographical references and index.
    ISBN 1–879105–75–6
    1. Aphasia—Popular works.   I. Title.   II. Series.
    [DNLM: 1. Aphasia—rehabilitation.   2. Aphasia—diagnosis.
   3. Aphasia—etiology.   WL 340.5 L991c 1997]
   RC425.L96   1997
   616.85'52—dc21
   DNLM/DLC
   for Library of Congress

                                              97–29700
                                               CIP

Contents

GETTING TO YOUR DESTINATION

TRAVEL AIDS AND GUIDES

Foreword

The books in the Coping With Aging Series are written for men and women coping with the challenges of aging and disease, and for their families and other caregivers. The authors are all experienced practitioners: doctors, nurses, social workers, psychologists, speech-language pathologists, pharmacists, nutritionists, audiologists, and physical and occupational therapists.

The topics of individual volumes are as varied as are the challenges that aging and disease may bring. These include: hearing loss, low vision, depression, impaired mobility, intellectual decline, speech and language impairment, disordered swallowing, bowel and bladder incontinence, loss of independence, medications, and caregiver stress. The volumes themselves, however, share common features. Foremost, they are practical, jargon-free, and responsible. Each contains professionally valid information translated into language for people who are not health care providers so that they can understand. Each contains useful advice and sections to help readers decide how they are doing and whether they need to do more, less, or something different. Each includes lists of services, suppliers, and additional readings. Each provides evidence that no single person need cope alone.

None of the volumes can substitute for appropriate professional care. However, when combined with the care, instruction, and counseling that health care providers supply, they make coping with specific problems easier. America is graying at the same time its treasury is inadequate to meet its population's needs. Thus the Coping With Aging Series offers help for people who need and want to help themselves and the ones they care for.

This volume, *Coping with Aphasia*, is written by one of America's outstanding clinicians. Dr. Lyon has spent a career working with men and women struggling to improve from and cope with the deficits of listening, talking, reading, and writing that brain damage can cause. Early in his career he grew restless with treatment approaches that concentrated only on drills and other exercises to help the aphasic person talk better. He thought there were better and more complete ways to help aphasic people and their families and caregivers get on with the business, joys, and challenges of life. Much of what he has learned over the years is included in this volume. One of its major themes is that aphasic men and women and the persons who love them need not wait for recovery to act for themselves. This book is full of suggestions about how people feel and what to do from day one. Reading it may well make a difference.

John C. Rosenbek, Ph.D.
Series Editor

Molly Carnes, M.D.
Medical Editor

Preface

Someone you love or care about has lost the ability to talk and communicate with ease. This change likely occurred abruptly, without warning. It may have come at night when your loved one was asleep or, more visibly, before the entire family as you sat around the breakfast table. Whenever its arrival, life dramatically changed for this person you love, and all those who depended on his or her preinjured self. Whether this change happened days, weeks, or even months ago, you are likely still pondering what happened. And you're wondering how you might help restore meaning and value to life, not just your loved one's, or yours, but more importantly, *yours together!*

You probably know by now that he or she suffered a stroke; that is, blood to the brain was suddenly interrupted. You may know as well that the injured portion directly monitors the use of speech, language, and communication. You've likely been told that recovery will take time and that it is too early to predict an eventual outcome. Even worse, you may have heard from a specialist, possibly a doctor, nurse, or therapist, that talking or communicating may not return. You likely couldn't bear to entertain such a possibility! Certainly, you know something quite serious has happened. But to hear that speaking won't return simply doesn't compute. You eagerly wait each day, hoping that today may bring signs of improvement and that the person you once knew might reemerge. You find yourself wondering, "What does it mean" and "How does it feel" to have this, something people keep calling *aphasia?*

This book is intended to help you cope with the complexities of what aphasia brings to everyday life. Whether you are a spouse, caregiver, daughter, son, grandchild, parent, other family member, close friend, business associate, therapist, nurse, doctor, or patient, the chapters that follow contain information and practical suggestions for making this journey easier. We have referred to you throughout these pages as *a loved one*. Whether this label truly applies or not isn't important, our intent is to aid those who care deeply about the recovery and welfare of someone who has aphasia. Also, we commonly refer to you and your loved one as *a couple* in this book. Should that designation not be appropriate, please substitute "pair" or "friends" or whatever might be more appropriate.

This book comes to you in the form of a journey. From its beginning pages, you need to know that it is purposefully loaded with lots of "cushion," padding to make the bumpy road ahead more tolerable, soothing, and passable. We did this with you in mind! By cushion, we mean the pages ahead are loaded with *abundant amounts* of explanation, examples, specifics for coping, and ways of approaching and talking to others about aphasia. Within the many explanations that follow, there are embedded "themes" that prevail throughout this entire journey. Chapter 1, for instance, begins by highlighting six common, enduring characteristics of aphasia that, if internalized and kept in mind, will make your trip much easier and more likely to be successful. These characteristics are presented in the form of guidelines, or "truths" about aphasia that do not change or diminish over time—they are as valid the first day of onset as they are 3,000 days later. For this reason, it is important to study these carefully and keep them in the forefront of your thinking and planning along the way.

Aphasia's impact on life is not as constant as the guidelines highlighted in Chapter 1. What may concern you or your loved one most on the second day after injury is not what is apt to concern you at the second month. Whatever these latter concerns may be, they are apt to be quite different from those at the second year's anniversary of onset. Because of this, you will find that this book is arranged in the form of a chronology or an extended road map that will help direct you over time. At each major juncture along the way, from hospitalization, rehabilitation, discharge, aphasia's first anniversary, second anniversary, to years later, you will find explanations of what to expect and how to cope at that time. Besides laying out your routes over time, they are specific for each traveler. At each juncture, you are given a list of common concerns and potential solutions for the person with aphasia as well as his or her caregiver. Chapters 4 through 8 cover the time from hospitalization to 2 years following injury. Chapter 14 extends this period of time to decades through stories of people who have become master drivers of these roads.

Before proceeding on this journey, though, you need more than the guidelines in Chapter 1; you need to know what aphasia is and is not (Chapter 2), and an overview of how to prepare for what lies ahead (Chapter 3). Chapter 2 identifies both the apparent and "hidden" aspects of this acquired disorder. Chapter 3 provides indications of what you may find down your own road, and how to read and select preferred routes for those presented in Chapters 4–8. You do not want to begin your travels without this prejourney information.

Realize, too, that your journey is apt to span more than the 2 years highlighted here. The trip's duration, though, is not so important as is establishing and maintaining a quality to life as you make your way ahead. **Within these first years, you and your loved one are apt to establish a pattern of coping that will set the course for much of what follows. For this reason, what you do at first, and how you elect to do it, is extremely important.** Setting up the right traveling *habits* and *outlooks* will extend to all that follows. The truth is, it will likely take you and your loved one a minimum of a year to simply begin to *see* and *understand* this new countryside. This does not mean that you'll remain hopelessly lost or confused up until then—not at all! It simply means that you will need that time to come to begin *living with* aphasia, understanding its changes, and most importantly, determining what they mean *to you!*

Chapters 9 through 13 target this important step—improving your understanding of aphasia. Although they follow the "journey chapters" (Chapters 4–8), they actually are "side trips." You can read them at any time and in any order, depending on your needs, wants, and interests. They directly address often-asked questions concerning aphasia, such as: "How does the brain normally handle speech, language, and communication?" "What changes in normal functions follow aphasia?" "What causes aphasia to occur?" "What problems might accompany aphasia with this type of injury?" and "What can be done to minimize the recurrence of such an injury?" Somewhere down the road, these questions are apt to greet you. When they do, pull over, select what you need, but don't worry or struggle through parts that don't address your needs at that moment.

At the end of this book, we tie together this trip's "realities" in stories of several pairs of travelers who have already made this trip (Chapter 14). For some readers, it might be more valuable to begin with this chapter rather than to end with it. There are a variety of personal accounts of people negotiating their own journeys and routes. You see, **this is one of the most fundamental truths about this journey: it is not the same experience and it does not follow the same routes for any two people!** It differs for each person who chooses to travel beyond the dilemmas posed by aphasia. However, like the people discussed in Chapter 14, your journey is apt to share certain common themes. Our sole purpose in writing this book is to do this: to share what some of these commonalities might be! In the end, though, where *you* do and what *you* do will be determined solely by you!

Finally, at the end of this book are four appendixes with extensive supplemental information. The first appendix is a glossary of medical and technical terms you are apt to encounter along the way; the second contains lists of printed material that you might wish to consult; the third lists national, state, and international stroke or aphasia agencies; and the fourth is a cursory view of assistive devices and materials for people with aphasia.

So, here we are, at a point where you are seeking more information and advice about the future, and we want only to share with you what we might to make your journey easier and more fulfilling. Years from now, you are apt to look up and find yourself in an entirely different countryside from where you are now or were before aphasia ever appeared. If, for example, you previously resided in the high mountain valleys, you may find rhythmically swaying prairie grasses before you, bending back and forth like a never-ending inland sea. Your natural instincts, at times, may be to say, "This doesn't look or feel right . . . this isn't what I know, and certainly not what I like! Where are my fields of wildflowers and the high mountain lakes?" On these occasions, try to reserve judgment until you have had some time to look more closely. There are wildflowers and lakes on your prairies, and you need to be aware that, although, the scenery may differ, beauty will still abound around you. **Often what you and your loved one will need most is the time to find it and to see it.**

Give yourself permission right now to start looking for something that, at this moment anyway, may not feel humanly possible.

> An attorney with aphasia once told me:
>
>> I wasn't a very nice or thoughtful person before my injury. I was always too involved in what I thought. With aphasia, it forced me to "shut up" and listen to others. I don't talk much anymore. I can't! But I listen hard and I understand people better . . . something I never did before!
>
>> I like who I am as a person *now* better than the person I was before!

If resuming life now with aphasia is ever to dominate over "being aphasic," then transitions like this man's are essential. That is what this book is all about: helping you and your loved one make transitions back to living productive lives again! The pages ahead are "chock full" of suggestions for ways of negotiating some of the more challenging and treacherous parts of this trip. Even if only a few help you or your loved one, they might provide just enough of a "push" to help you traverse the remaining parts. Whatever your course, the aim here is to restore beauty, purpose, and value to living daily life, whether that countryside contains prairie grasses or high mountain peaks. **Above all, you need to know that there is beauty *still before you*, and that this trip is worth your effort to find it!**

Acknowledgments

The seeds of this book began long ago when I moved from a university setting to a post as a clinical researcher at the VA hospital in Long Beach, California. I arrived with years of experience in remediating the communication of adults with aphasia and I was eager to search out other lasting solutions to the challenges of aphasia. What was most striking and influential in this new work setting was the presence of two young colleagues, Marianne Simpson and Sandra Davidson-Baxter. To my surprise, these speech-language pathologists devoted as much time and focus in their treatment to addressing the needs of the whole person, as they did to remediating their communication deficits. Over the years, these clinicians had devised peer forums for both patients and caregivers to normalize the living of life in spite of aphasia's presence. Positive and life-altering outcomes emerged regularly from these groups, and it was these results that provided the original impetus and direction for the themes of this book.

It is not surprising, then, that years later I was excited to begin writing this text with Marianne Simpson. Unfortunately, an unforeseen happenstance in Marianne's life interfered with her continued participation. Her inspiration, though, never diminished; much of the form, spirit, and thought of this book originates from years of shared clinical contact—decades ago!

Several other colleagues and friends strongly influenced the make-up of this book as well: Aura Kagan, Roberta Elman, and Nina Simmons-

Mackie. All are stellar clinicians who have devoted their professional careers to helping people confront their challenges with aphasia. Through conversations, documented works, and the sharing of their clinical interests and practices, they have provided me with valuable notions and insights. Aura's imprint stands on all suggestions regarding personal and social competency, finding pursuits in life that permit individuals to "forget" aphasia's daily presence, and seeking out "protected" communities in society where life's functions may once again resume. Her daily participation in such a community, a treatment center for people with aphasia as well as the people who attend to their long-term needs, speaks powerfully to the legitimacy of her suggestions. Roberta's presence is equally strong and influential, and is more broadly distributed throughout the entirety of this book. She has been a close confidante for over a decade; her clarity of thought and dedication to refining ways of making the lives of people confronting aphasia better have influenced key concepts here. She, too, devotes her daily practice to treating and being with the people she is committed to helping. Nina's insightful observations of people with aphasia in everyday interactions have changed the form and priorities of suggestions here. Her research in real-life settings suggests we may need to spend as much time merging the lives of those couples, families, and friends impacted by aphasia as we do repairing their communication. Although the mechanisms for doing so are just starting to emerge, Nina has been instrumental in reshaping a treatment dialogue about what is most needed and how best to proceed toward those targets.

The influence of the works of David Luterman and Mihaly Csikszentmihalyi stand out as well. Luterman has written extensively and cogently about counscling families dealing with communication impairments in everyday life. His thoughts about the traumatizing effects of these injuries and how we must orient our thinking toward "empowerment" of such individuals are central to this book's themes. Csikszentmihalyi is the originator of the concept known as "flow." He has written extensively about the properties of this life phenomenon, and about how all of us, whether shackled with permanent disability or not, must regularly "lose" ourselves through involvement in life to keep its form meaningful, rewarding, and pleasurable. It is precisely this quality of "flow" that is often most absent and most sought after by those coping with the enduring effects of aphasia.

There are many more "contributors" to this book, too many to name or acknowledge in full. Most notable are the hundreds of patients, spouses, and families from whom I've learned over the years. In fact, it is their collective story that constitutes the heart of this book, the actual "journey" itself. In addition, there are numerous professionals, caregivers, friends, and family who have added to its form and content, either directly or indirectly. In this regard, I extend a special thanks to: Terry Wertz, Jackie Hinckley, Sally Byng, Nancy Helm-Estabrooks, Cindy Neis, Sue Bowles, Hans H. Wängler, Martha Taylor Sarno, Ruth Coles, Ellen Bernstein-Ellis, Susan Barnett, Kevin Kearns, Audrey Holland, Pat Arato, Larry Boles, Kelly Mahoney, Peg Lemme, Carole Pound, Jack Damico, Bonnie Brinton, Freny Daruvala, Barbara Lyon, Bob Marshall, Sandy Milton, Denise Cariski, Susie Parr, Barbara Shadden, Martin Fujiki, Carol Ryff, Florence Blanc, Leonard LaPointe, Carol Frattali, and Karen Klein. And as with any list, it is by no means complete! There were many others who both mattered and contributed. I acknowledge and thank them all!

I owe, as well, a special thanks to Jay Rosenbek. He not only provided me with the opportunity to share this perspective, but he steadfastly supported and encouraged this book's themes and their realization from onset to completion. I'm indebted to him for his constancy and his dedication to seeing this project through.

Finally, this book would not exist had it not been for the enthusiasm, care, and careful eye and editorial pen of Marge Blanc. It is my greatest reward to return home nightly to her wit, charm, and presence.

This book is dedicated to

all

who have made and are making this journey!

❖ CHAPTER 1

What to keep in mind

The old adage that a thousand mile journey begins with the first step is worthy of consideration now. Your journey toward a renewed life begins with the realization that aphasia is usually enduring, but coping with it is within your means and abilities. Unlike other afflictions that you or your loved one may have experienced, where a 3-week regimen of antibiotics would restore health, aphasia typically comes and it stays! No amount of medication or rehabilitation is apt to return life to its preinjured level. Simply coming to grips with this fact, that your loved one's aphasia and its related disabilities will linger on and on, takes time. It usually takes months, if not years, to truly understand and integrate these realities into daily life.

As is often true of any challenge of long duration, your patience and stamina is about to be tested! For this reason, setting a course that promotes endurance and consistency is the single most important factor in getting where you want and need to go. As part of building stamina, "getting in shape" for what you are about to encounter is the first step. What complicates the process, though, is that aphasia often arrives without warning and without any time to prepare. Suddenly, you are thrust out a door and down a road with an agenda and schedule totally unrelated to your prior needs, wishes, or abilities. In the beginning, you are apt to struggle simply to keep the car on the road, a road that looks and feels totally different from any you have ever traveled before.

You are likely a few miles down the road already; you probably have managed just fine; or at least, you've survived! In fact, you may be amazed at how you've managed to do so much in so little time! You probably didn't know you had it in you. Quite likely, though, most of your energy and actions up to this point have been more reflexive than planned. They have come more from having *to react* to the perceived threats before you and their newness than having any long-range plan of action. Even so, in your current heightened sense of being, your stamina may seem to be the least of your worries. However, you need to know that as daily life starts to return to a more predictable course of operation, and one likely very different from before, you are apt to begin to notice increasing fatigue! It is usually a case of trying to keep the many changed parts of daily life in some semblance of order. You aren't used to any of this! Although you didn't have a chance to "get in shape" before this began, now you do! This chapter sets about putting together a general plan to help you do just that.

Part of building stamina at first depends on removing certain myths about aphasia, while incorporating certain governing "truths." In this chapter, we try to provide you with some of the latter, guidelines that if observed and adhered to over the entirety of this trip, will keep you on a preferred path and moving in a preferred direction. The actual exercises for building strength and endurance, though, don't really begin until Chapter 4. However, everything you will be provided along the way fits within these "truths," and if you can incorporate them now, the rest of the trip will be that much easier.

(1) Aphasia is well known and understood!

Life tends to present us occasionally with unexpected, and even tragic, moments and events. A certain percentage of these we are able to "sort out" and make sense of, while another portion tends to remain a mystery throughout life. Aphasia, though, is not one of the latter! It has been described for thousands of years. There are written accounts of its exis-

tence in Egyptian, Greek, and Roman civilizations. What is more pertinent to you, though, is that there is a well established body of literature
and information currently available about aphasia and how to cope with
it and its consequences. This literature comes in varied forms: newsletters, pamphlets, books, videotapes, audiotapes, and most recently . . . the
Internet! **No matter where you are, in location, thought, or need, there
is a vast amount of "help" sitting out there for your inspection and
reaction.** Appendixes B, C, and D provide lists from which to begin.

(2) You are not alone!

Because coping with aphasia is a way of daily life for over a million
Americans today, and millions more throughout the world, you need to
know that you are not alone on this journey. Many others are either making this trip simultaneously with you or have already done so. In fact, in
most states and large cities in America, and in most populated centers
world-wide, you can find ongoing support groups for people with aphasia and their families. Sometimes these support groups are in the form of
larger groups open to anyone who has suffered from a *brain attack* or
stroke, whether they have speech, language, and communication difficulties or not. Even in the latter case, however, there is usually a sufficient membership of stroke survivors to ensure that some in the group do
have aphasia (see Appendix C).

Besides forums where you might meet others with aphasia, there are
regional and national agencies in America that provide literature and/or
newsletters pertaining to the nature of and recovery from aphasia and
stroke (see Appendix B). In this country, the National Aphasia Association serves as a centralized agency willing to provide lists and literature
of this nature (P. O. Box 1887, Murray Hill Station, New York, NY
10156–0611; [800] 922–4622). Appendix C lists central agencies in
other countries that serve this same role.

The main distinction to keep in mind now, though, is that you are never
alone on this journey. **There are plenty of others traveling along with
you whether you see them or not; they are there! As a group, they
represent one of your strongest resources on this trip, as you gather
information and begin to make choices.** As you will see, we will keep
pointing you in their direction as you travel the road ahead.

(3) Getting to your destination is not a race!

With as much pain and anguish as aphasia brings, it is not surprising that most sufferers strive to "fix" it as soon as possible. Because of its protracted nature, though, any solution typically evolves slowly over time. You cannot get to your chosen destination on this trip by simply racing helter skelter ahead. It simply won't work. Most likely, you could not endure the physical or emotional hardship that maintaining such a pace would bring. Even if you could manage to race ahead, you likely would miss key landmarks along the way. In the end, you would find yourselves spending more time retracing your past route to relearn what was overlooked, than if the two of you had simply proceeded at a nice, steady, and comfortable pace from the outset. **Rest assured . . . you need plenty of time to observe and reflect as you travel. In fact, it is what you and your loved one learn along the way that determines where you go next. So give yourselves lots of time to absorb and adjust.**

Other people who have made this trip, and their suggestions, are likely to aid you. We provide ways of finding out this type of information. Finding a lasting solution depends more heavily, though, on you creating your own "information." Achieving this likely relies on an active interplay between what once was, what now is, how you and your loved one handle adversity, what assistance you get along the way, what you and he or she want, and how strong and enduring your desire is to pursue those ends. **Only the two of you can truly shape your own course and its ultimate outcome. That process takes time . . . you cannot do it quickly and still do it well.**

(4) Time is your strongest ally!

Because aphasia tends to come and stay, it is not uncommon for people with aphasia and their caregivers to view any permanent loss of function with apprehension and resentment. With this perspective, every passing day may come to stand as a reminder of what hasn't returned or may not return in the future. With this perspective, time down the road can come to feel more like an "imposed sentence" in life, than your ally. **The truth is, tomorrow and each day after are your strongest allies in molding a harmonious and comfortable existence later! Instead of looking at what isn't working and worrying whether it will ever work again, it is crucial to look at what is working right now, and how with each additional day, you might "add onto" whatever that might be.**

Know from the beginning that getting better is something that can, and will, continue for as long as you and your loved elect to work to have it continue! Getting better is as simple as that . . . as long as you continue to try . . . you *will* continue to get better! It may not involve "perceptible changes" in underlying skills later in life, but that does not eliminate continuing to find new ways of making better or more complete use of what still does work. For this reason, you need to begin framing time from this moment on as your friend, not your enemy . . . it is only through time and using it to your advantage that you and your loved one can make life resonate again.

(5) A lasting solution is not your sole responsibility!

Finding solutions to aphasia's many dilemmas involves more people than you alone. Too frequently, it is the caregiver who either knowingly or unknowingly assumes too much of the burden. Certainly, supporting and standing by your loved one throughout the recovery process is absolutely crucial, but taking on the responsibility of "fixing" his or her underlying dysfunctions is neither advisable nor realistic. You cannot "fix" what he or she cannot, and you cannot be responsible for what he or she is unwilling to do or to try. All you can do is offer to foster what is desirable and possible, as long as that offering fits within your own wishes and physical, mental, and emotional limitations.

Things *will* occasionally break down along the way on this trip, and when they do, it is not your fault that they did, nor is it your responsibility to make sure they resume working again. **Just as life was a shared process before aphasia, so too, it needs to be a shared process now.** Much is written in Chapters 4–8 about precisely how to keep life's responsibility "shared" between you, your loved one, and others.

(6) Harmony and balance in life are a realistic goal!

The most difficult "truth" to accept about aphasia is often this one. Quite likely, it just doesn't seem possible that life could ever again approximate the harmony and balance that were there prior to injury. You are probably "right," in some ways, in thinking that it won't be precisely the same as it once was. But you are "wrong" in thinking that finding and restoring a sense of comfort and ease in life is simply not possible because of aphasia. **If there is a recurring theme that you will find lavishly sprinkled across of the pages of this book, it is that daily life need not be *less* simply because aphasia is a part of its equation.** Although this is a "nice notion," it is much harder to make it a reality. That, though, is what this book is all about . . . helping you achieve a *new reality!* By the end, we may not have restored harmony and balance to their fullest potential, but we most certainly will have provided a basis on which to assure their presence and future growth.

Take a break! Take a few deep breaths and just sit back and reconsider the above guidelines as a whole. Rid your mind of something that feels hopelessly "broken!" The truth is, it's not as "broken" as it seems . . . but it's going to take *time* to allow you and your loved one to rework matters to your own advantage. Certainly what stands before the two of you is not insignificant or minor . . . but years from now, when both of you have had sufficient time to place it in its proper perspective, you'll know that this moment was neither as formidable nor as irreconcilable as it now feels.

Continuing on from here

Before setting out, you need to make a couple more quick stops. The first is to get yourself oriented to what aphasia is and isn't. As much as you need to know what aphasia is, you need equally to know what it is *not!* Too often, it is the latter confusion that causes the greatest disruptions in trying to restore harmony and balance to life. The second stop is to get oriented to what you will need to know and what you are apt to encounter down the road you are about to travel.

Now, just keep your vehicle within the above guidelines and us in your rear view mirror. Together, you will manage what lies ahead just fine!

CHAPTER 2

What aphasia is and is not

Many years ago when I was young in my profession, I invited the wife of a person with aphasia to attend an early treatment session with her husband and me. I was eager to show her ways of getting around the communication difficulties he was experiencing. She seemed outwardly delighted with each new possibility introduced. I would explain a particular strategy, demonstrate its use, and then she would attempt the same strategy in a slightly different context. For the next hour, she and her husband successfully interacted with an ease not experienced since the onset of his aphasia. I remember coming away with a special feeling of gratification because of what we had accomplished.

Earlier in the day, I had arranged to meet privately with this wife after our treatment session. I wanted to review what had happened and to discuss the weeks ahead. Given how well the session had gone, I looked forward to talking with her about developing these new ways of communicating. Besides wanting to compliment her on how well she had done, I was anxious to know how comfortable she felt with these new methods. Once a hospital volunteer had escorted her husband to his next appointment, I began our conversation about our meeting. Within seconds, I noticed tears starting to come to her eyes. I stopped and asked what was troubling her. She hesitated for a moment and said:

"Isn't it awful? His mind no longer works! He's no more than a child! It's unbearable for me to watch because he was such a gifted, creative man, and now just look at him."

As much as I wanted to console her, I was completely shocked. What had caused her to make such inferences? They were so far removed from any reality of mine that it took me a brief moment before I could capture her perspective. Then I realized where the problem rested. It was not with her, or with her husband's condition. It was with me! Unintentionally, I had failed to fully explain what aphasia was. Although the impairment to her husband's language and communication was severe, he most certainly had not lost his mind, nor was his mind reduced to that of a child.

This scenario depicts one of the most common fallacies associated with aphasia: the tendency of others to confuse one's inability to communicate with one's ability to think. **Aphasia, by itself, does *not* interrupt the integrity of thought; instead, it robs its victim of ready access to the words needed to express that thought.**

Painting a different picture of what aphasia is

If you have ever traveled to a foreign country where the language was totally unfamiliar and the native people didn't speak English, you've likely experienced something akin to aphasia. If you haven't, here is how that experience parallels what your loved one is currently facing.

Not understanding or being understood

You have just arrived in a South American country for the first time. You do not know the language, but you are excited about the possibility of learning it. With your translation guide close at hand, you begin negotiating your first obstacle: renting a car. To your surprise, the man at the rental desk greets you with a rapid barrage of words, none of which seem to have anything to do with renting a car. He seems to want something totally unrelated. You find yourself gesturing for him to slow down. Possibly, you think, a word or phrase might emerge from his speech if only he would talk slower. But none do. His words, whether fast or slow, simply make no sense. Next, you try to answer in your own words, but to your surprise, none of these make sense to him. He simply stares at you quizzically, shrugs his shoulders and disappears into the back room. You stand there frustrated and confused over what is happening. You hadn't anticipated this. You knew your command of his language was limited, but you hadn't expected him not to understand any of your words! As you wait, you keep trying to figure out, "What did this man want?" Not only did your words seem meaningless to him, but it does not seem likely that you will soon know what he wanted.

Disrupting language, not thinking

While standing in line, you start wondering how the remaining 2 weeks are going to be. There are far more complicated issues than this one awaiting you. *What if no one understands?* You start to feel "lost," and somewhat "inadequate" in handling matters. Then, in the middle of this thinking, you realize that this is *only* a communication problem! Your mind and thinking are perfectly intact and at your full disposal. You know who you are, where you are, and what you want. The problem is simply that your two languages don't mesh.

Communicating in other ways

You reach into your travel bag and dig out a pencil and pad. You copy the proper translation of "rental car" onto a sheet, add your name, driver's license number, the make of car you requested, and your confirmation number. To finish it off, you draw a quick sketch of a four-door sedan at the bottom. When the agent returns, your *revised communication system* works! It was the confirmation number for the car that he had wanted. Not unlike your loved one with aphasia, you have just tried to interact with someone who couldn't understand your use of language, yet all along, you knew perfectly well what you wanted to say.

Changing how you use communication

As your trip continues, the risk of being viewed "aphasic" alters your own mode and style of communication. Aware that your understanding and use of language is worse than anticipated, you purposefully avoid interactions with others. When you do communicate, you try to prepare well in advance. You limit your spoken attempts only to key words in the message. You shift, instead, to a much greater reliance on gestures. If these adjustments fail, you quickly produce your language guide and point to the desired word or phrase. On certain occasions, you find yourself drawing or sketching basic needs and wants.

Dealing with feelings of reduced self-worth and inner strength

It is also likely, as you change your communication mode and style, that your image of yourself weakens. You are not nearly as self-confident or self-assured communicating with others in the jungles of South America as you were at home. You begin withdrawing from social settings and interactions. As you start to avoid talking to others, you notice that the quality of your trip begins to change. Not only are you not doing all the things you had wanted, but you are aware and constantly frustrated over your limited ability to communicate. You try to compensate by taking more time and practicing, but most people do not understand you and they are too busy to stop and try. You begin to question whether coming alone on this trip was such a good idea. With your restricted activity and growing isolation, uncharacteristic doubts begin to arise about your personal strength and abilities.

This brief scenario of traveling to a foreign land captures many of the facets in daily life that your loved one is likely confronting at the moment, although this breakdown in communication is in his or her own native language. He or she has no other language to fall back on, no one "back home" to call and explain the frustrations to. Next, we describe the main distinctions between your hypothetical dilemma and those that accompany aphasia in one's own language.

Acquiring aphasia

Your loved one's aphasia was not brought about by traveling to a foreign land. Instead, it probably happened at home and was caused by an interruption of blood to the brain. This interruption occurred in a specific region of the brain, the part that governs language. When blood is stopped to any part of the brain, the affected person is said to have suffered a *cerebral stroke* or *brain attack*. When that stroke affects the ongoing use of language, the result is called *aphasia.*

Aphasia is but one of many consequences of cerebral stroke. Your loved one may have others as well, like partial or complete loss of movement or sensation on one side of his or her body, usually the right side; reduced vision; difficulty swallowing; or incontinence of bowel or bladder. Some of these impairments, if they are present, may be as concerning to you as his or her aphasia. Chapter 12 details the types and nature of other problems that may accompany aphasia. For now, though, we turn our focus to what your loved one's aphasia is and is not.

Facing interrupted language when thought and memory remain largely intact

When aphasia results from cerebral stroke, it usually describes the disrupted process of language while thought and memory remain largely intact. The gentleman in the opening scenario of this chapter could not make his basic needs known to his wife, but internally, he knew his intended message well. **Once the brain stabilizes after injury, aphasia typically spares one's basic abilities to think, reason, and remember while impacting one's understanding or use of spoken, written, or gestured words!**

In the initial days and weeks after injury, however, the type of insult to the brain that causes aphasia *can* interfere with thinking and recall. When this occurs, thinking typically returns gradually over a period of days or weeks. In some instances, it can take longer . . . up to several months. When it does take longer, it usually means that the extent of injury to the brain was extensive or that multiple injuries occurred. When injury includes both sides of the brain, thinking may not return to what it once was.

Feeling trapped in one's thoughts

Difficulties with talking, writing, or gesturing constrict one's ability to express basic ideas, feelings, worries, or desires. It is not that your loved one doesn't wish to share his or her thoughts, but rather, that his or her language "machinery" no longer permits such exchanges to occur.

Feeling less able to act

In the beginning weeks, aphasia often immobilizes or numbs the inner soul. The person with aphasia may try to act but something more basic and fundamental prevails. Many sufferers often sit in somewhat of a "protective cocoon," attempting to put sense and purpose back into something that feels totally raw, empty, different, scary, and isolating. This protective window of inaction is common. Probably in the bigger picture of what has happened and what will be needed, it is actually a kind of blessing in disguise. During this period, interactions are often confusing and exhausting for everyone. Because of this, lots of quiet time in the beginning may not be so detrimental.

Over time, your loved one's strength and ability to act will start to re-emerge. Yet, be prepared for this to come gradually over a period of weeks or months. In fact, it is apt to take even longer before your loved one feels strong enough to "grab the reins" and try again to direct his or her own destiny. As the inner drive slowly returns, however, his or her willingness and desire to venture out and to do more will likely follow. **Know that these changes in personal well-being often lead to greater ease and success with communication.**

Facing diminished feelings of well-being

When communication ceases, other basic functions of daily life, ones that have defined who and what we are suffer too. Recall your trip to that foreign land and how you started doubting yourself and your abilities when communication wasn't possible. As much as physical appearance, social or business stature, or economic wealth, it is the presence or absence of communication that affects how we live and what we seem capable of doing. Depending on the severity of injury, and your loved one's perception of its consequences, adjustments in his or her well-being are likely to follow.

Retaining one's past character

Self-image and self-esteem often suffer considerably with aphasia. Little, though, commonly changes in "the core" of who the person was. If your loved one was loving, caring, and attentive to family before, the same inclinations are apt to be true now. If your loved one valued the environment, conservative politics, or celebrating birthdays, these emphases are likely still there. What may change, though, is how these preferences in life are expressed. Outwardly, they may not be acted on in the same manner or to the same degree, but inwardly they likely still exist. **Aphasia doesn't, as a rule, change one's pre-aphasic character. What were your loved one's fundamental preferences, likes, and dislikes, still are. Instead, what is altered is how he or she views life's possibilities and his or her inner self.**

Adopting change while striving for quality of daily life

Unlike getting on a plane and returning home where you can speak your language again, aphasia, if it lasts over several days, is usually irreversible. Its permanency, though, does not mean that further improvement isn't possible. It is! In fact, in the initial stages of recovery, your loved one is likely to improve whether he or she cares to or not! Months later, however, the visible signs of improvement are apt to lessen. When this occurs, it does not mean that further change is no longer possible. It is! Rather, it simply means that you and your loved one may need to work more creatively within the sphere of what does work.

Be prepared for lasting difference! But be prepared, as well, for continuing to make more out of life regardless of its form. Lasting differences from aphasia are not *all* bad. Certainly, some are. But remember the attorney with aphasia who came to view listening to others as an improvement in life far beyond his pre-injured insights or abilities. There are silver linings in dark clouds; you simply need to know where to look and what to do when you find them. The "journey chapters" ahead do just this.

Misperceiving what is and is not possible

When aphasia occurs, it brings with it many misperceptions. We've encountered several so far: thinking that thinking isn't working, thinking that all of language is absent if talking is, and thinking that one's character or personality is totally different. But none of these misperceptions is as devastating as being thought of as "unable" to act in one's own behalf.

Aphasia and the other complications that accompany it tend to confuse people about what is and isn't possible in life. Without question, brain injury associated with aphasia tends to alter one's ability to perform basic functions, especially in the early going. In some cases, the extent of injury can severely compromise these abilities. Be advised, however, that there are few things in daily life that, with time and your loved one's willingness to try, can't be re-established at least in some modified or partial form. If injury is severe, participation may be highly curtailed in terms of ease, skill, or proficiency, but even then, much is still possible. If your loved one swam, cooked, gardened, played tennis, jogged, bowled, put jigsaw puzzles together, or engaged in some other favorite activities, there is likely some altered form of that which will still work now.

Maybe your loved one's version of "jogging" is currently confined to standing on a treadmill, fully supported by you or others, and simply trying to put one foot in front of the other. Perhaps you or your loved one would not refer to this type of participation as "jogging," but regardless of label, some "active" pursuit of a similar or related form *is* possible. Pursuing such an activity now, however, means knowing how to carefully and safely match current skills with current interests. **Being able over time to act in one's own behalf is an essential ingredient in making life work again, for both of you. If the pursuit is approached properly and given sufficient time, no impairment has to strip your loved one of his or her dignity or right to act in his or her own behalf.**

Recognizing that the injury of aphasia extends equally to you

Aphasia's impact extends well beyond your loved one. Just because he or she is the "injured" party does not mean that you aren't, or that you should devote more of your time and effort to resolving his or her issues than to addressing your own. True, the outward manifestations of injury rest solely with your loved one. It may be difficult, given current levels of dysfunction, not to feel as if you should completely "attend" to, or abdicate to, his or her needs. However, you are traveling a common journey, as you will soon discover. Its ultimate outcome depends on how well you attend to both parties' needs, and not just your loved one's. Chapters 4 through 7 specifically acknowledge this important reality by identifying and treating the paths of the person with aphasia and his or her caregiver (a loved one) separately. Chapter 8 takes on a different format and merges the coping suggestions into a single outline, but even so, this is done with you, as a couple or pair, in mind. For the two of you to reach your desired destination, you need to be equally attentive to both of your incurred "injuries" from aphasia.

In summary, then, aphasia impacts the use of language but, as well, it alters much of life. In an abbreviated way, you might say that it changes communication and feelings of well-being. Changes in language rest within the injured party while changes in well-being extend to everyone closely involved. We next explain how language and feelings of well-being differ.

Language features of aphasia

Aphasia interrupts a coding system of words that your loved one has known and used since childhood. Unlike traveling abroad where spoken words may be totally new and foreign, the inaccessible words denied to the person with aphasia often retain some familiarity. However, having a recognizable "ring" does not assure that they are understood or properly used. It does mean, though, that the basic parts of language still exist in your loved one's mind, even if he or she cannot "get to" them.

Facing interrupted access to language, but not losing it

Remember the wife who thought her husband's mind had been reduced to that of a child's. From what she could observe, his word usage was suggestive of a four- or five-year-old's message. She worried that he had "lost" his mind. We've already commented on how this wasn't the case, but it is equally important to know that his internal language was not reduced either. Even if the words he used might suggest so, the dictionary of words in his head was likely still as full as before. It was more a case that he simply couldn't access and "retrieve" the words that might best align with his adult message. Instead, the words he could get to were those of a child.

Generally speaking, aphasia does not *remove* language. The primary parts of your loved one's language system likely remain. Instead, it is the connections between these parts that tend to break down. When he or she goes to get a word to express a thought, access to his/her word dictionary becomes blocked. Your loved one knows the word "daffodil," and can readily distinguish daffodils from four or five other types of flowers. In fact, in some instances, he or she may have just said that word moments earlier in a slightly different context. But at this particular moment, the circuitry simply will not let him or her in. The word he or she seeks is not "gone" or "lost," it simply isn't retrievable at this time. Because of this, your loved one may elect to substitute the word "flower" instead. It is not really his or her choice and he or she knows this, but given the current blockage, it at least points the listener in the right direction.

In much the same manner, but with a more severely impaired language system, the husband in the earlier story sought to tell his wife what he was thinking. Unfortunately, the words "available" to him compared more closely to those of a child than his old self. It is understandable that she thought he had reverted to the level of a child, but her inference was wrong. In all likelihood, he still had the words he wanted to say; he just couldn't get to them.

Experiencing impairment in all areas of language use

Your loved one is likely to exhibit declines in all areas of language: listening, speaking, reading, and writing, and even in language-related gesturing. The degree of impairment, though, is apt to vary considerably from one language area to the next. A common scenario may be a person whose listening skills are impaired except in simple everyday exchanges, and whose speaking and writing is severely affected. As a result, this individual may be able to get the "gist" of simple conversations but is unable to respond in words, whether spoken or written. In contrast, there might be another person with aphasia who cannot understand what is said but who can recognize, or even write out, simple printed messages. In both of these cases, though, "some" impairment exists in all areas of language use if they are carefully assessed.

Not seeing impairment when it exists

It is not uncommon that a husband or wife might feel that his or her loved one understands "everything," and that only his or her talking is impaired. The truth, though, is that listening skills are almost always somewhat worse. Sometimes the degree of change is quite minimal. On other occasions, however, it can be quite substantial and still remain hidden from others. One may wonder how such misperceptions occur, especially when the impairment is significant.

Recall that many people with aphasia retain a sense of how language works even though their own language systems don't function properly. They know, for instance, that you've asked a question even though they didn't understand what it was. As a result, their manner of interacting may outwardly suggest they understood when, in fact, they didn't. For example, you may tell your loved one about a conversation with a neighbor:

> "I saw Ms. Riley this morning. She was on the way to the store. She asked how you were doing. Evidently, Frank (her husband) would like to visit. But I told her it was too soon. Maybe in another week or so, don't you think?"

As you tell this story, your loved one watches intently, hearing the tone of your voice, and "getting a feel" for your message. In truth, though, he is failing to understand key parts. Maybe he knows who the message is about, but what happened or why it did is not clear. It doesn't matter, though, because from the tone of your voice, your facial expressions, and delivery, he is happy to go along with whatever you think. You interpret his affirmation, though, as *confirmation* of having understood your message in its entirety. The latter, however, did not occur!

It is precisely for this reason, a possible "hidden" breakdown in language, that specialists (e.g., speech-language pathologists, neuropsychologists, and doctors) test listening skills in isolation. As part of their test battery, they are apt to ask your loved one to answer questions, too. However, their formulation and focus is quite different. They select questions that are short in length and require both "yes" and "no" answers to confirm one's understanding. For example: "Are you married?" and "Are you single?"; "Is your wife's name Betty (actual name)?" and "Is your wife's name Alice (fictitious name)?"; "Do you write with a toaster?" and "Do you write with a pen?"; "Does a cork sink in water?" and "Will a stone sink in water?" If your loved one can distinguish *both* sides of a set of questions quickly and accurately, there is a greater likelihood that his or her listening skills are relatively intact. Usually, though, as questions become more difficult, most people with aphasia require more time before answering, and errors occur.

Communicating in spite of language impairment

Sometimes certain areas of language may appear too severely impaired to be used for communication. For instance, it might be that your loved one's writing abilities are dramatically altered. He or she is unable to write short notes, grocery lists, or checks. Even simple, familiar words, like table, chair, and door, are either misspelled or lack letters. However, you notice that when your loved one is unable to say a word, he or she occasionally attempts and is able to write out the beginning letters of words. Since you often know the topic, the use of writing in this manner is quite helpful in deciphering your loved one's communicative intent. With a different person who has aphasia, it might be that another area of functioning, like gesturing, is the best way to aid communication. For instance, maybe pretending to sip from a teaspoon of hot soup helps this person to say "soup." **Because each person with aphasia is apt to be different in his or her language and communicative abilities, it is important to have an experienced speech-language pathologist determine which of these areas might strengthen interactions with others.**

Finding varied degrees of language use

From the last section, you know that aphasia may affect listening, reading, speaking, writing, and gesturing to varying degrees. In other words, your loved one's reading may be more involved than listening, or writing more than speaking. It is also likely that his or her aphasia differs in some way from that of others who may "appear" to have much the same problem. Although people with aphasia share certain similarities, each person's language profile is a bit different from the next; no two people with aphasia are exactly alike!

For example, one person with aphasia might talk in complete sentences but omit all meaningful words. When describing a Western (movie), he or she might say:

> "Well, they were on these things and getting going *(talking about riding horses)*. One of them got . . . you know . . . *(gestures being shot and dying)* . . . and then someone came over and . . . you know . . . *(gestures holding somebody up with a gun)*."

Another person with aphasia describing the same movie might not say any complete sentences and use only single, meaningful words:

> "cowboys . . . riding . . . shot . . . dead . . . holdup."

Chapter 10 describes the major "types" of aphasia. For now, though, realize that your loved one's language, although impaired, is not identical to that of others with aphasia. Some features are similar but others are not. Once again, an experienced speech-language pathologist can aid you with these distinctions and their importance to everyday communication.

Retaining "some" use in all language areas

Whereas aphasia disrupts all areas of language use, it typically spares "some" function in each as well. The remaining parts that do work, though, may be hard to recognize at times, especially when the person's aphasia is severe. Even in such cases, aspects of listening, reading, speaking, or writing exist, but do not aid normal communication. For example, your loved one may be able to say familiar courtesies, like "Hi," "Bye," or "OK," yet not be able to utter a meaningful word in a normal conversational exchange. Overlearned tasks like counting, saying the days of the week, reciting nursery rhymes, or singing familiar songs may elicit lots of recognizable words from him or her, yet none of these words are accessible in everyday conversation. Also, it may be that your loved one can readily repeat short words when given a model, like "bed" or "bathroom," and yet seconds later, not be able to name these same items when shown pictures of them. **So, although speaking may "work" at times, and under varying conditions, use may not transfer freely to everyday conversation. Nevertheless,** *some* **use of speech remains, and this principle of partial use likely applies to all other language areas as well. Thus, your loved one is apt to be able to perform in all areas of language use** *to some degree.*

Continuing to change even when language impairment is severe

Even when a language area is severely impaired, persistence in seeking change often yields *some* gain, especially in the early going. Even later, well beyond the year following injury, certain individuals continue to experience change, although at a much reduced rate and of a smaller magnitude. Even so, some of these later changes in function may be far more significant to their users than earlier ones. One person with aphasia, whom I have known for nearly a decade since his injury, still practices his "talking" every day. He began by not being able to repeat familiar, short words like "pan" or "hat." To do so, he required two or three slow presentations and careful attention to the mouth of the speaker. Now, he readily repeats multiple words and uses many of them spontaneously in his everyday conversation. His speech still is not functional for expressing basic needs. But to him, his talking is remarkably different and better with each passing year. He insists that he will talk in short sentences in the years ahead. Given his perseverance and the determination to do so, the likelihood of achieving more recognizable and usable speech remains a strong possibility.

Well-being features of aphasia

No matter what your relationship is to the person with aphasia, the fact that you are reading this book indicates your involvement. As introduced earlier, aphasia is not specific to *a* person; it injures all those close at hand. At first, the changes are too many to contemplate. One finds oneself reacting rather than acting, trying to keep life moving forward rather than fracturing. Daily harmony is more a wish than a reality. These aspects of aphasia extend well beyond the language impairment. They involve the consequences of what this impairment brings to daily life. They are as much of what aphasia is as the physical injury and impairments themselves.

Revamping your loved one's concept of self

Much has been written about life satisfaction or "quality of life." It seems that we all, whether brain injured or not, require constant amounts of certain ingredients in order to flourish inside. **Seemingly, a mixture of self-determination, self-acceptance, self-growth, purpose or direction in life, and others who care about us and we about them, are essential. For the person with aphasia, most of these sustaining forces to daily life diminish, especially in the beginning years.** For some sufferers, key ingredients of well-being may appear totally depleted. When this is true, loneliness, withdrawal, depression, and even anger can linger on, not for days or weeks, but months. Just as your loved one's language and communication are partially repairable, so too is his or her personal anguish. As you'll soon note, the chapters ahead (Journey Chapters 4 through 8) devote as much time to addressing these aspects in life as they do to addressing your loved one's communication difficulties. For now, though, it is important simply to note that the elements making up well-being *are an undeniable part of the handicap of aphasia.*

Facing your own challenges

We have already highlighted how your loved one's aphasia extends to you. As well, we've urged you to accept the legitimacy of your own needs and challenges in this process in order to make life better for both of you. **From the beginning, it is crucial that you not only acknowledge your own legitimacy, but that you act in your own behalf as much as, if not more than, you would to aid your loved one.** Getting where you need to be years from now depends as much on this action as anything you might do to further your loved one's recovery. Each of you needs *your own well-being* supported in order to keep this process of recovery moving in the direction it needs to go.

Determining aphasia's influences on thinking

One of the hardest adjustments for family and friends is sorting out aphasia's influence on thinking. When aphasia is quite severe and normal communication nonexistent, it often becomes difficult to judge what of your message was and was not understood, and how well the person with aphasia was able to interpret the portion that was. Should your loved one's language and communication be severely impaired, you need to know that his or her thinking is probably not as impaired as it may seem. Aphasia alone usually does not impair thinking over the long haul.

Recalling again the husband with aphasia in the opening scenario: he had a severe aphasia. Initially, he showed no sign of understanding any of my simple spoken questions such as: "Where you are?" "Where do you live?" or "How many children do you have?" Yet, when shown a map of the United States and given other nonspoken cues that oriented him to my topic, he readily pointed to a small Pennsylvania community where he was raised. When shown four pictures of people doing work, he quickly identified his own occupation. And by having me draw stick figure sketches of a family, I soon knew how many children were in the family and how many were boys or girls.

What complicates this picture is that your loved one's thinking may be compromised in the beginning hours or days of aphasia. The first section involving concerns of the person with aphasia in Chapter 4 speaks to this issue and how best to confront it. If your loved one's injury is recent and communication is sparse, you may wish to skip ahead to that section right now. However, if your loved one's injury is weeks or more old, it is more likely that his or her thinking may be better than it outwardly appears.

Understanding Aphasia

You now have been exposed to the basics of what aphasia is and is not. It is a language problem induced by brain injury that affects all of life, not just your loved one's but yours and all others who care for him or her. It is not a disorder of thinking or recall, nor is it a disorder of changed personality. But a *truer understanding* of your loved one's aphasia is still months or more away, especially if it is of recent onset. The important part is that you've begun to deal with it. **Try to remember that the core of your loved one is still there . . . unchanged. Outwardly, things may look much different; inwardly they probably are not. His or her mind and the structure for inner language are there. It is just that the interconnections that support retrieval of that language are faulty.** Give yourself a moment to reflect back on your own questions, thoughts, and feelings about aphasia. When you are ready, you can turn to the next chapter and begin to read what you need to know about the road ahead.

CHAPTER 3

What to expect and how to read the road maps ahead

An important part of your journey is getting a feel for the entirety of the trip. Taking a look at the bigger picture will help you to avoid some unexpected surprises along the way, and give you and your loved one a better chance of reaching your ultimate destination. Be advised that a common experience on this journey is finding oneself hopelessly lost at times. Whereas this may not be a problem when you have others nearby to help redirect you, it can be frightening when caught alone on a seldom-traveled strip of country road. Staying oriented to where you are, though, is not as hard as you might think. Once you know which routes are possible, what to watch out for, where to target your travel, and when to alter your route, then traveling the road ahead is apt to look far more inviting. Giving you such *a plan of travel* is the purpose of this chapter!

It all begins by laying out a huge map so you and your loved one can inspect all the likely routes and types of terrain you are apt to encounter. From here, you and your loved one can start to decide which routes might serve *your needs* best. Many successful ones have been traveled before, and there are others awaiting your exploration.

Overviewing the journey

This is a long journey you are about to take. Don't be fooled into thinking it's anything less! Because it takes a long time, however, does not mean that it need be extremely harsh or punishing. It simply means that it takes time to find and make the "right" choices for you . . . ones that allow life to work, and to feel harmonious and comfortable again. Given how "broken" life is apt to feel at the moment, you may doubt that you can make this journey easily. However, try not to let its chaotic or unpleasant appearance contaminate your view of what might be. Confusion and strain are the rule in the beginning, and they often emanate from all the *unfamiliar* settings, people, and rules that abound! However, this foreignness will not endure, and months from now you will establish a more predictable and comfortable pace. For all the reasons listed in Chapter 1 (keep scanning these!), this journey is well worth your while. Furthermore, getting there safely is well within your means and capabilities.

Making it to your destination requires a steady pace, a persistent attitude, and a willingness to risk whatever exists for something even more! As long as you and your loved one can keep these ingredients strong and active, you will successfully reach this trip's conclusion. The "journey chapters," 4 through 8, are there to keep your anguish level low and the level of these ingredients high. Know, too, that it is not wrong or impermissible to occasionally pull over and stop. You will find plenty of places to do so. These stops are not just to rest and catch your breath, but to reflect on where you have been and where you need to go next. In this regard, realize that this journey is not about getting to a single destination down the road. It is far more involved than that. It is about slowly accepting the life changes from the past to the present, and then transforming the current situation into a working reality of personal choice and pleasure. As a result, you may travel through the same locations many times and for many different reasons before one or more may come to feel like the place you ultimately want to be.

Finally, know that this journey need not consume the remainder of your lives. Yes, portions of what has changed will likely endure forever, but it is important that this transformation become *a natural and positive force* rather than one that constantly weighs heavy on your shoulders. Traveling these roads can be fun, and must be, in order for life to really resume. Down the road, "living life with aphasia" needs to replace "being aphasic and trying to live life."

Getting "a feel" for the travel ahead

Arriving where you want to go requires starting where you are, and adding "mileage," slowly and judiciously. This building process probably involves two major emphases along the way: (1) *making skills that* **aren't** *working work better* and (2) making *skills that* **are** *working, work more completely and functionally*. During the first 6 to 12 months of this journey, the first emphasis often tends to predominate, that is, trying to "fix" skills that aren't working. Somewhere near a year postinjury, the emphasis begins to shift toward functionally expanding the skills that do work.

Making the most of the trip ahead actually requires a steady dose of both of these emphases from the beginning. It means supporting and *encouraging every morsel of function* that may be derived from skills along the way, while *never shutting the door* on the possibility that more skills may evolve. In truth, these emphases are not separate, but parts of a single entity . . . adding function depends on making full use of what is working, and making full use of what is working depends on developing skills that weren't working before.

For example, maybe your loved one's speech is quite limited at the moment, but he or she can write out the beginning parts of words. By emphasizing writing whenever possible (making use of what is working), you notice that more spontaneous words are appearing in his or her everyday speech ("fixing" skills). Since he or she can write the beginnings of many words and then say them (what is working), you realize, too, that he or she might be able to use these rough notations to make grocery lists and shop independently (a function previously unknown). In the first case, basic skills are increasing . . . your loved one is talking better. In the second case, enhanced function is evolving from making better use of existing skills . . . your loved one is now grocery shopping without your assistance. Both types of emphasis are continuously important to the routes ahead.

Looking more closely at what lies ahead

There are many different ways of viewing the road ahead; two stand out as important in helping minimize your anguish while keeping you on a preferred course. One guideline deals with how to cope most effectively with your loved one's needs in a modern health care system. What makes this road map so difficult to read, is that the current routes, especially in America, happen to be experiencing major revisions . . . they are "under construction." Standard services provided in past years, in both private and governmental sectors, are no longer there, and new ones are still being revised and modified. Basically, the incentive at the moment to building new routes is singlefold: to reduce medical and rehabilitative expenditures. We, in America, are in a terribly tenuous and uncertain period of health care reform. Even if these changes do not apply to your area at the moment, should you be a reader from another province or country, it is likely in a world where systems are moving closer together that they will in the near future. What reverberations there are apt to be in your location is hard to predict, but you may well want to pay attention to whatever different route(s) may be evolving in your own locale.

A second way of viewing the road ahead, one separate from how health care might affect your loved one's recovery, is how to make daily life return to its fullest potential. As one might expect, this second route guide is more personalized, self-styled, and enduring. Because of this, how it unfolds is more influential in determining the quality of your lives years from now.

Today's health care in America

Nothing creates a sense of isolation more than being placed in situations where the rules are unknown, the pace rapid, and the pressure intense. When aphasia arrives, it typically brings all of these circumstances with it. Until recent years, the course of management for people with aphasia in medical and rehabilitative settings was predictable. Of late, though, this road has been uprooted by a federal debate to nationalize health care. Although action at a federal level now appears unlikely, health care reform has not disappeared. At this very moment, state governments and the private sector overseeing such care are working feverishly to implement cost-saving changes that would preclude further federal intervention. Because of this, health care systems and regulations vary considerably throughout America at this time. Thus, depending on where you live, treatment of your loved one's aphasia may differ substantially.

To understand this variance, look briefly at opposing ends of the delivery service continuum. At one extreme there may be little change from past years, although such pockets of traditional care are quickly disappearing. If this is the case for your area, Figure 3–1 lays out likely routes for your loved one's course of treatment. Notice that main treatment components are specified according to where, when, and why they exist. For the moment, do not worry so much about understanding each box and its interconnecting lines. The significance of this information is discussed in a later chapter. For now, simply *overview the entire format for services* and *how they interrelate.*

You can see that in the past, one's stay in the hospital or rehabilitative setting was apt to extend over months. Any earlier release typically occurred *only* because existing skills, both physical and communicative, were sufficient to permit the injured person to be seen at the hospital as an outpatient. Note, too, that the length of treatment was determined by the degree of improvement in therapy. As long as the person with aphasia was making consistent and substantial gains, therapy continued. When improvement slowed or "plateaued," plans for discharge followed. Placement outside the hospital or rehab center consisted of several options: an extended care or nursing home, a residential care facility, or one's own home. Chapters 6 and 7 define these settings and how discharge typically followed. Basically, though, if the person with aphasia was not able to care for him- or herself unaided, placement favored an extended care or nursing home facility. Those individuals who could manage self-care well, but not totally unaided, were candidates for a residential home. If function permitted near-independence, then returning home was a more likely choice. Discharge to one setting did not preclude later transfer to a more independent setting should functions continue to improve and permit.

At the opposite end of the treatment continuum is a quite different set of options (Figure 3–2). This route reflects current revisions currently underway or in effect in this country. Years from now, some other models are apt to evolve from this one. Again, don't concern yourself with understanding every component part; simply scan this figure in relation to component parts in Figure 3–1.

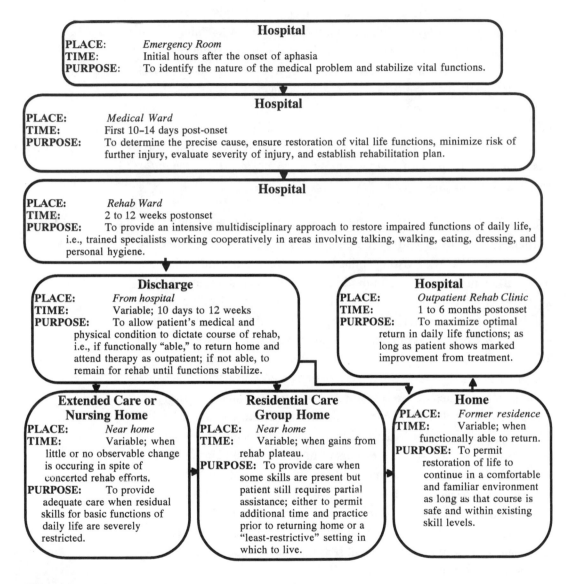

Hospital
PLACE: *Emergency Room*
TIME: Initial hours after the onset of aphasia
PURPOSE: To identify the nature of the medical problem and stabilize vital functions.

Hospital
PLACE: *Medical Ward*
TIME: First 10–14 days post-onset
PURPOSE: To determine the precise cause, ensure restoration of vital life functions, minimize risk of further injury, evaluate severity of injury, and establish rehabilitation plan.

Hospital
PLACE: *Rehab Ward*
TIME: 2 to 12 weeks postonset
PURPOSE: To provide an intensive multidisciplinary approach to restore impaired functions of daily life, i.e., trained specialists working cooperatively in areas involving talking, walking, eating, dressing, and personal hygiene.

Discharge
PLACE: *From hospital*
TIME: Variable; 10 days to 12 weeks
PURPOSE: To allow patient's medical and physical condition to dictate course of rehab, i.e., if functionally "able," to return home and attend therapy as outpatient; if not able, to remain for rehab until functions stabilize.

Hospital
PLACE: *Outpatient Rehab Clinic*
TIME: 1 to 6 months postonset
PURPOSE: To maximize optimal return in daily life functions; as long as patient shows marked improvement from treatment.

Extended Care or Nursing Home
PLACE: *Near home*
TIME: Variable; when little or no observable change is occuring in spite of concerted rehab efforts.
PURPOSE: To provide adequate care when residual skills for basic functions of daily life are severely restricted.

Residential Care Group Home
PLACE: *Near home*
TIME: Variable; when gains from rehab plateau.
PURPOSE: To provide care when some skills are present but patient still requires partial assistance; either to permit additional time and practice prior to returning home or a "least-restrictive" setting in which to live.

Home
PLACE: *Former residence*
TIME: Variable; when functionally able to return.
PURPOSE: To permit restoration of life to continue in a comfortable and familiar environment as long as that course is safe and within existing skill levels.

Figure 3–1. The road of the past.

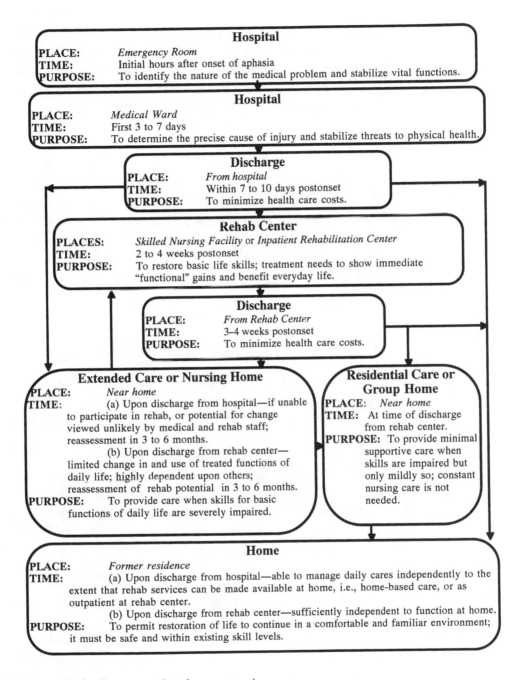

Figure 3–2. Current road under construction.

What is quickly apparent is that: (a) hospital stays are apt to be of a much shorter duration, (b) if rehabilitation (rehab), occurs, it is apt to be in a separate, less costly, intermediary facility outside the hospital, (c) duration of rehab is apt to be much shorter and depend on the ability of the person with aphasia to acquire functional, life-sustaining skills quickly, and (d) discharge is apt to be twofold, first from a hospital within days of onset and second from a intermediary care center weeks or months after that. Discharges in general occur sooner and serve to reduce the quantity and cost of services.

While health care changes serve to help unburden a financially taxed system, they also mean less time and fewer direct services for your loved one's rehab. When the main emphasis is on reducing costs, it is likely that "short cuts" may occur. More than ever before it is incumbent on you to become familiar with your loved one's needs and to become his or her advocate. Besides the legitimacy of the needs your loved one has, they are often *yours as well!*

Finding and making your own route

The road to adjusting to aphasia and its related disabilities is different for each traveler. By this, we do not just mean for each person with aphasia, but for your loved one and yourself as well. Although the two of you may be in the same vehicle and on the same roads a lot of the time, your views and reactions to the various landscapes and terrains is apt to differ. Tables 3–1 and 3–2 lay out common perspectives experienced by people with aphasia and their caregivers, respectively. Note that the term "caregiver" is used throughout the journey chapters, even though we know you may not be an actual caregiver. The term is meant to be taken broadly to include anyone reading this book who loves and cares for a person with aphasia. The descriptions in Tables 3–1 and 3–2 represent a "middle ground" of past travelers and may or may not be specific to you or your loved one. Collectively, though, these profiles may provide a reference point from which to plan your routes ahead.

The journey before you divides into five distinct time periods: hospitalization, rehabilitation, leaving formal care, one year later, and two years later. For each of these time periods, there is a journey chapter (Chapters 4–8). To help preview these periods, we've tabulated the descriptions in Tables 3–1 and 3–2 by: how the problem is perceived (sense of problem), how change is seen at that time (point of reference), how future change is viewed (looking ahead), and ways for aiding you at that time (guides). To begin with, examine these two tables separately by scanning their general features. Don't concern yourself with the guide section initially. Simply examine the problem, point of reference, and each traveler's view of what lies ahead.

Go back once more now and compare each traveler's impressions by time periods. Start with hospitalization and look at the afflicted person's likely perspective and then the caregiver's. Move to rehabilitation, the next period, and do the same. If possible, keep your focus on the evolution of the journey rather than on individual differences.

Now go back once more and examine the guide sections for each traveler. Don't worry if the abbreviated suggestions don't seem complete or fully interpretable at this time. Their inclusion serves simply as an introduction in order to highlight general directions that you might wish to consider. The many particulars involving suggested guidelines are detailed in Chapters 4 through 8. For now, simply try to derive a sense of coping options considered by other travelers. These overviews are for your benefit, to allow you to get a sense of the road ahead. How best to select and negotiate specific routes is addressed later as we move into the journey chapters themselves.

Reading the road maps ahead

You need to know that Chapters 4 through 8 look different from the ones you've read so far. Don't be deceived by their new appearance. They are just as reader-friendly and personal as these first chapters. They have been purposely structured as special kinds of "road maps" so you can quickly locate the aspects of the journey you most relate to or need help with. Because they follow a different format, we want to be sure you are well familiar with it before proceeding.

How the road maps ahead are laid out

Following a standard introduction to each period, journey chapters present a list of common features experienced or observed in people with aphasia and their caregivers. Identified as *profiles*, these lists are to help

Table 3–1. Overviewing the road as experienced by the person with aphasia- -guides to making the journey easier and more fulfilling.

TIME PERIOD	SENSE OF PROBLEM	POINT OF REFERENCE	LOOKING AHEAD	GUIDES FOR HELPING

Hospitalization (1 to 2 weeks postonset)	• confused
	• aware something "out-of-the-ordinary" has occurred
	• unsure of *what* or how bad the problem is
		• likely without a referent . . . too "sick" and disoriented
		• if able to do so, thinking of the way life was before aphasia
			• likely not focused on what lies ahead; too "sick" to do anything more than be affected by the current confusion	• strive to maintain a calm, positive, warm, and self-assured manner while around loved one
				• talk less, reach out more . . .
				  -touching
				  -smiling
				  -reassuring

Rehabilitation (2 weeks to 3 months postonset)	• less confused but still not totally "grounded" • as rehab progresses, more aware of injury • likely to begin to sense the seriousness of the problem • even so, still thinks that problem will resolve itself completely with time	• the way life was before aphasia	• exhibits mild to moderate concern over what this may mean • inwardly, far more concerned; likely scared and worried about implications • hard to imagine daily life in present state of dysfunction	• constant and frequent doses of encouragement to move ahead • acknowledge aphasia's presence and basic nature • begin stressing the value of time as an ally and the likely "gradualness" of recovery • keep communues simple, to the point, and within loved one's ability to understand and respond • distinguish between "caring for" and "doing for" your loved one; strive to avoid the latter

Stage			
Leaving formal care . . . starting a "new" daily routine alone (3 to 9 months postonset)	• alert to surroundings • becoming oriented to the fact that a "lasting" problem exists • likely discouraged that recovery hasn't been faster and more complete • hopeful that more will return with time	• the way life was before aphasia	• beginning to sense that improvement is not going to be automatic or fast • likely telling self, though, that all will be "back-to-normal" in a few more weeks, or at worst, months	• establish and maintain an adult-to-adult relationship . . . if not always possible in form, at least in spirit • avoid assuming responsibility in full for your loved one's well-being or daily routine • permit and encourage loved one to act in his or her own behalf to the degree possible and safe • seek out and use community resources, e.g., aphasia/stroke groups, aided transportation, daycare, senior centers, noncredit adult classes
One year later (12 months postonset)	• revising self-image to include aphasia • still resisting notion that problem will remain as severe as now • aware of steady gains but change is far less than envisioned • possible bouts of depression as awareness of aphasia's	• starting to judge change from the time after injury • noting that current status is "much better" than at 3, 6, or 9 months postonset • however, still highly aware that performance is far below pre-injured levels	• rate of change is beginning to slow • starting to understand that aphasia is *NOT* going to fully resolve over time • likely more worried and concerned about what this means for the immediate and long-term future	• acknowledge and console loved one over possible long term functional deficits • stress, if possible, that his or her value to you is *NOT* tied to performance in any of these areas • reassure that value is in the person he or she *is* • realize that functional restrictions typically do *NOT* preclude participation in daily life . . . only how well and how much might be done

(continued)

33

Table 3–1. *continued*

TIME PERIOD	SENSE OF PROBLEM	POINT OF REFERENCE	LOOKING AHEAD	GUIDES FOR HELPING
One year later (12 months postonset)	permanency increases • struggling with self-image and con-fidence in altered state • increased tendency to turn to and rely on others			• promote involvement and personal ownership in activities of choice • such participation must be of loved one's choice . . . avoid directly "forcing" involvement • as encouraged earlier, if loved one is unwilling to act in his or her behalf, remain supportive of the person but resist "doing for" him or her in daily life what he or she is capable of
Two years later (24 months postonset)	• aphasia becoming a part of self and daily life • small, gradual gains continue • improvement likely more apparent to people directly involved with loved one than to outsiders • if engaged in life, starting to "accept"	• fading comparisons to preinjury skills and abilities • usually, noticing changes in comparison to levels of function weeks or months ago	• finally internalizing, possibly coming to "accept," that aphasia is never going to resolve completely • if engaged in life, likely moving onto new challenges in spite of aphasia • if not engaged, likely viewing life as not	• maintenance and expansion of the guides from a year ago is "key" to continued personal growth and well-being • it is never too late to change focus or become more actively involved in one's own destiny • long-term success of loved one's recovery is directly related to incorporating aphasia into self-concept and proceeding with life in spite of it

aphasia
- if inactive, likely experiencing enduring bouts of anger, depression, and self-pity
- Level of dependency on others tied to personal well-being

possible because of aphasia

- proceeding ahead requires loved one, of choice, to grab the reins and assert a direction, or desire . . . which when acted upon restores purpose and meaning to his/ or her daily existence

Table 3–2. Overviewing the road as experienced by the caregiver—guides to making the journey easier and more fulfilling.

TIME PERIOD	SENSE OF PROBLEM	POINT OF REFERENCE	LOOKING AHEAD	GUIDES FOR HELPING
Hospitalization (1 to 2 weeks postonset)	• in utter shock • immobilized by dramatic change in loved one's appearance and function • worried about the seriousness of the injury • unclear what the implications may be but optimistic that injury will repair itself over time	• how loved one was before injury	• initially concerned solely with loved one's survival • as initial days pass and medical condition stabilizes, more focused on recovery, what to expect, and how to obtain such information	• keep in the forefront . . . aphasia a condition not just of **your loved one** alone . . . it is yours as well • accordingly . . . treat yourself with kindness, a forgiving attitude, and lots of latitude throughout the course of this journey • to the degree humanly and medically possible, resist spending every waking moment at your loved one's side • when present, outwardly reflect warmth, hope, and a positive and caring attitude • when absent, inwardly make your emotions and thoughts the priority • remember . . . time is not an adversary but rather an ally
Rehabilitation (2 weeks to 3 months postonset)	• struggling to put the parts of life back into some	• how loved one was before injury	• likely aware that recovery will take time and progress	• concentrate on the moment rather than months away • sort out what of daily life is and

working "whole"
- getting oriented to what has happened and the proposed course for treatment
- overwhelmed by foreignness of what's happened and quantity of new information
- still hoping that life will return to "normal," i.e., the "way-it-was-before" aphasia's arrival

Leaving formal care . . . starting a "new" daily routine alone (3 to 9 months postonset)

- feeling better over the progress made in rehab
- alarmed, though, that therapy is ending
- urgently sensing that "there's got to be more"
- worried over inability to attend to

- judging progress two ways:
  - amount of improvement since injury
  - amount still needed to return loved one to pre-injured self

- confused and worried over the future, especially now that therapy is ending
- feeling the need to push the system, loved one, and self for more
- optimistic that further gains are

is apt to be gradual
- may have heard as well from an informed source that:
  - communication will never be possible, or as it was, again
  - what gains occur are apt to evolve in the first 6–12 months

is not important at this specific-moment in time . . . find ways to temporarily postpone what isn't
- avoid letting your identity "merge" completely with the perceived needs and demands of **your loved one**
- consciously devote time to keeping **your** own life distinct, operational, and enriched . . . even if it means **not** attending to "every" aspect of your loved one's routine
- a healthy and lasting recovery requires **both** of you to be mentally, physically, and emotionally well and cared for

- this juncture in the road likely sets the tenor and course for much of what's to follow
- everyone must find one's own most comfortable path . . . there is no single solution
- coming to successfully link what "was" with what "is" often requires several key components:
  - keeping interactions adult-to-

continued

Table 3-2 continued

TIME PERIOD	SENSE OF PROBLEM	POINT OF REFERENCE	LOOKING AHEAD	GUIDES FOR HELPING
Leaving formal care . . . starting a "new" daily routine alone (3 to 9 months postonset)	• what will be needed at home • sensing that maybe a full recovery is not realistic		possible and will follow	adult, not adult-to-child -supporting and caring for loved one's continued improvement yet promoting a self-determined and self-sustaining routine -actively searching out new and acceptable ways of fulfilling your own personal needs
One year later (12 months postonset)	• initial encouragement over treatment gains giving way to discouragement. . . not only has aphasia *not* gone away, gains are now slower and less distinct • as aphasia's permanency registers, increased concerns over how to cope with daily life in this state	• still judging progress in two ways: -amount of improvement since injury -amount still needed to return loved one to preinjured self • if the latter method is prevailing, greater tendency toward discouragement	• beginning to revise thoughts about future . . . starting to entertain what to do if loved one's condition does *not* improve substantially beyond current level of dysfunction	• strive to stay positive at a time when *your* expectations for further change may tend to fall short . . . . -rely on past guides to keep your focus, direction, and momentum moving ahead -try not to emphasize what isn't working but rather what is -recalibrate change . . .from a societal scale of normalcy to any improvement in your loved one's performance over time

38

- actively look for and pursue methods that might add onto, rather than subtract from, the activities of daily life . . . not just for your loved one but for yourself as well

- hopeful, though, that a favorable turn of events may still reverse matters

Two years later (24 months postonset)

- settling into a routine for coping with daily life
- new routine notably different
- likely still struggling to make parts fit and feel comfortable
- responsibility for loved one's daily routine likely needs to be equally shared by now in order to prevent feelings of entrapment
- your opportunities for personal fulfillment and growth are equally important to establishing healthy routine

- combined referents as before
- however, because change seems so minimal now and because overall performance is far from preinjured condition, attention to change likely to diminish

- likely not expecting much, if any, further change in loved one's condition
- focusing on what might make life better given residual skills
- if extracting some "beauty" out of daily life now, likely optimistic more will follow
- if unable to find value in daily life now, likely growing weary and impatient

- if your daily routine and thoughts are less about aphasia and its imposed restrictions and more about what you do and will do, you are right on course
- if this is *not* true . . . i.e., your loved one's aphasia still dominates most of daily life's routines . . . know that it's never too late to start building a different operational base, that is, learning to look for, see, and use the beauty in the landscape at hand
- this journey isn't over until the struggles of living daily life are far less prominent than the pleasures derived
- remember . . . aphasia does *not* preclude having or living life as you so choose

orient you to what others often felt or observed when they were near this point in time. Figure 3–3 displays a sample layout of one of these profiles.

The next section of each journey chapter summarizes the **primary concerns** of travelers, once again from the separate perspectives of the person with aphasia and the caregiver. To ensure some consistency through the course of the journey, we have chosen to place them in categories according to "theme." Table 3–3 lists the categories and a brief description of each.

Figure 3–4 contains a sample page of how primary concerns appear in journey chapters. Note that they appear in the form of a briefly stated concern or question, that is, what the person may be wondering or worrying about at that time. Also, these categories have been arranged according to their commonly perceived importance, the most concerning issues first with lesser issues following. You and your loved one's concerns and questions may differ either in type or order of importance, but some commonalties are likely to occur. Select from these lists those concerns which parallel your needs and wants; leave the others until they do concern you.

The third section of each journey chapter contains comments that address the previously identified concerns of the person with aphasia, while the fourth section provides comparable specifics that address the concerns of the caregiver. The ordering of content in sections three and four mirrors the ordering of primary concerns. Each concern or question is considered from two perspectives: first, with respect to any "information" you may need to understand or know about its nature (WHAT TO

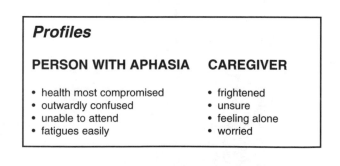

Figure 3–3. Sample page containing profiles for person with aphasia and caregiver.

Table 3–3. Categories of concerns with descriptions.

CATEGORY OF CONCERN	DESCRIPTION
Health	pertaining to the physical wellness of your loved one
Thinking	pertaining to your loved one's ability to think, reason, or remember
Communication	pertaining to exchanging information and staying connected with your loved one
Emotions/Feelings	pertaining to emotions or feelings; may be in reference to your loved one or yourself
Family/Friends	pertaining to maintaining ties with family and friends
Recovery	pertaining to the restoration of lost or impaired functions
Employment	pertaining to your or your loved one's ability to work
Finances	pertaining to current monetary obligations and meeting costs associated with medical or rehabilitative services

---

Primary Concerns

PERSON WITH APHASIA   **CAREGIVER**

Thinking   **Health**
1-What has happened?   1-What caused this?
2-Where am I?   2-How stable is he/she?

Health   **Emotions**
1-Am I going to live?   1-Is he/she going to live?
2-How bad is my injury?   2-What if he/she . . .?

Figure 3–4. Sample page displaying primary concerns.

KNOW), and second, with respect to what "action" you may want to consider in terms of coping with it (WHAT YOU MIGHT DO).

To expedite locating content within journey chapters, we've provided you with a number of short cuts. First, in the upper margin of each page you will see which person's concern is being addressed: the person with aphasia or the caregiver (a loved one). Second, all concerns are boxed and appear initially in the margins of pages. Third, categories with more than one concern are all numbered; numbers found in the margin of pages correspond with previously numbered concerns. Fourth, shading differentiates help whether you are within a "**WHAT TO KNOW**" or **"WHAT YOU MIGHT DO"** section. The latter are shaded; the former are not. Figure 3–5 displays a sample page highlighting the use of these formatting aids.

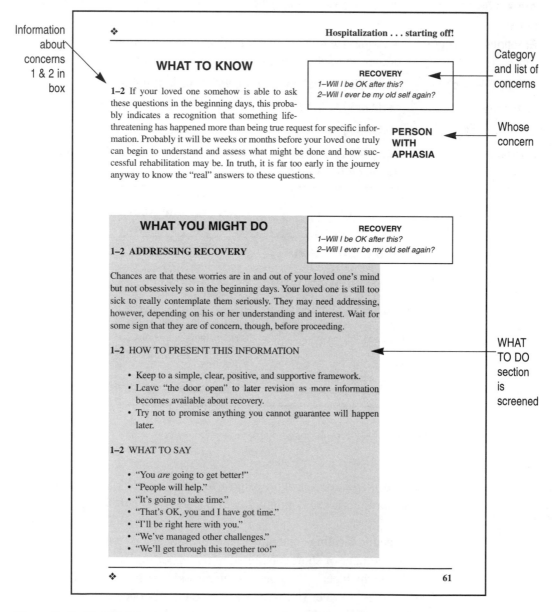

Figure 3–5. Sample journey page.

Proceeding from here

Now we are ready to help you travel down that road together. Perhaps you and your loved one are already many miles past the beginning point, that is, past hospitalization, rehabilitation, and even some months of living with aphasia on your own. Skipping ahead to wherever you are in your journey makes perfectly good sense. However, if you are a year or more beyond aphasia's onset, it may prove helpful to at least scan selected parts of Chapters 5 through 7, before jumping to wherever you might be. Sometimes not taking an important route in the beginning can cause you to get miles off course later on. To reach the place where you ultimately want to go, you may need to back up and retrace some old routes differently in order to prepare yourselves for what we might be suggesting next.

Realize that from the minute you turn onto this road, the trip ahead is yours, nobody else's! Yes, there are others who have made it who can help you now. We'll attempt to do the same. **But ultimately where you go and how this journey evolves depends solely on you and your loved one. This trip's form or content don't need to work for anybody but you.** So from the very beginning, pay particular attention to the thoughts that resonate the most with you! Do all you can to promote the parts that do, and worry less about the parts that don't. Ultimately you will want to fashion a unique and personal form of living life that allows you and your loved one not to feel entrapped by aphasia. Rather, your goal will be to live your own form of life in spite of aphasia. So start that engine . . . and let's go find out what works best for you.

CHAPTER 4

Hospitalization . . . starting off!

Your introduction to the hospital likely came abruptly without warning. It may have started with an unannounced ride to the hospital's emergency room. You stood quietly and in shock while medical personnel attended to your loved one. Somewhere within you, you kept asking: "How could this *really* be happening?" "It *must* be a bad dream!" You hoped that somehow this dream would end and that life would return to normal. Well . . . enough time has passed to know that the hurried trip to the hospital was *not* a dream, nor was its aftermath. Now, the operative parts of daily life are strewn all about as you struggle to find something . . . anything . . . that feels familiar, and *works*.

Very likely, nothing about the process of hospitalization is apt to feel familiar . . . it occurs in a setting and with a set of rules that probably are new, foreign, and even *scary!* But hospitals are not without predictable ways of operating, and the more you know about these, the easier this part of the journey is. Before elaborating on hospitals' patterns of operation, you need know some common features of these beginning days

---

after injury. **For most spouses, and other loved ones of the injured person, these days are usually** *the most confusing, the most emotionally jarring, and the most mentally depleting* **of the entire journey. When trauma of this magnitude occurs, even though it is largely of an emotional origin, you and your body are experiencing a form of** *emotional shock*. **Just because the physical injury involved your loved one, and not you, does not mean that you are immune from its emotional injury.**

Chances are that your normal thinking and reasoning processes are not fully accessible or functional at the moment. Your body and mind feel partially numbed as if injected with some megadose of a deadening agent. Previously simple tasks, like deciding where to go and what to do next, are simply too much. Because of this, you need to be especially aware of the presence of such changes, and also forgiving of yourself. You likely need to give yourself a little time to recapture a sense of feeling and groundedness. Rest assured that most likely none of the hours or days "lost" to your own recovery will jeopardize what needs attending to at the hospital.

In certain rare instances, though, important "life-or-death" decisions may be required in the beginning hours or days after injury. If this is true for you, give serious thought to seeking assistance from others: close family, friends, clergy, and/or medical personnel. This is probably *not* a time to try to assume the full burden for stressful and weighty decisions. Look to others to aid you until some normalcy returns to your own body, mind, and spirit.

The more likely scenario, though, is that your loved one's medical condition is beyond anyone's control or power to remediate. That is, there is nothing known to science, medicine, or humans that can either stop or reverse the injury that has already happened. Instead, you and your loved one are at the mercy of the powers that be. For now, you must simply wait, and allow life to run its natural course.

Know, too, that being in a state of emotional shock is often disconcerting. Your mind wanders aimlessly about, filling and refilling with related and unrelated segments of the past hours or days. You keep rummaging through these details in search of something that might help. When nothing does, you try again to redirect your thought to the moment at hand, but quickly it drifts back to where it just was. As disconcerting as this circular quagmire may be, it is actually invaluable in the process of moving matters forward. **This period of mental inefficiency and confusion is apt to force you to "wait, watch, and listen" until basic levels of reason re-emerge. Knowing this, you can, and should, excuse yourself for not being at the "top of your game." With a brief period of adjustment to what has happened, you will be on your way again!**

So, take a few days, get your bearings, and when you are ready again . . . so are we. If by chance, you have arrived at this particular juncture without reading the preceding chapters, go back and do that right now! In fact, even if you are still trying to sort matters out, a simple overview of aphasia's nature is apt to be medicinal. In any case, you need the information in Chapters 1 through 3 to understand what comes next. Don't proceed without it.

Profiles

PERSON WITH APHASIA

- experiencing state of most compromised health
- possibly unable to sit, walk, attend to self-care, or communicate
- outwardly appearing confused
- inwardly frightened
- less able to initiate or participate
- fluctuating ability to attend
- easily fatigued
- possibly incontinent of bowel and bladder
- likely at risk to eat or drink

CAREGIVER

- frightened and scared
- unsure of how to proceed
- feeling overwhelmed and vulnerable
- possibly not feeling up to the challenge
- feeling alone
- worried
- possibly having some feelings of guilt

Primary concerns

PERSON WITH APHASIA

Thinking
1–What's happened to me?
2–Where am I?

Health
1–Am I going to live?
2–How bad is my injury?

Emotions
1–I'm scared . . . stay close, OK?
2–I need you . . . please help!

Communication
1–Why can't people understand me?
2–Why can't I understand them?

Recovery
1–Will I be OK after this?
2–Will I ever be my old self again?

CAREGIVER

Health
1–What has happened to my loved one?
2–What caused this?
3–How stable is his or her medical condition?
4–What might I expect in the days and weeks ahead?
5–How can I help?

Emotions
1–Is my loved one going to live?
2–What if he or she doesn't?
3–Will our lives ever be the same?

Communication
1–Why can't my loved one communicate?
2–Will he or she be able to communicate again?
3–What can be done now?
4–How can I help?

Recovery
1–How and when will my loved one get better?
2–Who can help and what will they do?
3–How can I help?

Family/Friends
1–What should I tell them?

Employment
1–What should I tell my loved one's employer?
2–What should I tell my employer?

Finances
1-How much is all of this going to cost?

WHAT TO KNOW

THINKING
1–What's happened to me?
2–Where am I?

1–2 In the beginning week or weeks of injury, all your loved one's brain functions are likely to be somewhat diminished. He or she may not know

PERSON WITH APHASIA

where he or she is, the time, date, or even who you are! Even though the "true" injury is likely confined to a limited region of your loved one's brain, the one that regulates language and communication functions, a protective mechanism in his or her body often diminishes the flow of blood to the entire brain. This short-term reduction in blood flow results in "whole brain" disturbances that often leave sufferers mentally confused and disoriented to place, time, and person.

1–2 Another name for whole brain disturbance is ***mental status change***. Although memory and thinking typically decline during this period, people with aphasia often remember later how confused and unclear their thinking was! Months later, it is not uncommon to hear: "I simply could not understand what was happening! People were moving about quickly and talking. But I couldn't figure out what they wanted. All I knew was that it must be something pretty bad . . . the doctors' faces looked very serious and I remember wondering whether I was going to survive!"

1–2 Not too strangely, when people are suddenly thrust into a new situation where nothing makes sense, fear is apt to follow. Nothing is more alarming than suddenly recognizing that everyday functions are absent, yet not knowing why! Sometimes changes in one's mental status actually help buffer the recognition of such losses. However, even when this is true, most people with aphasia are aware that something dramatic and life-threatening has just happened. Your loved one may not have a *full appreciation* of what has happened or its severity for several weeks, but he or she is probably terrified by what he or she can see and sense.

1–2 Fear in the early-going is not confined to the person with aphasia. It immediately permeates the lives of everyone else close to him or her. Perhaps having witnessed the consequences of your loved one's injury firsthand, your first worries were probably about his or her survival. Depending on your personality style, this fear may or may not have been readily apparent. However, if it still exists and is quite visible, it makes sense to try to consciously "mask" such worries while in your loved one's presence. Although his or her understanding of words may not be good, the look on your face is likely a "neon sign" of what has happened

PERSON WITH APHASIA

and what its consequences may be. Quite likely, you do not have the answers to many questions yet, so it is important to avoid unconsciously conveying any feelings of pending doom or tragedy. Such signals may only complicate your loved one's tenuous medical or physical status.

1–2 Your worries and concerns, though, need not go unaddressed. If you feel overwrought with anxiety at the sight of his or her physical status, then remain "bright" while at bedside and take frequent breaks outside his or her room. To the degree you can, save your own moments of personal despair until you are alone or in the company of selected others, like family, friends, or clergy. Later, when you know more about your loved one's status, you will be able to be more forthright in sharing your emotions with him or her.

THINKING
1–What's happened to me?
2–Where am I?

WHAT YOU MIGHT DO

1–2 READJUSTING YOUR PERSPECTIVE

Before addressing your loved one's concerns, it is important to readjust your own perspective. While it may not be easy to witness dramatic differences in his or her apparent ability to talk, communicate, think, reason, or remember, initial severe limitations in the beginning hours or days often *do not* reflect severity of injury! Try not to jump to conclusions, especially negative ones keep in mind that it is still very early and a lot is apt to change in the days ahead, especially with regard to thinking, reasoning, and remembering.

1–2 WHAT TO REMEMBER

- Your loved one has not lost his or her mind.
- Instead, whole brain functions probably are temporarily compromised.
- Such changes are typical at this time.
- Thinking, most parts of reasoning, and memory should gradually return in the weeks ahead.
- The exception may be if your loved one has suffered multiple injuries to the brain.

If so, a more lasting impairment to thinking is possible. Even then, though, gains from initial levels of function are still likely.

- Because of mental status changes, he or she may not understand simple, everyday facts or happenings.
- Try not to be personally hurt if your loved one doesn't know you . . . with a little time, recognition of place, time, and person will likely return.

1–2 HOW TO USE YOUR APPEARANCE TO AID YOUR LOVED ONE

- Approach your loved one warmly and positively.
- Use an embracing smile.
- Try to project a feeling and sense of confidence . . . as if "you have matters in hand!"
- Reach out and touch your loved one often.
- Hold his or her left hand . . . the right side may not be fully operative or sensitive to touch.

1–2 WHAT TO SAY AND HOW TO SAY IT

- Use a calm and reassuring voice.
- Speak normally, do *not* shout.

  If your loved one's hearing was OK before the injury and he or she is not understanding your message now, it is likely due to the brain injury, not a sudden loss of hearing. Talking louder won't help!

- Keep your sentences short and to the point.
- Separate main points, i.e., allow extra time between words and thoughts for your loved one to think, process, and react.
- Present your points slowly, e.g.,

  what has happened: "Jim, you've had a stroke."

  where he or she is: "You're in the hospital."

  who you are: "Remember me? I'm your wife, Betty."

  what's happening: "You'll be here for a few days. The doctors are running tests."

- If your loved one is alert and attentive, writing out critical words and numbers, e.g., the time of day and dates, or people's names, in big letters and numbers on a tablet may possibly help.
- Repeat the important parts of messages several times.

  Holding onto new information is probably very difficult at this

PERSON WITH APHASIA

**PERSON
WITH
APHASIA**

time. Do not assume that if you tell your loved one something that it will be retained and intact over time. You likely will need to repeat it numerous times until any retention occurs.

1–2 WHY TRY TO COMMUNICATE WHEN YOUR LOVED ONE'S THINKING ISN'T WORKING

- Hearing a familiar voice is reassuring, calming, and often therapeutic.
- Interacting with a familiar person tends to diminish your loved one's anxiety and fear.
- Communicating is more than just exchanging information; it helps bond people together.

  More important than hearing "facts," your loved one needs to feel and know that you are there and supportive. Because he or she is likely quite frightened, reassuring him or her with your presence and a consoling voice likely goes a long way in making matters better.

WHAT TO KNOW

HEALTH
1–Am I going to live?
2–How bad is my injury?

1–2 Assuming his or her mental status permits, your loved one is apt to have these questions in the forefront of his mind whether he or she is able to express them or not: "Am I going to live?" and "Just how bad is my injury?" Depending on your loved one's abilities to think, reason, and communicate, you likely need to address these issues to *some degree!* However, the extent to which you do needs to be carefully gauged in the beginning, especially if thinking or understanding of spoken words is restricted.

1–2 Recall that people with aphasia initially have difficulty understanding speech and yet may outwardly "appear" to understand everything! When this is the case, even the simplest words may sound familiar but not be understood. If you add to this that thinking and memory might be compromised, any reliable exchange of information is apt to be tenuous at this time. What might be shared in the morning, even if partially understood, may not be recalled moments or hours later. Also, because your loved one's talking likely isn't as functional as his or her understanding, any attempt on his or her part to respond to your explanations may only complicate matters.

1–2 For these reasons, it is advisable to keep explanations brief at first, and to limit them in number. If this feels unnatural to you and very different from your relationship before, try to use more non-spoken messages instead of words . . . touching, reassuring your loved one with gestures and maintaining an embracing smile sprinkled with short encouraging phrases: "You rest . . . I'll be close by." "Everything's OK." These messages often work the best!

WHAT YOU MIGHT DO

> **HEALTH**
> *1–Am I going to live?*
> *2–How bad is my injury?*

1–2 COMMUNICATING WITH LOVED ONE

The objective here is to lessen your loved one's fears and anxieties, not to convey *a lot* of information. Details can be added later when his or her thinking and language permit. Your prime concern now needs to be reducing his or her worries and confusion. **If talking and trying to communicate only add to the problem, stop talking! This type of exchange can wait until a time when he or she *is* able to understand speech.**

1–2 WHAT TO KEEP IN MIND

- Keep your content simple, clear, brief, positive, and reassuring.
- Keep your comments general, rather than specific.
- Just deal with broad facts . . . no details or speculation.
- Convey a sense of hope.

1–2 HOW TO SAY IT

- "You've had a stroke."
- "It's too early to know why."
- "You're doing OK."
- "Just rest."
- "We'll talk later."
- "We'll get through this!"

**PERSON
WITH
APHASIA**

1–2 HOW TO PROCEED WHEN UNDERSTANDING IS RELATIVE-LY INTACT

- Only address matters further if your loved one requests it.
- Highlight only the parts of his or her condition that might lessen his or her concern or worry.
- Present each part as before—point-by-point—keeping it simple and clear.

  "You've had an injury to your head."

  "It is completely over."

  "It is *not* getting worse."

  "Your condition is stable."

- Continue *only* if your loved one seems attentive and interested.
- Again, writing out key words may help.

EMOTIONS
1-I'm scared . . . stay close, OK?
2-I need you . . . please help!

WHAT TO KNOW

1–2 It is not surprising that your loved one may feel depleted, vulnerable, and in need of help. All of a sudden, previously simple activities either are impossible or require considerable effort and support. Talking, eating, going to the bathroom, dressing, and walking are no longer available like they once were. Whether your loved one can express it or not, you can sense his or her desperation, anguish, and pain over absent and disordered functions. While he or she is in this tenuous state of being, you likely are aware of his or her crying out for your presence, assistance, and commitment to help.

1–2 Your immediate heartfelt impulse may be to step forward and announce: "Don't worry, dear, *I'll* take care of everything . . . you just concentrate on getting better!" There is no question about the inherent value of being able and willing to do this, that is, to make an unconditional pronouncement of your love and support. He or she very much needs this now and continuously throughout the many miles ahead. As well, you may not be able to inhibit *your* need to attend to every part of your loved one's compromised state. However, it is important to know the potential harm that may come from well-intended but excessive attentions in the early going. Not only might your assistance be more

**PERSON
WITH
APHASIA**

than your loved one actually needs, it may "entrap" you in a form of support that can be neither maintained nor easily withdrawn later.

1–2 In the next chapter, Caregiver-Recovery, we distinguish between "caring for" versus "doing for" your loved one. The crux of this difference is knowing that your loved one's ultimate well-being miles down this road depends on his or her re-emerging and developing ability to act in his or her own behalf. Whatever you can do along the way to promote this outcome, the less you'll need to do later. For now, though, you likely *do not know* what your loved is capable of doing, nor can you stop yourself from providing what "might be" needed in this emotionally laden state of new injury. It is important, though, to begin developing a philosophy you can carry with you down the road ahead, one that supports well-being without excessive attention to what doesn't need your support. Much more on this subject will be presented in the chapters ahead.

1–2 One way to begin facilitating your loved one's resumption of control over life is to start removing yourself periodically from his or her side. Take frequent half-hour breaks when he or she is napping, or involved in another activity or test. Go outside and get some fresh air. From the very onset of injury spending some time away from your loved one is apt to be as therapeutic for you as it is for him or her!

WHAT YOU MIGHT DO

> **EMOTIONS**
> *1–I'm scared . . . stay close, OK?*
> *2–I need you . . . please help!*

1–2 REASSURING YOUR LOVED ONE

Steady doses of reassurance are important throughout this journey, but especially so in the beginning days and weeks after injury. Reassurance, though, involves more than words. It is likely that your demeanor and frame of mind will carry more weight than spoken words. If possible, come to him or her with strength, composure, and the appearance of being "in control" of matters and life.

1–2 WHAT TO SAY

- "I can see the concern in your eyes and face . . ."

PERSON WITH APHASIA

- "I'm sure this is difficult and scary!"
- "Your doctor says you are doing fine at the moment, don't worry."
- "I'm right here, and I'll remain so!"
- "We'll make it through this, I promise!"

1–2 WHAT TO CONSIDER

- Be outwardly strong, warm, and positive.
- Give no sign, in these first days, of fear, discouragement, or failure.
- Try not to remain too long or to do too much with your loved one:
    give yourself frequent breaks:
        it is *not* essential that you be present every moment.
        try leaving once he or she is asleep or at other appointments.
        get used to stepping away and letting him or her "manage"—it's important to recovery!
    go outside . . . change your environment . . . get out of the hospital.
    push your thoughts in other directions:
        something pleasant.
        something unrelated.
        something fun.
        something positive.

COMMUNICATION

1–Why can't people understand me?
2–Why can't I understand them?

WHAT TO KNOW

1 Aphasia interferes with sending and receiving words. Depending on the type and severity of your loved one's aphasia, you may wish to take a "side trip" here and examine his or her profile in more detail in Chapter 10. The hospital speech-language pathologist should be able to help you select the sections of this chapter that apply to your loved one's injury. In general, though, you need to know that the greatest difficulty talking is apt to be occurring right now! It is not unusual for speech to cease or for it to be impaired beyond recognition. When unrecognizable, it is because the proper words cannot be found, or because the words selected are either wrong or distorted. Regardless, the spoken message fails to communicate the basic needs of the person with aphasia.

1 Some people with aphasia "know" that their talking isn't working. Even so, out of a longstanding habit of communicating with speech, they cannot stop trying. In the beginning, these speakers start their message, only to abort the effort shortly with signs of frustration or dismay. Some of these impaired talkers quickly reduce the frequency and length of their spoken messages. Still others continue to talk much as they have been, but with dissatisfaction over not being able to express their needs. If their impaired speech persists, frustration with it is apt to lessen gradually over time, but dissatisfaction with not being able to talk may linger on for years.

1 It is possible, too, that your loved one may not be aware that his or her speech is even impaired. When this occurs, it may be due to mental confusion, inability to monitor his or her own speech, or both. Such speakers may deliver a cluttered, unclear message and look at you as if you should have understood them. Should this form of unrecognizable speech exist, do not act as if you understood the message when you did not. Trying to explain that you did not, though, may or may not work. Even if it does, you likely will need to repeat this explanation in the days ahead. If your spoken explanation didn't register, you may want to try a nonspoken gesture, like shrugging your shoulders, holding your hands up, and shaking your head back and forth. If you cannot make him or her understand even then, do not persist. Seek out the hospital's speech-language pathologist for his or her suggestions.

2 When your loved one's understanding of other people's speech is impaired, communication becomes even more challenging. Usually it means:

- interpretation of spoken messages breaks down . . . words simply don't compute!
- there may be little or no awareness on his or her part that understanding is even compromised.
- your loved one's speech may be totally unrecognizable.

Should these features describe your loved one's communication, you may want to skip ahead to Chapter 10 and read the sections devoted to Wernicke's or Global Aphasia.

2 The most encouraging news for people with aphasia who struggle to understand spoken words is the promise of improvement. Whereas impaired speech typically improves over time too, problems with under-

**PERSON
WITH
APHASIA**

standing often improve first and more quickly. In fact, most people with aphasia eventually come to understand and recognize simple messages within a familiar context or setting. A large percentage of these individuals eventually are able to understand and follow everyday conversations. Yet, when understanding is severely impaired, improvement is apt to be far more gradual, that is, extended over months and years, not days and weeks. Should your loved one face severe difficulties with understanding, you'll likely need to learn other ways of conveying messages besides talking. For now, though, realize that you've got plenty of time to adopt these methods as you travel further down this road and learn more.

2 The hardest task for caregivers when their loved one's understanding is severely impaired is remembering what the problem is. Quite often, it seems as if the mind itself is not working. Remember, though, that fictitious trip you took to South America in Chapter 2. You knew exactly where you were, what you wanted, and where you planned to go next. It was just that you couldn't comprehend the messages from the native people. Well, people with aphasia know about themselves and the world around them too. It is just that spoken words may carry little, if any, meaning. Should your loved one seem puzzled over your messages, do not assume his or her mind is *not* functioning well. It likely is!

COMMUNICATION
1–Why can't people understand me?
2–Why can't I understand them?

WHAT YOU MIGHT DO

1 INTERACTING WITH YOUR LOVED ONE ABOUT COMMUNICATION

Addressing this concern depends on your loved one's ability to understand simple speech. If understanding is poor, you may need to postpone these suggestions to a later time. But even when understanding or thinking aren't perfect, attempts at sharing often help. Your loved one may not "get" all parts of your message, but will still benefit from your effort to connect the two of you. With repeated presentations and additional time, a better understanding is likely to emerge.

1 WHAT TO SAY

- "You have suffered a stroke."
- "It has damaged your brain, especially the part that controls talking."
- "I know *you know* what you're trying to say."
- "This isn't easy."
- "But we'll manage."
- "It will get better with time."

1 IF UNDERSTANDING YOUR LOVED ONE'S MESSAGES REMAINS A PROBLEM

If you find yourself constantly confronting an angry communicator because you cannot grasp the meaning of his or her message, then consider the following:

- "I'm sorry, but I don't know what you're saying."
- "Your words are *not* making sense."
- "*I am* trying to understand."
- "I know this is hard, but it's *not* easy for me either."
- "Let's rest for now, we'll try again later."

1 WHEN YOUR EXPLANATIONS DO NOT HELP

- Quite likely, your loved one's understanding of speech is *too* impaired.
- Refer to suggestions in the next section.

2 WHEN UNDERSTANDING IS SEVERELY COMPROMISED

When both talking and listening are not effective for your loved one, you will need to explore other ways of conversing. Depending on the severity of your loved one's comprehension problem, the preferred way(s) for doing this may be simple or complex. Confer with the hospital's speech-language pathologist for suggestions on to how to proceed.

2 IF *SOME* UNDERSTANDING IS POSSIBLE

- Review communication suggestions in earlier sections in this chapter.

PERSON WITH APHASIA

PERSON WITH APHASIA

Person with aphasia: Thinking.

Person with aphasia: Emotions

- **Never talk in front of your loved one or allow others to do so as if he or she weren't there.**

   Overall understanding may not be good, but occasional words and phrases may still be interpreted correctly. People with severe aphasia often remember others telling grim tales about them or their condition in the early days of recovery. Never risk such a breach of trust. Talk to people in your loved one's presence as if he or she understands *everything*.

- When communicating, use fewer words, focus on key terms and omit smaller parts of speech.
- Talk slowly and deliberately, use pauses between words and phrases.
- Pair key words with corresponding hand and facial gestures, i.e., movements that reinforce your words.
- Let your loved one know that *you know* that he or she has trouble understanding words, *not* hearing or thinking.
- Never act as if you do understand his or her speech when you don't.
- Try to provide assurances that his or her condition will improve over time.

2 IF YOUR LOVED ONE CANNOT UNDERSTAND SPEECH

- Rely mainly on facial expression and hand gestures.
- Focus on just staying personally connected, i.e., reach out, touch, and warmly embrace your loved one.
- When talking, use one or two words at a time.
- If talking only increases confusion and alarm, eliminate it altogether.
- Kindly and reassuringly use hand gestures to discourage your loved one's attempts to talk.
- Keep the mood positive and strong . . . as if you *know* things will get better!

2 IF NONE OF THIS WORKS

- Do not prolong any exchange that doesn't feel positive.
- If you can't get your loved one to quiet down with gestures, leave the room momentarily.
- Discourage communicating through words and search out the hospital speech-language pathologist for other options.

WHAT TO KNOW

RECOVERY
1–Will I be OK after this?
2–Will I ever be my old self again?

1–2 If your loved one somehow is able to ask these questions in the beginning days, this probably indicates a recognition that something life-threatening has happened more than being true request for specific information. Probably it will be weeks or months before your loved one truly can begin to understand and assess what might be done and how successful rehabilitation may be. In truth, it is far too early in the journey anyway to know the "real" answers to these questions.

PERSON WITH APHASIA

WHAT YOU MIGHT DO

RECOVERY
1–Will I be OK after this?
2–Will I ever be my old self again?

1–2 ADDRESSING RECOVERY

Chances are that these worries are in and out of your loved one's mind but not obsessively so in the beginning days. Your loved one is still too sick to really contemplate them seriously. They may need addressing, however, depending on his or her understanding and interest. Wait for some sign that they are of concern, though, before proceeding.

1–2 HOW TO PRESENT THIS INFORMATION

- Keep to a simple, clear, positive, and supportive framework.
- Leave "the door open" to later revision as more information becomes available about recovery.
- Try not to promise anything you cannot guarantee will happen later.

1–2 WHAT TO SAY

- "You *are* going to get better!"
- "People will help."
- "It's going to take time."
- "That's OK, you and I have got time."
- "I'll be right here with you."
- "We've managed other challenges."
- "We'll get through this together too!"

CAREGIVER

WHAT TO KNOW

1–4 You probably know some of this information. Other parts of the answers, though, are likely still unclear or vague. It will take you days or weeks to obtain even "preliminary" answers. It will take much longer to fill in the details, depending on your interest and motivation, and the time to do so. Once again, depending on your needs and interests, there are several "side trips" ahead that you may wish to consider. Chapter 9 provides a detailed explanation of how the normal brain handles speech, language, and communication; Chapter 10 explains how brain injury involving aphasia alters these functions; Chapter 11 explains the causes of injury. If the above questions are foremost in your mind, you may want to pull over and selectively scan this information now, or when time permits.

1–4 In the beginning, these questions may seem almost unapproachable, not just in terms of their complexity but, more basically, in terms of how to get accurate and reliable answers. You may feel displaced and intimidated by the hospital setting. As you've likely observed already, "important people" scurry about in this place with a heightened intensity and urgency. It is apparent that they are attending to many other sick people besides your loved one. You may question in this atmosphere how critical your questions are, when they should be asked, and how.

1–4 In the simplest terms, your *questions and worries are important* and *they do deserve attention!* In the totality of all that happens within a hospital, attending to the concerns and questions of the family is a critical part of the service provided. You should not view yourself as an imposition or obstacle, although at times the behaviors and reactions of some professionals may seem to suggest that.

1–4 What is *most important* in trying to address your concerns is knowing "how." That is, to be successful in getting the information you want, you need to work *with* rather than *against* the tendencies and preferences of the health care professionals involved. To do this, you first need to understand who oversees which services. Generally, services on medical wards rest with two key providers: physicians and nurses. Below is a summary of what each does in this setting. Physicians focus on identifying the cause of the problem, minimizing its effects, restoring what was lost, and minimizing further injury. Nurses provide life-sustaining care and provide health care functions. **CAREGIVER**

PHYSICIAN	**NURSE**
• determines what caused the medical condition	• oversees and carries out health care services: monitoring vital signs dispensing medications maintaining diet, i.e., food/fluid intake attending to personal hygiene, i.e., bathing and toileting
• determines if anything can be done to reverse or stabilize the condition	
• if so, treats the condition	
• determines if there is any continuing risk to the patient's well-being or survival	• determines which health care services will be required at discharge
• if so, provides treatment to minimize the risks of further damage	• aids patient and family in ensuring that optimal health care is maintained inside and outside the hospital

1–4 To help maintain a good working relationship with physicians and nurses, you need to prepare yourself to interact with people who likely bring quite different orientations and preferences to the interaction table. Some may discuss your concerns and worries in-depth while others may provide only a brief sketch of the essentials that they view as important at that time. When an answer is short, it doesn't necessarily mean that the physician or nurse is disinterested in your loved one's physical well-being. Chances are that *time* is the real issue. Time in a hospital is the most precious and guarded commodity. As a result, messages from physicians and nurses may often seem cryptic and confusing.

1–4 Nevertheless, you have a *right* to a full explanation of what has happened. More importantly, you need to know the status of your loved one at the moment and what might be expected in the days and weeks ahead! A crucial issue, though, is how to approach these professionals to get answers to your questions, and remain on good working terms. Specific suggestions follow in the next section of this chapter.

1–5 You may feel at times that not everything is being done for your loved one that could or should be. You are probably right! Hospitals obviously are not devised to serve a single person, but many! It is likely

CAREGIVER that the extent of attention and care your loved one receives in the hospital may be far less than you would typically provide at home. But before "rocking the boat" over what is *not* being done, ask yourself: "Is the care my loved one is receiving *satisfactory?*" If so, it may well be in your and your loved one's best interest to leave the unattended facets of his or her care alone for the time being. Being perceived as a constant thorn in the side of those who are trying their best to provide quality service may only alienate the very people you most want to work with. If, on the other hand, the level of care is *not satisfactory*, consult the suggestions that follow in the next section.

5 As far as your helping at the hospital, know that *nothing* is required of you! In fact, "helping" often means removing yourself from the hospital environment. If your loved one's medical condition is stable, there is actually little you can do! As stated earlier, being present every minute of the day likely is not very beneficial to your loved one, you, or the people trying to best serve him or her. People with aphasia tire very easily at first, and permitting large blocks of time for him or her to rest when not engaged in medical procedures is important. Your presence may only interfere with this. Being away helps you as well by giving you time to get refocused and to attend to issues outside the hospital.

5 Should you *elect* to help with certain self-cares while in the hospital, be sure the professional in charge knows of and supports your involvement. Any helping is apt to require some specific training. Bedside feeding, for instance, may require you to attend to your loved one's positioning, types of food, order of presentation, and bite size. If you are not carefully trained, your good intentions might very well make your loved one seriously ill. Review the steps in a particular procedure with the proper personnel before proceeding!

WHAT YOU MIGHT DO

1–5 GETTING ANSWERS TO YOUR QUESTIONS

Getting answers to these questions involves learning about the hospital and preparing ahead. In a system where time is at a premium, the more organized you are, the more willing and cordial you'll find the medical staff. Often, the better your relationship with these professionals, the more likely it is that your concerns will be taken seriously and attended to.

HEALTH

1–*What has happened to my loved one?*
2–*What caused this?*
3–*How stable is his or her medical condition?*
4–*What might I expect in the days and weeks ahead?*
5–*How can I help?*

CAREGIVER

1–4 HOW TO ARRANGE MEETINGS

- Ask the physician(s) and nurse(s) how they would prefer to handle your daily questions and concerns.
- Typically, nurses are more accessible than doctors. However, each should have designated times in their daily routines when your questions might be addressed. Realize that allotted times are apt to be brief. That is, plan for no more than 5–10 minutes daily. The ward clerk can probably assist you in contacting your loved one's primary physician or nurse.
- Comply with each professional's schedule—even if it means changing your own.
- Remain composed and polite but do *not* neglect your needs. Keep looking for a common ground from which to interact and work together.
- Within reason, hold professionals to an agreed on plan.
  Certainly, unexpected and urgent matters may arise in the hospital that necessitate canceling or delaying appointments. However, this should be more the exception than the rule. When it isn't, inquire if there isn't another way or time to ensure your needs do get met.

1–4 HOW TO PREPARE FOR MEETINGS

- Carry a pocket notebook with you.
- Write down your questions and concerns ahead of time.
- Order these questions and concerns according to importance.

CAREGIVER

- Don't worry if you cannot state your questions in medical terms . . . work on keeping them clear and precise.

1–4 HOW TO MAKE THE MOST OF THESE MEETINGS

- Enter meetings with a positive attitude and from a position of shared "equality."
- Concentrate hard on *listening* to the details of what you are told.
- Don't hesitate to ask for clarification of terms or procedures.
- Verify, that is, restate in your own words, what you think you were told.
- Note key points.
- Don't move to the next question until you are satisfied with the answer to the last one.
- Parts of some answers may be unknown. Ask when that missing information might be known.
- Try to stay on the topic.
- Summarize key points at the end of the meeting, to be sure your understanding is clear and correct.
- Confirm when and how you'll convene again.
- Ask for any printed materials that might help you to understand their key points better.
- Take a few minutes afterwards and write down main points.
- Keep good records. Maintain weekly logs of key developments. Besides aiding you in remembering what was said at any point in time, these help in judging change and progress over time. Make it a habit to write down events over time. This will serve you well now, but especially in the months and years ahead.

4 WHEN THINGS ARE NOT WORKING AS YOU HAD HOPED

- Start by questioning the act or policy, not the person involved:
  For example: "Could you tell me how patients' baths are handled?"
  Rather than: "You people haven't given my husband a bath in three days; what's going on here?"
- Ask politely if there might be anything that could be done to change matters.
  "I know how busy you are."
  "It's just that he has had a bath every day of his life."
  "I know that's asking too much now."
  "How about every other day?"
  "Perhaps I could help?"

- If matters don't change and if you remain equally discontent, you may wish to speak with a hospital administrator. All employees, including nurses and doctors, have supervisors to whom they must answer.

5 HOW MIGHT YOU ASSIST

- Ask the professional in charge how you might help.
  Again, there is apt to be little that you can do specifically that isn't already provided.
  Whatever assistance you do add, it needs to work "with," rather than "against" the existing structure. If you have a specific function in mind, it is not inappropriate to ask whether and how you might assist with it.
  Comply with whatever ruling is handed down.
  Be sure you know what to do, and how to do it, before proceeding.

CAREGIVER

WHAT TO KNOW

EMOTIONS
1–Is my loved one going to live?
2–What if he or she doesn't?
3–Will our lives ever be the same?

1–2 Just as people with aphasia wonder about their survival, caregivers typically agonize over their loved one's longevity and what life would be like without him or her. These are all natural reactions to the abrupt, unexpected, life-altering changes that have just happened. In this context, you needn't ever question their legitimacy!

1–2 Such questions, though, may seem pointless, or even "negative." Your natural tendency may be to want to say: "My loved one *is* going to live and our lives together *will* return to a level of quality!" Remaining positive when life is challenging and the facts are few is a tremendous boost if you can "pull it off." However, even if you can, this feat is apt to be fleeting, there one moment and gone the next! Don't expect more and don't punish yourself for *not* being able to hold a constant, bright face. Even if your loved one's survival in the immediate future seems well assured, the traumatic injury has sent shock waves to the very core of those closest to the injured party; quite likely, this may be the first time you've ever directly addressed your loved

CAREGIVER　one's mortality. That your optimism is fleeting and fluctuating is no surprise!

1–2　You may even wonder: "If this could happen so quickly and without warning, what is to say it won't again!" Or even, "If this could happen to him or her, am I not equally at risk?" Once your loved one's current condition is stabilized, everything will be done medically to discover its cause and minimize the risk of its recurrence. Also, whatever caused your loved one's injury quite likely is unrelated to any pending health risk of yours, although this may cause you to be more cognizant of such matters. Thus, the many questions that may be spinning off from your own emotions are apt to be like "after-shocks" from an internal earthquake. They are natural and to be expected. Before they are entirely over, months or years later, your view of life and self are apt to be quite different.

1–2　Try to remember that your loved one's aphasia probably is more *yours* than his or hers at this moment. Of the two of you, you are the one most likely to be able to see and sense the brutality of all that has happened. Quite possibly, your loved one's impaired thinking and perceptions have buffered him or her from what is abundantly clear to you! As a result, your body and mind are apt to be protectively trying to "shut down," or provide a cocoon in which to escape all the emotional shock and pain. This is not such a bad thing. It is a reflexive mechanism to allow *you* time internally to readjust and to resume life again. Although it may not feel right or of your own choice, you need to recognize it for what it is, and try to work with it rather than against it.

3　Quite likely, life as you defined it before this injury *is gone!* Yes, there are a small number of sufferers from aphasia who return to a near-normal state following injury. Many of these victims, though, still feel an enduring "sting" from the consequences that remain, however subtle they may be. Know too, that even though recovery is rarely complete, some of what was lost will return. However, in its revised form, it is apt not to seem or feel the same to you or your loved one. More importantly, you need to know that not all of the new parts are necessarily worse! They are different, but there is often good to be had no matter how bad they may seem initially! Over the course of this journey, your progress can be gauged by how well you have come to find good in what seems apparently bad, and harmony in what seems totally dysynchronous.

3 Recall, too, that people with aphasia are not doomed to lives of lesser quality. Certainly, skill levels are likely to be more restricted. Being *less able* to perform, though, does not automatically mean that participation in life is over, or that what remains cannot come, over time, to have value. In fact, in certain areas, there may be a greater appreciation and a better sense *of living* following injury. However, it is too early to try to address these concerns now. You need to work first toward establishing an operative base beneath yourselves. Later in Chapters 6, 7, and 8, we will lay out step-by-step progressions for helping to make life productive and meaningful again.

CAREGIVER

WHAT YOU MIGHT DO

1–2 COPING IN THE EARLY GOING

EMOTIONS
1–Is my loved one going to live?
2–What if he or she doesn't?
3–Will our lives ever be the same?

Coping successfully with one's emotions is as important as finding lasting solutions to physical ailments. Emotions may seem less tangible, but they are no less important. They typically change over a course and through an evolution of their own. As we proceed, we'll frequently revisit them. In general, they often contain core components of what must be revised constantly throughout the journey if life is to include meaning and purpose again.

1–2 WHAT TO RECOGNIZE

- The fact that you are in a state of emotional shock!
- A state of shock is *not* a time to try to think constructively or act decisively.
- You are not "a wimp". . . feeling vulnerable is not only all right . . . it's normal at times such as these. . .and essential!

1–2 WHAT TO DO

- **Give yourself permission to pull over on the side of the road and let the dust settle.**
   Getting yourself grounded is the first order of business. This means allowing a sense of feeling to return to your legs, arms, and body even if it takes days or weeks.

CAREGIVER
- **Don't try to override your emotionality with reason. Let your emotions reign.**
- **You may find the company of family or a close friend particularly helpful in the beginning.**
  Having important others to just listen may be as therapeutic and calming to you as your bedside manner is for your loved one. You needn't shoulder the enormity or complexity of aphasia alone.

1–2 HOW TO KNOW WHEN IT'S SAFE TO MOVE AHEAD

- Feeling the blood slowly returning to your arms and legs.
- Starting to look out the "car window," even though you may not know where you are.
- Starting to *trust* your instincts, while knowing it will be some time before you feel like yourself again.

1–2 WHAT TO DO WHEN YOU DO FEEL "MORE IN CHARGE"

- Single out what seems *most important* at this time.
- At first, take small steps in dealing with whatever is at the top of that list.
- Divide what is needed into "tenths."
- Try out a tenth at a time, and then re-evaluate how you *feel*.
- Focus more on "the doing" of it, and less on the outcome.
- Be especially kind to yourself.
- Keep adding on gradually until you are up to speed.

3 LOOKING AHEAD

You don't know what the road may bring miles and miles from where you are. It is not wrong to "hold out" until you know more about your loved one's condition before you proceed. There are certain basic adjustments that you are going to need to attend to regardless of his or her condition or recovery. If you feel adventurous, you may want to start contemplating these and how best to achieve them in your own way.

3 WHAT ADJUSTMENTS WILL BE NEEDED DOWN THE ROAD

- Relinquishing or giving up the past.

> This adjustment is major, and time consuming. It seldom comes easily or automatically. It starts, though, with simply recognizing the importance of not letting what once was stand in the way of what might be.
> - Searching out the good in what feels bad or unwelcomed.
> - Promoting that good over any more pervasive feelings of gloom or despair.
> - Keep slowly emerging from that cocoon you protectively spun months ago.

CAREGIVER

WHAT TO KNOW

COMMUNICATION
1–Why can't my loved one communicate?
2–Will he or she be able to communicate again?
3–What can be done now?
4–How can I help?

1 Quickly, once more, Chapter 10 details the types of communication breakdowns associated with aphasia. If this first question looms large in your mind, ask the hospital's speech-language pathologist to guide you in selecting the most pertinent information as it relates to your loved one's condition. You may find that in order to truly understand his or her communication difficulties, you first need to understand the concepts of speech, language, and communication and the differences between them. You may need to know first the functions underlying each of these terms and how they function for normal communicators. The "side trip" in Chapter 9 provides you with these explanations.

2 As far as whether your loved one will be able to communicate later, the answer is "yes." However, the degree of ease and proficiency in interacting with others varies considerably among people with aphasia. Roughly half of all individuals with aphasia regain their ability to communicate basic needs, wants, and thoughts through talking. However, the other half is not able to do this through speech alone. Many can make their basic needs known through a combination of speech and *other forms* of expression, such as voice inflection, facial expression, gesture, writing, drawing, and pointing. These individuals with limited speech also depend on normal interactants who are familiar with, and able to converse in, their "modified" communicative system.

2 Whether your loved one will be an independent communicator, that is, a person who is able to converse well enough not to need the support of

CAREGIVER others, is difficult to know *with certainty* at this time. In the beginning days after injury, a majority of people with aphasia cannot communicate without support. Which of these individuals will later become independent talkers, though, depends on a number of factors. These factors are reviewed in the next journey chapter (see Person with Aphasia: Recovery). For now, though, know that it will take several months and likely a trial period of communication therapy to determine whether the independent use of spoken words will return or not.

3 A speech-language pathologist will likely come and see your loved one in the first several days of hospitalization. The purpose of this visit is apt to be twofold: (1) to determine whether he or she is able to eat and drink safely and (2) to assess the basic nature of his or her communication problem, its severity, and whether treatment might help. Quite likely, the injury to the brain has not just impaired communication alone, but also the more vegetative functions, such as the muscle movements of mouth, lips, tongue, or throat. These temporary dysfunctions may interfere with eating food and drinking liquids. Another "side trip" in Chapter 12, entitled "Eating and Drinking Difficulties," details these concerns and how they are typically addressed.

3 An initial assessment of your loved one's communication dysfunction necessitates that your loved one be somewhat alert and interactive. Sometimes, in the beginning days, the shock of injury to the brain may preclude this. If some formal or informal testing is possible, it is apt to target the type(s) of communicative injuries and whether treatment might help. You need to know, though, that if treatment is recommended, it may or may not begin now. It often depends on how rehabilitative services will be provided. Chapter 5, Rehabilitation, walks you through the processes of how and when these decisions are apt to be made.

4 Your role may be somewhat limited in the beginning days after injury since your loved one's stay in the hospital is apt to be brief, and only a matter of days. Even so, you can help prepare for what lies ahead by seeking out the hospital's speech-language pathologist for information about your loved one's communicative status at this time, and an overview of how treatment may or may not be provided. Again, it may take this professional a couple of days to complete his or her initial assessment.

WHAT YOU MIGHT DO

1–2 COPING WITH IMPAIRED COMMUNICATION

COMMUNICATION
1–Why can't my loved one communicate?
2–Will he or she be able to communicate again?
3–What can be done now?
4–How can I help?

There are many reasons communication may fail in the beginning days of aphasia. Like mental status issues, some of these may change dramatically in the weeks and months ahead. For this reason, it makes sense to learn simple strategies to aid general communication at first, and to postpone long-term solutions until you know whether they are necessary. Be aware that some of the difficulty your loved one is having communicating is because of an *inability to understand spoken messages*, even if it does not appear this way to you.

CAREGIVER

1–4 DEFINING COMMUNICATION THERAPY

• Ask the hospital's speech-language pathologist for answers to the above questions, and for any specific suggestions for improving communication at this time.
• Ask how treatment might proceed.
• Ask how you might aid this process.
• Ask for any additional literature on the subject of aphasia.

1–4 GENERAL SUGGESTIONS OF WHAT **YOU** MIGHT DO

• Review communicative suggestions from the earlier sections in this chapter, such as Person with Aphasia: Thinking, and Person with Aphasia: Communication.
• When talking, use slow, deliberate, clear, simple, speech.
• If talking doesn't work, try adding gestures, drawings, or printed words.
• When listening, focus on the entire message, not individual sounds or words.
• Don't act as if you understand when you don't.
• Use "yes/no" questions rather than open-ended ones,
  Example: "Is this about lunch?" versus "Tell me what you want?"
• Start your questions at a general level rather than too specifically,
  Example: "Is this about you and me?" versus "Are you talking about where we're going next summer?"

CAREGIVER

> • Keep verifying what you think your loved one is saying.
> • Don't remain on a topic when the exchange isn't working or is stressful:
>> Postpone it until later.
>> Seek suggestions from the speech-language pathologist.
>
> **1–4** WHAT ELSE TO DO
>
> • Try not to get too far ahead in your thinking.
> It likely will be months until anything definite is known about your loved one's communicative potential.
> • Accordingly, it will take some time to know what the best long-term communication plan might be.
> • Know that there are effective ways of coping with communication and life should talking not return.

RECOVERY
1–How and when will my loved one get better?
2–Who can help and what will they do?
3–How can I help?

WHAT TO KNOW

1 Recovery from aphasia and its associated dysfunctions typically is a slow, long, and arduous process. Most sufferers experience steady improvement over the first 6 to 12 months. Although the rate of gain is apt to slow after the first year, improvements still follow months and years later. Physical gains in involved limbs are apt to come sooner and faster than talking, writing, or communicating. One often hears expressions of dismay over the "snail-like" pace that recovery takes: "Why is this taking so long?" "Why must I work so hard to attain so little?" "Why are little things still so hard to do?"

1 In spite of recovery's protracted nature, improvement typically extends for as long as the injured party persists in trying to make matters better! For some, that duration is a lifetime; for others it may be considerably less. If it is less, then the decision to stop trying needs to be out of personal choice, and not secondary to fears, misperceptions, events, or the opinions of other people. If it is out of informed choice by the person with aphasia, then the decision needs to be respected and accepted.

2 The medical specialty that oversees recovery from aphasia and its associated dysfunctions is called *rehabilitation*. Rehabilitative services involve a variety of professionals with differing specialties. Table 4–1 contains a list of these people and their respective domains and duties. Make yourself familiar with these professionals and their functions. Although their duties may vary slightly depending on whether they are in a hospital or a specialized rehabilitation (rehab) setting, they provide much the same functions as outlined here. Also, even though your association with these individuals in a hospital setting may be brief, it is important to establish contact with them. They often represent your loved one's strongest advocates for ensuring recovery.

CAREGIVER

2 Rehabilitative services commonly begin within days after your loved one enters the hospital. As with communication, the initial focus of these services is on assessing the type and severity of injury and the potential for recovery. Again, your role at first is to try to determine what course and formula for rehabilitative services is apt to be followed. Give each specialist several occasions to meet and interact with your loved one. Then, make an effort to learn about their findings and recommendations. Be aware that rehabilitative services most likely will *not occur in the hospital*. Instead, your loved one will be transferred to a rehab center where the level of medical care is still sufficient, but not as intense or formal as it was in the hospital.

2 Do know that your loved one's formal rehabilitation and his or her recovery are two separate entities. That is, your loved one will be discharged from rehabilitative services well before his or her recovery is ever completed. You may wonder why this is. The answer is that the gradual nature of return of function does not "afford" for full compensation in today's health care system. Because payment is denied after a rather arbitrary point in time, however, does not means that further change is unlikely. It is common to hear from people with aphasia that they are improving *years after* formal rehabilitative services have stopped!

3 The best way to assist your loved one at this point is to become well informed about rehab and its potential course. The health care professional who is responsible for setting the direction and tempo of rehab is your loved one's physician. In today's health care environment, reimbursement for such services typically requires a doctor's prescription. When the physician concludes that benefits from treatment have run their expected course, such services are usually terminated.

Table 4–1. Members of a rehabilitation team and their key functions.

REHAB MEMBER	FUNCTION
Physician	is the rehab team leader.
	oversees all medical care.
	coordinates rehab treatment plan.
	is responsible for direction and outcome of rehab.
Nurse	oversees daily health care directives.
	is the prime provider of daily health care needs.
	interacts with family about health care functions now and in the future.
Speech-Language Pathologist	oversees assessment and treatment of voice, speech, language, and communication.
	is likely a prime provider, or team leader, in assessing and treating swallowing difficulties.
	screens other functions that may impact communicating, like thinking or memory.
	interacts with family to help coordinate and maximize optimal use of communication in real-life.
Physical Therapist	oversees assessment and treatment of physical mobility and movement of the lower extremities (legs).
	stresses resumption of function, from sitting upright in bed or a chair to transferring from a bed to a wheelchair, and walking.
	evaluates and recommends modifications to living environments which will maximize motility and independence.
	interacts with family to coordinate a plan for optimal function in real-life.
Occupational Therapist	oversees assessment and treatment activities of daily living and movement of the upper extremities (arms, hands).
	stresses resumption of functions such as dressing, grooming, personal hygiene, and eating.
	is probably involved with difficulties in swallowing.
	interacts with family to coordinate a plan for optimal function in real-life.
Social Worker	oversees family, social, vocational, and financial concerns of the patient and family.
	directly assists in matters involving placement of patient following hospitalization and rehabilitation, or any social complication that may interfere with the implementation of this plan.

REHAB MEMBER	FUNCTION
Social Worker *(continued)*	interacts with family frequently to be sure that the necessary social and financial support to carry out rehab's recommendations are in place.
Dietician	oversees patient's dietary needs.
	assures that adequate liquid and food intake are maintained within the constraints of the patient's medical and health requirements.
	interacts with family as to how to meet such needs in real-life.
Psychologist	oversees assessment of higher cognitive and perceptual functions of the brain.
	is often directly involved in determining the patient's mental status to be able to act competently in his or her own behalf.
	may be helpful in assessing and helping with mood changes associated with head injury.

3 Because the physician has ultimate control over rehab's presence and course, it is important to know where your loved one's doctor stands on such issues. Some doctors, for instance, are highly supportive of rehab's therapeutic value and advocate strongly for its inclusion after hospitalization. Others may favor prescribing a short trial period of treatment and seeing whether such services produce change. Still other physicians question rehab's practical value at all. Find out where your loved one's doctor stands on this issue. If it is toward the nonsupportive end of the continuum, you may wish to start searching for a physician who is more favorably inclined to support these services beyond hospitalization.

3 It is important as well to determine whether your health insurance covers rehabilitative services and, if so, to what degree. For instance, most primary private insurers, such as Blue Cross/Blue Shield, and governmental health care providers, such as Medicaid or Medicare, allow for all forms of rehabilitative services and for varying numbers of treatment sessions. Find out precisely what your loved one's health care provider allows. Besides knowing the range of services possible, determine who is responsible and what is necessary for such services to be provided. Most likely, you want assurance that the most service possible will be offered within the limits of your loved one's insurance provider.

CAREGIVER 3 It is likely to take a minimum of a few days for rehab team members to visit and assess your loved one for the first time. It also takes 3-4 days before the medical team has a better sense of what caused the injury, its severity, and whether rehab is an immediate consideration or not. However, even before this time has lapsed, it does not hurt early on to inquire about a time table for procuring this information. Certainly, by the end of the first week of hospitalization, some "preliminary" version should be available.

3 You will need to compare projected plans for rehab services with what your loved one's health care plan allows. Some significant discrepancies may appear. For example, the health care provider may allow for 90 days of intense rehabilitation following injury while current plans may be to discharge your loved one immediately to a nursing home without such services. You need to question quickly why this particular "non-rehab" choice was made. Very simply, it may be up to you to monitor and advocate for your loved one's optimal care, especially in the early going!

RECOVERY
1–How and when will my loved one get better?
2–Who can help and what will they do?
3–How can I help?

WHAT YOU MIGHT DO

1–3 PREPARING YOURSELF FOR REHAB'S COURSE

The actual process of beginning rehab is likely a week or more away. Within the first week following injury, though, some plan is apt to be initiated by the doctor in charge. Whether it will get implemented, though, is a different question. Recall that until a few years ago, people with aphasia in America often received 1 to 3 months of intense rehabilitation in a hospital. This is no longer the case. More likely, your loved one will be moved to an intermediate or long-term care center for rehab. Although this process is apt to be intimidating because it involves unfamiliar territory, scouting ahead may save you and your loved one a lot of anguish later on.

3 WHERE TO BEGIN

• Ask the ward clerk who your loved one's social worker is.

In the beginning days, social workers are often far more accessible than your loved one's physician and often are an active member of the rehab team. Because of this, they often know a lot about standard hospital policy and procedures. This professional is apt to know how rehabilitative services are typically managed in this facility, when discharge is apt to occur, and places to which patients are often discharged.

CAREGIVER

- Arrange an appointment with the social worker.
- Have in mind probing whether projected rehabilitative services mesh with coverage limitations from your loved one's health care provider.

3 WHAT TO ASK

- How long will your loved one likely be in the hospital?
- Where will he or she go after that?
- How are rehabilitative services typically handled?
  in the short run (the next week)
  in the long run (the next month)
- How might you best prepare for what lies ahead?

3 WHAT TO DO NEXT?

- Meet briefly with your loved one's physician before the end of the first week of hospitalization.
- Ask him or her to specify the recommended course of rehab.
- If the physician does not provide many details, then ask:
  Which impaired functions will receive treatment?
  When and where will that treatment begin?
  How long will it last?
  What if more treatment is still needed . . . what options are there?
  If further rehab is *not* going to be recommended, why?
  What provisions, if any, exist for such services later on?
- You need not feel intimidated by the doctor, nor need you be hostile or abrupt either.
- Keep an up-beat, interested attitude, but don't feel "the lesser person" in the exchange because this information may be unknown or new to you.
- You do have a legitimate right to be there and ask these questions!
- Good luck . . . and hang in there!

FAMILY/FRIENDS

1–What should I tell them?

CAREGIVER

WHAT TO KNOW

1 Close family/friends are apt to experience the same initial shock you did. They may wish to rush immediately to your loved one and you with whatever support possible. Depending on your personal style and circumstances, you may wish to welcome their efforts at this time or not. However, there are a number of subtleties here to consider.

1 One of these is your loved one's current medical and physical condition. People with aphasia often are too sick and exhausted in the beginning days of injury to entertain or interact with others for any duration. They may appear interactive at first, but the slightest effort, either mental or physical, often depletes their total reserves. They often lack endurance and drift between periods of sleep and restlessness. Because of this, demands placed on them by visitors are simply too much. In addition to lacking reserves, some of these adults simply do not want loved ones, whether family or friends, to see them in their current state of injury or dysfunction. Of equal concern, even if the afflicted adult wishes to see family or friends, is how well visitors may react to seeing their loved one in such a compromised position. Thus, it is often best and advisable to discourage visitations in the beginning days and weeks. Not until your loved one's condition has stabilized somewhat, is it likely that visits may add more than they detract.

1 There are, however, some good reasons for visitations early on. If your loved one's medical condition is tenuous, and his or her survival uncertain, you may welcome and need the presence and help of family and close friends. This is not just for their emotional support, but to help you sort through and make important health care decisions. If your loved one is sleeping or marginally cogent, it's quite likely that his or her medical condition would be not be adversely affected by having others present. Such visitors, though, need to know and adhere to the earlier admonishment: Never talk about your loved one or his or her condition as if he or she were not present. If something needs to be discussed that you might not care to have him or her hear, do step out of the room and attend to it privately.

1 Keep in mind that you likely will welcome the support of others further down the road. Maintaining "some" ties now will help establish a bridge to these contacts later. Occasional updates provide some continuity and permit you to define realms and means of interacting and assisting that others might provide.

1 Finally, for some caregivers, the immediate support of friends and family may be very important. If you wish to have others around you, by all means avail yourself of their comfort, strength, and advice. Remember that your emotional needs are possibly the *most* important ingredient in the recovery equation right now! If these needs of yours are pressing, attend to them! It is vital to you and your loved one. You may, though, want to keep these contacts to meeting places outside the hospital, simply because of the amount of confusion and demands on your time while there.

WHAT YOU MIGHT DO

FAMILY/FRIENDS
1–What should I tell them?

1 TALKING TO FAMILY AND FRIENDS

It is more *your needs*, than your loved one's, that should determine the presence and role of family and friends in the beginning. If you elect to have their support, it may be best to try to meet separately away from the hospital. This may seem impossible in the first days . . . and it probably is. But as you approach the end of the first week and if your loved one's survival is not in question, brief meetings outside the hospital may be good therapy for you. Your loved one will be perfectly attended to in your absence.

1 WHAT TO FOCUS ON

- In general, you may want to keep your explanations brief.
- Discourage their visiting the hospital now.
- Tell them you'll let them know when and how their participation might help.
- Be honest about what you need now. If it is a shoulder to lean on, it is fair to seek it out and accept it.

1 WHAT TO SAY

- "He or she apparently has had a stroke."

CAREGIVER

> • "It's too early to know any of the specifics."
> • "He or she will be hospitalized for while."
> • "When I know more and time permits, I'll let you know."
> • "I appreciate your interest and concern, it's just too early to visit."
> • Possibly . . . depending on your needs: "I could sure use a friendly face, though. I'd love to have you drop by the house tonight."

EMPLOYMENT

1–What should I tell my loved one's employer?

2–What should I tell my employer?

WHAT TO KNOW

1 You are going to need to notify your loved one's employer about the injury. Depending on the relationship of this person to your loved one, it will likely determine the tenor and extent of information exchanged. Minimally, though, you need to request further time to evaluate the seriousness of your loved one's injury and his or her ability to return to work. In the days or weeks ahead, however, this employer will likely require preliminary answers to these very questions.

1 The outlook for returning to work following brain injury *is not encouraging*. Exceptions do exist, but they often involve people with minor injuries and/or an employer who wishes to accommodate their employee rather than the system. Consequently, a high percentage of people with aphasia never return to work, at least not in their previous work capacity. However, at the present time, it is probably premature to know whether some form of work might be possible. Ideally, it would be best if such decisions could be postponed until rehabilitation is completed.

2 There are simply too many demands on your time at the moment to try to juggle obligations at the hospital and work, too. Besides feeling the need be near your loved one, you likely will need time to prepare for all that lies ahead. However, you do *not* want to entertain or make any long-term modifications in your employment at this time. If possible, negotiate several days to a week off to give yourself some time to adjust to what has happened and to establish a plan for how to proceed from there. Quite likely, maintaining your employment is an essential ingredient in a long-term plan. There are ways of doing so and still attending to your loved one's needs.

WHAT YOU MIGHT DO

1 INFORMING YOUR LOVED ONE'S EMPLOYER

> **EMPLOYMENT**
> 1–What should I tell my loved one's employer?
> 2–What should I tell my employer?

CAREGIVER

You are probably going to have to face a final decision about your loved one's employment before rehab ends. However, the longer you can postpone this eventuality, the better. Many people define themselves through their work and even if it appears highly unlikely that returning to one's past employment is possible, it may help the recovery process to leave that door partially open.

1 WHAT TO SHARE

- Again, keep your explanation brief.
- Indicate that your loved one's ability to return to work is unlikely in the weeks ahead.
- Indicate that a more reliable answer will follow after a full assessment and trial therapy.
- Discourage the employer from visiting at this time, explaining that your loved one is "too sick" to have visitors.
- Assure this person you will update him or her as you are better informed.

2 ARRANGING TIME OFF

- Consider taking a couple of days off in the beginning to reduce the multiple demands on you.
- Don't make any permanent change in your work schedule or employment until you know more.
- Guard against using all of your vacation or annual leave now . . . you'll need additional breaks down the road.

CAREGIVER

WHAT TO KNOW

1 Admission into a hospital seldom occurs without some established and guaranteed method of payment. However, if the expense of hospitalization is a prime concern, the easiest solution is to arrange to meet with the social worker overseeing your loved one's case or a hospital financial advisor. Usually, a case worker is assigned to each patient on a medical ward; the financial advisor is likely located in the hospital's admissions or accounting section.

1 If your loved one's money is in a bank account where you are not a legal co-signer, you may want to pursue a legal document called a ***Power of Attorney***. This designation permits you to act in your loved one's behalf until he or she can resume such duties. A Power of Attorney does not require a court order yet it permits you to pay any outstanding bills or other forms of indebtedness. The social worker can assist you in pursuing this designation.

WHAT YOU MIGHT DO

1 RESOLVING EXPENSES

You need to review precisely what your loved one's health insurance covers. If it pays only a portion, or if a sizable deduction must first be met before coverage begins, there are typically ways that subsequent payment can be arranged. This is *not* a time to add to your already-sizable burden in daily life by worrying about incurred medical expenditures. Make an appointment to speak with hospital personnel immediately if these matters are highly concerning or troublesome. Do not let them fester.

1 WHERE TO BEGIN

- Arrange a meeting with a hospital's social worker or financial advisor.
- Bring your loved one's health care insurance policy to this meeting.

1 WHAT TO ASK

- "What will his or her costs be?"
- "How and when are charges incurred?"
- "When will payment be expected?"
- "Is a deferred payment plan possible?"
- "How does such a plan work?"
- "If a deferred payment plan is not possible, what other options are there?"
- "How does one apply for such aid or programs?"

Pulling over on the roadside

The first, and "most traumatizing" portion of the journey is likely behind you. This is not to say that all of the terrain and road ahead is smooth riding, it is *not!* In fact, some sections that lie ahead are quite rugged and treacherous. However, these rough sections of road need not bog you down at the moment. Take a few moments and pause, just reflect on all that you've *successfully* negotiated so far. In spite of a terrible and wrenching ordeal over the past 7 to 14 days or longer, you and your loved one are *still alive* and *still together*.

The exteriors of the world you once knew may be a bit tarnished but the interiors are still alive and vital. With time, these inner cores will serve you well. Quite likely, what has happened is that this unannounced and unwelcomed event has momentarily seized life's energies and control from you. Instead of feeling like the determiner of your own destiny, life's steering wheel seems to have slipped out of your grasp. On the section of road ahead, we begin by taking the first step in handing that control back to you and your loved one, by way of his or her rehabilitation.

Know that this is just the first step, and it is a crucial one! It is from here that we literally begin moving forward. We still have a lot of road to cover, but more importantly, we need to do it together—a step-at-a-time!

❖   **CHAPTER 5**

Rehabilitation . . . striving to improve!

You are at the first crossroads of this journey. Depending on your circumstances, you probably arrived here within the first several weeks of travel, and you may not feel totally prepared to venture on from here. The vividness of all that has happened is still reverberating inside. Bits and pieces of conversations with physicians, nurses, or other professionals drift in and out of your thoughts like segments from old movies seen over and over again. Each time one of these scenarios emerges, you try again to identify something new or important that might help you understand the confusing mix of terms, people, events, and emotional upheaval. You keep asking, "Will we ever get our lives back as we once knew them?" Most worrisome of all, you may feel as if you haven't gotten *anywhere* at all!

You *have* gotten somewhere, though! You probably know many of the basic facts surrounding your loved one's injury. As well, you are apt to have some insight into its cause, severity, and whether his or her long-term survival remains in question. This "new" information has helped put some order into something that was completely unfamiliar just weeks ago. Even so, you remain unclear about what these "new" facts *truly* mean. Now, standing at the first crossroads of this journey, a second wave of concerns begins to invade your thinking: "Can people *really* get better from this?" "If so, how?" "What does it take? "When will that begin?" "Who will help?" "How long will all of this take?"

These questions pertain to the area of ***rehabilitation*** (rehab), and you are not alone in wondering about them. By this time, they are apt to be *the* prime issues in your loved one's health care planning. As you learned in the hospital, physicians, nurses, and rehab specialists are all sorting through these concerns and making preparations. Although each probably has his or her own "educated guess" about your loved one's potential for recovery, the true answers still lie months or more down the road. What you have been told, though, is that *some* improvement is apt to follow almost immediately. How much more will come from therapies along the way is highly variable and depends on many factors, both within and outside your loved one's influence.

Whether rehab begins in the hospital or is moved to a separate rehab center, its initial course is apt to depend on two factors: (1) the assessed potential benefit from treatment, called ***prognosis***, and (2) the extent to which such rehab services are reimbursable. If your loved one's potential looks promising and payment permits, ***a trial period of treatment*** is apt to follow. Then, based on his or her reaction to such therapies, further treatment may or may not continue. The precise course of rehabilitation, though, may be more complex depending on the subtleties of the health care system in your area of the country or world (see Chapter 3). To effectively negotiate the curves in this road, you need first to know as much as possible about your loved one's potential for improvement and how the "rehab game" works in your area. Only then are you in a position to serve as a "flagperson" in making sure your loved one gains access to preferred routes. In certain rehab systems, financial incentive to health care providers is not always in how many services they provide, but how few. It may be incumbent on *you* to understand the possibilities to ensure that your loved one receives optimal services.

As you proceed down the road ahead, know that the scariest, most alarming moments of the journey are probably over, *behind you!* By this, we mean that the period of not knowing what was happening, or whether your loved one would survive has passed. For most peo-

ple, the intensity of this initial threat *will never* be equaled again. You have personally faced and endured a "near death experience." Coming this close to a loved one's mortality tends to change the act of living daily life forever. When survivors rethink how they lived life before, and how they will live it in the future, one of the frequent changes is that death no longer holds the same ominous or foreboding stranglehold it might have before. There is often a stronger commitment to live each moment fully, rather than postpone life's pleasure to a future date.

This revamped sense of life and self, as important as it is, will *not* free you from the challenges ahead! These challenges are simply a part of the journey. The bumpy, winding roads directly before you are inescapable. But for each rough section you are apt to encounter, know that there are as many opportunities to find personal growth and success as there are chances to encounter disappointment or failure. The difference is in how you and your loved elect to see, experience, and travel these rough sections. That's the second aim of this chapter, to guide you through a restorative process that will make traveling them much easier. **Keep in mind that simply *moving forward* is 9/10ths of the struggle. Each step in an intended direction brings you closer to where you ultimately want to go, but it also gives you the momentum and strength to keep going.** These "collective steps" lead to miles, and these "collective miles" lead to personal growth and ways of redefining and living life. It is worth the effort . . . keep pressing forward . . . we'll be right there with you through the rough sections ahead!

Profiles

PERSON WITH APHASIA

- improving slowly in overall health
- becoming aware of time, surroundings, and people although not back to normal
- knowing that something "significant" has happened; likely displaying increased concern about the consequences
- becoming more oriented toward self and levels of dysfunction

CAREGIVER

- lessening concerns about loved one's survival
- orienting better to daily operation of hospital or rehabilitation center but still not fully comfortable
- focusing better on matters at hand (than at first)
- worrying over your ability to oversee recovery when knowledge is minimal

- gradually improving in communication, likely more in understanding than talking
- eating an oral diet again, probably confined to soft foods and thickened liquids
- beginning to work on simple functions involving body movements, e.g., sitting, transferring from bed to wheelchair, and standing
- starting to work on self-cares, e.g., dressing, bathing, and using the toilet
- having minimal endurance . . . fatiguing easily
- performing inconsistently, i.e., good at one moment . . . remarkably poorer moments later
- family and friends asking about him or her and whether they might stop and visit

- trying to learn more about your loved one's condition and how best to proceed
- experiencing partial denial, i.e., either questioning if this is truly happening or, more likely, bargaining that everything will soon be back to "normal" in a month or two
- experiencing bouts of anxiety and fear when faced with all the realities before you
- struggling to keep life outside the hospital or rehab center operational while attending to your loved one's needs inside
- occasionally feeling vulnerable and in need of a helping hand but reluctant to involve others

Primary Concerns

PERSON WITH APHASIA

Recovery
1–Can anything be done to help me?
2–When will it start?
3–How long will it take?
4–Will I be my "old self" again?

Feelings about self
1–I'm *not* worth much to anybody or anything like this!

Relationship
1–How can you still love me?

CAREGIVER

Recovery
1–Treatment is *finally* beginning . . . now we can turn this thing around!
2–What should I expect from rehab and recovery?
3–What can I do to help this process?

About your loved one
1–He or she *looks* and *acts* so different. Is this change temporary or permanent?

2–I sure wouldn't blame you if
you didn't . . . I don't like
myself like this either!

Communication

1–What is *wrong* with my talking?
It is *absolutely* terrible! e.g.,
Some words come out while
others won't!
Some words come out and then
moments later, they won't!
The harder I try to say a
word, the worse it gets!
2–How do I improve my ability
to talk?
3–What's going to happen if my
talking doesn't improve?

Health

1–Tell me again . . . what caused
this?
2–I'm not in any danger of dying,
am I?
3–What's being done about this?
4–Could it happen again?

Family or Friends

1–Please, don't let others see me
like this, OK? . . . maybe later,
when I can talk!

Emotions

1–I can't believe this happened to
me . . . it's *not fair!*
2–I don't deserve this!
3–Why do I feel like I'm
constantly on the verge of tears?

Employment

1–I *cannot* work like this . . .
what's going on in this arena?
2–I hope I can still return to work
someday!

Communication

1–What can be done to improve
his or her talking?
2–How can we make our own
communication better?

Health

1–How much can my loved one
do physically?
2–What else do I need to know at
this time?
3–Is there any chance that this
injury might reoccur? If so,
how do we prevent it?

Emotions

1–He or she looks so unhappy
. . . I just wish I could "fix it!"
2–My inability to do more totally
drains me emotionally.

Daily Life

1–I've managed to keep things
together . . . but I don't know
how long I can keep juggling
demands at work, home, and
the rehab center!

Family or Friends

1–I appreciate their concern!
2–What is the best way to
respond to them?

Employment

1–How can he or she return to
work . . . maybe I should tell
his or her boss right now!
2–How am I going to work . . .
and attend to him or her?

RECOVERY

1–Can anything be done to help me?
2–When will it start?
3–How long will it take?
4–Will I be my "old self" again?

WHAT TO KNOW

**PERSON
WITH
APHASIA**

1 During the first days or weeks after onset, compromised mental status and physical health likely interfered with your loved one's ability to grasp the seriousness or extent of injury. Now, though, improving abilities to perceive, reason, and attend have likely sharpened his or her perspective of the injury. A better understanding may not always yield "good news." Months or years later, many sufferers recall early traumatic moments during hospitalization when they realized for the first time that a previously simple task, like buttoning or unbuttoning a shirt or blouse, was no longer possible. Such moments can be humbling and elicit a plea for help.

1 The answer to this first question, "Can anything be done to help me?" is a simple "Yes!" In fact, the first step in treating your loved one's dysfunctions is *not* necessarily to try to repair them, but rather to reassure him or her that there *is* hope and *a reason to make a sustained effort*. The first order of business often consists of steady therapeutic doses of reassurance . . . sort of daily vitamins . . . that prompt your loved one to want to participate in spite of his or her diminished level of functioning. Nothing is more medicinal in restoring hope than knowing that experienced, trained help is close at hand. As a result, rehab staff members typically make a concerted effort to see, or "connect with," incoming patients immediately on their arrival. They attempt to briefly assess your loved one's current functions, but more importantly, to reassure that they will do everything possible to see that optimal function returns, and to help your loved one and you cope with what may not.

1 Over the course of rehab, each specialist will attempt to move impaired skills closer and closer toward a restored state of functional use (see Table 4–1 in Chapter 4 for a review of rehab specialists and their roles and responsibilities). When carefully gauged and constantly applied, these specialized "nudges" often allow for a more self-sustaining level of function to emerge. In addition, this type of stimulation often builds confidence in existing levels of function and the idea that with continued work, even more might be possible.

2 "Treatment" officially begins not with *treating*, but with *assessing*. That is, each rehab specialist will likely perform a battery of formal or informal tests to determine where and how to begin therapy. Because some of this assessing may have been done already in the hospital, minimal testing may be needed on arrival in a rehab setting. Within days of your loved one's arrival, a full schedule of therapies should be up and running. Depending on your loved one's physical and mental ability to participate, such services will likely occur twice daily (morning and afternoon).

PERSON WITH APHASIA

2 Keep in mind that a majority of incoming patients enter rehab frightened about their current status, unclear whether treatment might help them, yet "open" to making a concerted effort. For these individuals, treatment will begin promptly and continue for as long as the person's effort, change, and reimbursement for services allow. There is a smaller group of sufferers, however, who view their newly acquired losses as too severe or debilitating to warrant trying to improve. These individuals cannot imagine even *trying* to rebuild from current levels of devastation, nor for that matter, living life like this! When this happens, it may be hard, if not impossible, at first for others to encourage them to try. They simply *refuse!*

2 Should your loved one fall in this latter category, do *not* panic! Strong reactive feelings to one's changed status are more of a "knee jerk" reaction than a well-considered or enduring rule. Rehab staff members know and recognize this; more importantly, they are prepared to deal with it! Usually, through steady doses of encouragement, coaxing your loved one along by singling out and promoting existing functions, these professionals can entice your loved one to try.

2 On rare occasions, though, people with aphasia simply elect not to try! When this occurs, ongoing rehab services may need to be postponed *temporarily*. The injured party *must*, of his or her own free choice, be willing to participate in therapy for treatment to be of any value. Beyond a point, you cannot, nor should you attempt to, "force" your loved one's participation. If this is your situation, reassessing his or her rehab status in 4 to 6 weeks is a reasonable option. Usually, with more time, decisions to not participate will soften. All you can do until then is to attempt to *foster a willingness to try.*

3 How long rehab will take is highly variable, but it is safe to say: "A long time!" It might be easier to look at the recovery process in two

**PERSON
WITH
APHASIA**

stages: what your loved one is apt to get back in the beginning months of treatment and what your loved one is apt to get back after such services end. *How much* and *how quickly* function might return during rehab are issues associated with several "prognostic" factors:

- *age:* the younger a person is, the more likely and rapidly the return of function. Rather than the person's actual age, the physical aging process is of greater importance; some people at 70 years of age look and feel 50; some people at 50 years more resemble someone who is 70.

- *extent of injury:* the smaller the amount of brain injury, the more likely and rapidly the return of function.

- *severity of aphasia:* the less severe the aphasia, the more likely and rapidly the return of function.

3 While the factors cited above often serve as an early guide for judging return of function, the most reliable indicators are:

- change (+) or lack thereof (–) from a trial period of treatment.

- presence (+) or absence (–) of a strong desire and will to change.

- change (+) or lack thereof (–) over time.

Even these, though, are not totally reliable. Some people with aphasia may take many months to really show significant signs of meaningful recovery. The "bottom line" is that, as long as the person with aphasia and the caregiver are both vested in making matters better, function will likely continue to improve, at least to some degree!

4 The question of becoming one's old self again was introduced in Chapter 4 (Person with Aphasia—Recovery), but at that time, it was probably just a vague notion or worry. With your loved one's increased alertness and a much better sense of injury now, this question is now a more pressing concern. **You already know that** *full recovery is unlikely.* **However, emphasizing this fact or even suggesting it is frequently counterproductive. To begin with, your loved one likely probably won't believe you—at least not initially—there simply is too much to concede in his or her own image of self and life. Second, even if he or she should "listen," this news may be more alienating than helpful.** As noted earlier, your loved one needs steady, frequent doses of encouragement in the early going! Hearing a discouraging message is

quite the opposite! If told the truth, he or she may react by saying: "Why even try?" Or worse, "How can I get back what I *know* I can when my loved one doesn't have any faith in me?"

4 Over time, your loved one will come to internalize his or her own version of dysfunction. That version will continue to be updated by experience. It is usually far better to let the *living of life* define this process and outcome, than for you to render a frank "pronouncement." Also, you do not need to view your silence on this issue as some form of dishonesty. Rather, your silence allows the best prognostic indicator to run its natural course. No one really knows for sure . . . only with time will we know that!

4 Related to not "telling the full story," is "telling a story that's not true." Definitely avoid the latter; that is, you *never* want to suggest or promise that a full recovery is possible! You can, and need to, describe the outlook for recovery as positive. But, it is a different issue to indicate that a full return to normal functioning is likely. Suggestions for how to do this follow.

WHAT YOU MIGHT DO

RECOVERY
1–Can anything be done to help me?
2–When will it start?
3–How long will it take?
4–Will I be my "old self" again?

1 EXPLAINING REHAB

It is important to keep your loved one as encouraged as possible. Although it is *not* your duty or responsibility to make him or her participate in rehab, how you approach and present this phase of the journey may greatly influence what transpires.

1 WHAT TO SAY:

- "There are trained professionals who know about your injury."
- "They can help you . . . if you only let them!"
- "The choice is yours . . . but the opportunity is *ours*."
- "I can *not* manage this challenge alone."
- "So please, give these people a chance to help you . . . and us!"

2 PREPARING FOR REHAB

Refamiliarize yourself with the rehab staff and their separate functions and duties. This information was presented in Table 4–1 (Chapter 4: Caregiver—Recovery).

**PERSON
WITH
APHASIA**

2 WAYS TO HELP

- If your loved one's communication allows, overview with him or her what is about to happen.
- Keep your explanations brief and positive.
- Specify how rehab works, and what to expect.
  Use an encouraging tone: emphasize that rehab professionals specialize in taking what is working and building on that rather than looking at what isn't working. Rehab requires some time and effort, but in the end your loved one is apt to be better off.

3–4 THE LENGTH AND EVENTUAL OUTCOME OF REHAB

Try to keep your loved one favorably disposed toward "working at" getting better and letting the future take care of itself. Keep the distinction fresh in your mind that rehab is *just* a beginning. Recovery typically spans a period of years and decades, and depends on a persistent will to seek change. The challenge at first is simply to get recovery moving in a positive direction.

3–4 WHAT TO SAY:

- "Getting better is going to take time."
- "All you can do now, is to try . . . stay with it . . . and give it your best effort!"
- "Don't not worry about how long it takes . . . we've got plenty of time!"
- "We'll just take it . . . regardless of what it entails . . . one step at a time."
- "In the end . . . we'll manage . . . we have before . . . and we will now!

FEELINGS ABOUT SELF
*1–I'm not worth much to anybody or
anything like this!*

WHAT TO KNOW

1 Becoming more aware of disordered abilities is apt to cause your loved one to devalue his- or herself. What contributes most to the revamping of his or her self-image is the striking contrast between what once was and what currently is. Now a form of being exists that your loved one never

---

associated with him or herself. Just as troublesome, he or she cannot help worrying about what these differences may mean or signify to others. This contrast of former and current selves is vividly etched in your loved one's mind.

PERSON WITH APHASIA

1 Not surprisingly, many sufferers enter rehab feeling that current levels of function are of little value, either to him or herself or to others. It does little, if any, good to try to contest these matters with your loved one in the early going. Arguing the inherent "worth" of what is present and working is apt to be seen as patronizing. He or she likely realizes the marked differences in function by now and is not about to discount them *as insignificant!*

1 A period of self-devaluation or self-deprecation is normal. In fact, such a period may only be starting at this point. As the contrast to the past becomes far more evident months down the road, so too, does diminished impressions of one's self. Few people with aphasia avoid having to confront feelings of personal devastation through bouts of doubt, anger, and depression (See Person with Aphasia—Emotions in this chapter.) As a caregiver, be prepared for these signs; they may begin at any time. Realize, too, that it may take time *to allow* your loved one to see "worth" in something that feels so devoid of promise or hope!

1 Gradually, the contrast between the past and present will begin to fade. What happens is that the person with aphasia accumulates enough time *living with aphasia* that the images prior to injury become supplanted with those since. It is a combination of not just seeing life through one's preinjured eyes, but finding value in the current moment, that permits this change to occur. Acknowledging existing function is often the first step, but it is adopting a *changed perception* of the inherent "value" of these functions that will determine whether your loved one's self-image will improve over time. Escaping aphasia's grasp and living life freely and independently means finding and accepting value in "what is" rather than seeing whatever exists at the moment as marginal or worthless.

WHAT YOU MIGHT DO

1 RECONCILING PAST AND PRESENT PERCEPTIONS OF SELF

PERSON WITH APHASIA

Resolving doubts about one's self is unquestionably one of the most challenging tasks of coping with aphasia. The extent of change, in the beginning, is typically enough to magnify the differences between past and present functioning and to bring all parties momentarily "to their knees." Often, though, the best solution is simply to permit this personal devaluation process to run its own natural course. There seems, in this case, to be truth to the old adage that sometimes one must go down in order to find one's way back up.

1 WHAT TO DO

- Acknowledge the practical differences in daily life and how they must be difficult to cope with.
- However, do *not* languish over or become fixated on these.
- Instead, keep your focus on gains since the injury.

  It is very important to begin judging improvement in relation to what existed at time of injury instead of what function was like prior. Even if your loved one minimizes your comparison by maintaining that current function remains far beneath past uninjured levels, do not acquiesce on your point. Simply smile and restate the obvious: "The fact is, you're better able now than you were at the time of injury . . . congratulations . . . and let's keep this going!"

- Avoid making light of current levels of functions.

  You want to avoid "joking" about his or her diminished skills in any form. In some rare cases, "making light" of one's shortcomings is a natural motivator for some people to act and do more. But usually, such individuals are the initiator of these disclaimers. You do not want to be that initiator at any time in the recovery process.

- Accentuate how your loved one's worth is bound to the person he or she is inside, not to any performance level.

  If you can, it may be advantageous to state that his or her current levels of function never need to change in order to retain your love and devotion. That is not to say that these levels won't continue to change; they will! It is only to make clear that your love is independent of your loved one's abilities *to perform in life*.

WHAT TO KNOW

1–2 Along with questions of self-worth, people with aphasia often worry about their physical or sexual appeal to their partner. With changes in facial appearance, movements of arms and legs, and communication, they commonly wonder if

RELATIONSHIP
1–How can you still love me?
2–I sure wouldn't blame you if you didn't . . . I don't like myself like this either!

their loved one will still find them physically and sexually desirable. Such worries begin to surface as the impaired adult becomes more aware of his or her changed abilities and appearance. As this occurs, the injured party may look to his or her partner for subtle signs that he or she still is still "attractive" or "desirable." If possible, you may wish to lay these worries to rest as soon as possible.

WHAT YOU MIGHT DO

RELATIONSHIP
1–How can you still love me?
2–I sure wouldn't blame you if you didn't . . . I don't like myself like this either!

1–2 STAYING CONNECTED

Adjusting to the physical changes related to aphasia and brain injury is not just a struggle for patients. Caregivers, too, often need time to adapt. It is possible that differences in your loved one's appearance and manner may initially alter your comfort and ease in being close or affectionate. Such a reaction in the early going is *not* uncommon. However, keep in mind that inwardly he or she is much the same person as before. You may just need a little time to recalibrate your own system. Again, don't be harsh or condemning of yourself. This issue and how to cope with it is discussed in greater detail in Chapter 6: Caregiver—Relationship.

1–2 REACTING TO PHYSICAL CHANGES IN YOUR LOVED ONE

• If possible, try to maintain the same degree of physical closeness as you did prior to the injury.

**PERSON
WITH
APHASIA**

An outward display of affection may require some work on your part as first. After a little bit of time and better understanding of what has happened, current functions are apt to "feel" and "mean" far less. If either party physically withdraws from the other, the consequences can be enduring unless the situation is repaired early on.

- At a minimum, display an interest in and personal warmth toward your loved one.
- Reach out frequently, touch and sit near him or her.

COMMUNICATION

1–What is **wrong** with my talking? It is **absolutely** terrible! e.g.,

  Some words come out while others won't!

  Some words come out and then moments later, they won't! The harder I try to say a word, the worse it gets!

2–How do I improve my ability to talk?

3–What's going to happen if my talking doesn't improve?

WHAT TO KNOW

1 Remember that the first weeks and months of aphasia represent the most challenging time for trying to communicate. Keep in mind, too, that disruptions are probably not due to a loss or absence of language, but to "faulty connections" within the injured brain. That is, people with aphasia usually have a clear sense of what they want to say, as well as a sense of the symbols they would like to use. The breakdown is that they cannot access or sequence these symbols.

1 To better understand this type of disruption to talking, think of your loved one's communication breakdown as being similar to an electrical motor with faulty wiring. All of the motor's parts are present and functional. The motor sits idle much of the time, however, because electricity cannot reach key connections inside the motor in the proper sequence. When these electrical signals occasionally do connect, the motor magically spins into motion and, for a brief period, it appears to work perfectly. The duration of operation, though, is apt to depend on the extent of damage to connecting circuits. If only minimal, the machinery may work a fair amount of the time. If severely impaired, it may work only on rare occasions and under special conditions. When it does stop running, though, do know that it is not due to its parts being faulty; rather it is due to a disruption in transmitting the signal.

1 When people with aphasia attempt to talk, they encounter a similar fate. That is, their electrical wiring (neural circuits) are not fully functional either. Each time they attempt to send a speech signal to their mental dictionaries to retrieve or order words, the signal gets blocked or misdirected. What causes these signals to go awry varies, but for many it is *the amount of internal noise* or *overloaded circuitry*.

PERSON WITH APHASIA

1 There are many ways that noise can get into, and interfere with, talking. For example, you may recall times in your past when you couldn't stop thinking of a certain recurring theme. Perhaps you had heard a popular tune on the radio while driving to work. You began humming the melody out loud and several hours later the same tune was *still there*, reverberating in your head. You then tried to consciously rid yourself of this "noise" by shifting your thinking to other thoughts or ideas, but minutes later the same tune was back pestering you. The persistence of something in one's head when it is no longer wanted, is just one type of internal noise that is prevalent in people having brain injury.

1 "Getting stuck" on something that was desired earlier but is no longer desired at the moment is known as *perseveration*. Whether purposeful signals get misdirected in a similar manner over and over again, or "overlearned" signals pop up when they are no longer desired, perseveration tends to interfere with language signals reaching their proper destination. Not surprisingly, then, much of aphasia therapy is built on devising effective ways of reducing or eliminating noise, like perseveration, so purposeful language might once again occur.

1 SOME WORDS COME OUT, WHILE OTHERS WON'T

It is somewhat common that people with aphasia might be able to say the days of the week (Monday, Tuesday, Wednesday, etc.) but not list major holidays (New Year's, Valentine's Day, Easter, etc.).
The reason for this: Days of the week are rotely learned. As a consequence, much less energy is needed to trigger the mechanism into motion than to trigger the mechanism to recall and name holidays of the year. Getting into one's "dictionary of holidays" is much harder than saying a sequence of words that naturally prompt one another, as in the days of the week.

1 SOME WORDS COME OUT AND THEN MOMENTS LATER, THEY WON'T

A person with aphasia might sing selected parts of a familiar tune, like "She'll be coming around the mountain," and yet moments later when

PERSON WITH APHASIA shown a picture of a woman driving a team of horses around a mountain, be unable to produce a single descriptive term or word about the picture.

The reason for this: Again, words in a familiar song context are much easier to retrieve and reproduce than the same words in a novel context. The words in a song actually help facilitate one another whereas the words needed to describe a picture are "unique" to that moment and situation. The latter challenge *adds noise* to your loved one's speech system and interferes with his or her transmission of the signal.

1 THE HARDER I TRY TO SAY A WORD, THE WORSE IT GETS

For most people with aphasia, any "demand" to say a word only increases the likelihood that retrieval may not occur! If someone asks a person with aphasia, "You get milk from a _____ ," it is possible that a desired word, "cow" or "carton" might follow. However, if, moments later, you hold up a picture of a cow or a carton and ask, "What is this?" a person with moderate to severe aphasia would likely be *unable* to say the same word!

The reason for this: Obviously, the inability to talk isn't because the word isn't present, but because there is an overload or "noise" in the speech transmission circuitry!

2 Improved talking is both possible and likely if vigorously pursued. Improved talking comes from both building new connections not present before the injury, and learning how to lessen noise and interference within the existing language system. The greatest success likely includes a combination of both of these methods. It is the speech-language pathologist who is best qualified to direct these efforts. As you begin to become more involved in rehab, you should develop some idea of what these treatment efforts might be (see Chapter 4: Caregiver—Communication).

3 Any concern your loved one may have regarding limited return of speech is likely more a fear than a true question at the moment. Certainly, the woes of not being able to talk or communicate are real, but it is too early for most sufferers to entertain the consequences of not being able to talk. Most believe, and rightfully so, that their speaking will improve with time. Too many, though, believe that it will return *to its former level of function*, which is *not likely!* **It may take several months to a year to *really* know whether your loved one's talking will once**

again support the expression of basic needs or more. In the interim, though, it may be advantageous to learn of "other ways" to communicate when talking is only marginally present, and how these ways might aid you as a couple now, and in the future (See Caregiver-Communication in this chapter).

PERSON WITH APHASIA

WHAT YOU MIGHT DO

1–2 COPING WITH IMPAIRED TALKING

- HOW TO PROCEED

- Carefully review how talking is impaired for your loved one. Ask the speech-language pathologist to specify these aspects of dysfunction. Also, ask which *type* of aphasia your loved one has and review its special characteristics in Chapter 10.
- Keep in mind that talking involves "re-routing" or "enhancing" the quality of the speech signal, not relearning it:

  Your loved one is *not* without words like a child trying to learn a language.

  Your loved one is without a "means" to get to the words that are already there in his or her head.

COMMUNICATION
1–*What is **wrong** with my talking? It is **absolutely** terrible!* e.g.,
Some words come out while others won't!
Some words come out and then moments later, they won't!
The harder I try to say a word, the worse it gets!
2–*How do I improve my ability to talk?*
3–*What's going to happen if my talking doesn't improve?*

2 WHAT TO SAY

- "You seem more aware of your talking problems."
- "Sometimes words come out, and sometimes they don't."
- "*I know* that *you know* what you want to say!"
- "Those words just won't come out, will they?"
- "Therapy should help that—it begins soon!"
- "Give it a chance and some time!"
- "We'll work this out together."

3 WHAT TO SAY

- "It's far *too early* to wonder about *how much* talking will come back."

| PERSON WITH APHASIA | • "Let's just work on improving from where we are."
 • "The therapist will help you, and us, communicate better"
 • "We'll go forward from here, OK?" |

HEALTH

1–Tell me again . . . what caused this?

2–I'm not in any danger of dying, am I?

3–What's being done about this?

4–Could it happen again?

WHAT TO KNOW

1–4 Although you've likely told your loved one basic answers to these questions, it is not strange that he or she might ask for clarification. *Lots* of repetition about such matters is commonly necessary. In fact, it is likely a good therapy for you as well. Your loved one needs to hear important "facts" more than once to internalize them correctly, and you need practice in "how" to share information clearly and concisely. Repeating important information, and occasionally adding to it, helps diminish natural "slippage" in retention that may come from brain injury. It also helps lessen your loved one's fears and worries.

1–4 Even if your loved one *appears* to be understanding most of your spoken messages, try to keep your explanations simple and to the point. Only if he or she requests *more* information or you can see worry or concern, is it advisable to keep adding onto explanations. Quite likely, you will need to readdress these issues continuously in the months ahead. With more time, you are apt to know much more about your loved one's health status, what is being done, and how best to communicate this information to him or her. Again, the rehab speech-language pathologist can assist you with these issues.

HEALTH

1–Tell me again . . . what caused this?

2–I'm not in any danger of dying, am I?

3–What's being done about this?

4–Could it happen again?

WHAT YOU MIGHT DO

1–4 KEEPING YOUR LOVED ONE INFORMED ABOUT SUCH MATTERS

For many, it is *not* so much the technical information that they seek as it is a sense that matters are being attended to. Keep this in mind when you explain health-related concerns to your loved one. On-going sharing of information is more about reassuring him or her than about conveying facts.

1–4 THINGS NEEDING CONTINUED ATTENTION

- The "retelling" of basic information to your loved one.
- Prime areas of concern are:
    current health status and stability.
    the cause of injury (consult Chapter 11 for more information).
    what is being done and why.
    what remains to be done and why (consult Chapter 13 for these details).

1–4 WHAT TO FOCUS ON

- Keep your messages positive and personal.
- Keep points clear, simple, and truthful.
- If questions still exist, stay with what is "known" . . . avoid wading through details.
- Assuming this is true, reassure him or her that nothing is too much or too grave to manage.
- Keep your tone upbeat and hopeful.

WHAT TO KNOW

> **FAMILY/FRIENDS**
> *1–Please, don't let others see me
> like this, OK?
> . . . maybe later, when I can talk!*

1 Remember that visits from others are *not* crucial in the early going. It is *not* strange or wrong to discourage people from visiting until after rehab is over. Your loved one's endurance and abilities to interact are likely marginal. He or she is likely quite aware and self-conscious about these reduced skills as a communicator. Permitting additional time for such functions to resume makes perfectly good sense.

1 If visits from others are desirable and of your loved one's own choice, it is important to "set the stage" rather than to just let them happen. Communication difficulties associated with aphasia are often humbling, frustrating, and humiliating. It is advisable to take time and do everything possible to minimize communication breakdowns *before* they occur. Basically, people unfamiliar with aphasia are "in the dark." And as you likely remember yourself, they are apt not to know what has happened, what they should do, or how best to interact. Providing a brief overview of how to communicate helps everyone feel freer and more at ease.

PERSON WITH APHASIA

1 At first, you may need to urge visitors to come, stay briefly, and keep their communication to a minimum. They may drop in, and say "Hi," spend a little time on current issues, and leave! Visitation periods of 15–30 minutes are often ideal, even when the injured party seems alert and interactive. Communicating takes *lots of energy* . . . on everyone's part. So begin with small doses in a controlled fashion!

1 Also, depending on your loved one's mental, medical, and physical condition, keep in mind that visitors might wish to channel some of their time into other activities besides talking, like reading aloud, playing cards, or telling light or humorous stories.

1 Finally, just because visits with family or friends may be curtailed in order to help your loved one, it does not mean that you cannot visit with these people separately. As suggested earlier (Chapter 4: Caregiver—Family/Friends), it is advisable to do so away from the rehab center. Your contact with close family or friends is often a healthy outlet; if desired, their input may be as well. You needn't sit and lament about your current woes, especially if that only adds to the on-going burden. Instead, it might be nice to shift your thoughts to other shared topics of interest besides your loved one's condition and future.

FAMILY/FRIENDS
1–Please, don't let others see me like this, OK?
. . . maybe later, when I can talk!

WHAT YOU MIGHT DO

1 IF VISITS ARE DESIRABLE TO YOUR LOVED ONE

Your loved one's endurance is apt to be less than is outwardly apparent! As a result, keeping visits brief (15–30 minutes) is advisable. Over time, you can come to better gauge whether such periods might be extended.

1 HOW TO PREPARE

- You need not present a lot of detail to visitors.
- Focus on key issues that are apt to be confusing: The problem is one of "getting into" his or her mental word dictionary, not a problem of thinking or memory.
  Urge visitors to simplify their use of words.

> Slow down and allow your loved one time to react.
> Remember that there is no value in talking loudly.
> Ask visitors to stay upbeat, but natural!
> Keep the atmosphere light and low key.

- Reassure visitors that understanding your loved one's speech is apt to be difficult.
- Indicate that such "breakdowns" are to be expected.
- It will be better if visitors can focus on staying connected as friends rather than trying to figure out each part of messages.
- Provide examples of how an interaction might proceed.

1 WHAT TO DO DURING VISITS

- Start by modeling the proper tone and manner of interacting.
- Try not to dominate, or "talk for" your loved one.
- Be a "facilitator," a pusher of "the communication swing." Let your loved one and the visitor do the interacting (Caregiver—Recovery details the use of rehab "swings")!
- Once the visitor and your loved one are comfortable with each other, let them interact alone.

WHAT TO KNOW

1–2 Becoming more aware of one's injury not only heightens a sense of the injury itself, but often a sense of its injustice. Your loved one may have worked hard and diligently to further him or herself and family. Now, without warning, all of the apparent benefits from these strenuous efforts appear erased. With this sobering perspective, it is quite understandable that your loved one may feel angry and dejected.

> **EMOTIONS**
> 1–I can't believe this happened to me . . . it's **not fair!**
> 2–I don't deserve this!
> 3–Why do I feel like I'm constantly on the verge of tears?

1–2 Strong emotional reactions to aphasia are common in the beginning. Those feelings may resurface and their intensity may continue to increase throughout the initial 6 to 12 months. Regular venting of such anger is often the best way of allowing victims to evolve out and beyond it. Most sufferers do come *to adjust* and *to forgive* the world for this injustice. They eventually come to realize that "fighting against" something that isn't likely to change is a wasted effort.

**PERSON
WITH
APHASIA**

Once beyond blaming *others* or *life*, they are freer to see and cope with their current state of function, rather than angrily fixate on what once was. However, when anger is extreme or shows no signs of lessening over time, you may need to seek the advice of a professional specialist. A rehab social worker or rehab psychologist are likely choices. Your loved one's physician may assist as well.

3 Injury to the brain can disrupt one's thermostat for gauging or reacting to life's challenges and stresses. Because of injury, people with aphasia may be moved easily toward displaying an inappropriate degree of tears or laughter. Such breakdowns often are not due to a psychological or emotional reaction to injury, but to physical, biochemical differences in the brain due to injury. When one's emotions are easily and inappropriately triggered, the condition is referred to as ***lability***. The nature and management of lability are highlighted in Chapter 12 (see section entitled Emotional Lability).

EMOTIONS

*1–I can't believe this happened to
   me . . . it's **not fair**!*
2–I don't deserve this!
*3–Why do I feel like I'm constantly
   on the verge of tears?*

WHAT YOU MIGHT DO

1 WHEN ANGER IS A NATURAL PART OF RECOVERY

Coping with your loved one's anger is often difficult if its source or future duration is unknown. Anger following aphasia is common, especially when it is directed toward the *unfairness* of what has happened. In this respect, anger is often a necessary step toward your loved one being able to put his or her injury into a workable, and ultimately acceptable, framework.

1 WHAT TO DO

- Work at accepting the therapeutic value of anger for your loved one, and if it is "within reason," try to work with it, rather than against it.
- Acknowledge only the unfairness of this turn of events!
- Maintain that, in spite of its unfairness, there still is something you can manage together!

   "Yes, it is *bad* . . . yes, it was *not deserved* . . . but no, it is not insurmountable!"

"Together we can stand up to this. Together, we can make things better. *We can!*"

- Try not to "force" acceptance of injury. Acceptance cannot be imposed. It must come of free choice over time.
- Let your loved one independently take that step toward "what is," and away from the feeling of unfairness at having "what was" taken away.

1–2 WHAT TO DO IF ANGER CONTINUES

- Seek professional advice from your physician, rehab social worker, or rehab psychologist.
- If possible, continue to support your loved one, but don't let his or her anger entrap you:
    avoid letting it dictate your lifestyle.
    avoid taking on the burden of making his or her anger dissipate.
- Arrange respites for yourself:
  arrange for your loved one to spend time occasionally outside the home:
    senior daycare centers.
    senior or aging coalition centers.
  find ways to pursue activities of your choice outside the home.

- Find peer-support groups for your loved one and yourself:
  Being around others who have dealt with this challenge is often beneficial. It is an ideal way of venting your frustrations while learning how others have coped with theirs.

3 WHAT TO DO

- Know that emotional lability is often modifiable.
- The best way to minimize its negative effects is to teach your loved one to direct his or her attention away from the unwanted emotion itself:
    For example, when inappropriately crying abruptly surfaces, ask him or her to squeeze an uninvolved hand as tightly as possible, or grab the arm of a chair. Diverting your loved one's attention away from the crying often helps pull the labile person out of his or her embarrassment.

EMPLOYMENT

1–*I cannot work like this . . . what's going on in this arena?*
2–*I hope I can still return to work someday!*

**PERSON
WITH
APHASIA**

WHAT TO KNOW

1 As awareness of one's surroundings increases, your loved one is apt to worry more about his or her employment status. It is reasonable that he or she would wish to know how work-related matters are currently being handled. Years ago, a patient of mine had withdrawn a sizable sum of money the day before his injury and "hidden it" in a secure location in his office in preparation for an upcoming trip. He remembered doing this, but couldn't remember precisely where he had placed the money. Despite severe aphasia at the time, this man could not rest until others understood his concern. Although this gentleman knew he could not return to his job then, he was terribly concerned that this matter be resolved.

1 If your loved one was highly involved with work before, it is likely that concerns will prevail. Accordingly, it is important to update him or her from time to time on general information about his or her work status. It is also reasonable that your loved one may want to know whether his or her boss has called, and what information was shared.

1–2 If work was *highly significant* in your loved one's life prior to injury, you may wish to be cautious about detailing "specifics" of injury to his or her employer at this time. The severity of impairments appear much greater now than it really is, and it is difficult to know precisely how much function might return with time and treatment. Even though the "odds" do not favor your loved one returning to work, it is likely preferable to forego a final judgment this early. You may want to state politely and truthfully that assessment and treatment have only begun, and that it will likely be several months before his or her potential to work are really known.

2 To prepare your own state of mind, you should know that unless the employer is willing to adapt the job and its responsibilities to match your loved one's eventual skills, returning to his or her former employment is unlikely. Besides modifying the job, the employer needs to be willing to alter its pace, demands, and performance expectations—at least in the early stages. Under these special conditions, it may be possible for a person with a mild aphasia to return to work and maintain some semblance of employment. However, the extent of time and effort required of both parties to achieve a working solution is usually substantial. Their motivation and dedication to finding a mutual solution must be strong.

Needless to say, few employers will do this. As a result, most people with aphasia fail to return to work.

2 Even if the chances of success are small, it is not out of the question that some *other* type of paid employment might be possible. Depending on your loved one's injury, age, and desire, it is reasonable that new areas of interest might slowly emerge. The first "story" in Chapter 14 is about a gentleman who was an optometrist prior to suffering a stroke at age 35. Although the stroke was mild in many ways, permitting him later to walk, talk, and participate in much of life, it was too severe to permit his work as an eye specialist. However, he previously had tended flower and vegetables gardens as a hobby. Over many transitional years, he slowly perfected these gardening skills to a point that they came to provide him with a paying clientele. Although payment was minimal, it was highly rewarding and advantageous to his personal growth; it helped him reclaim a "new" sense of self-worth and independence.

2 Finally, many more people with aphasia return to unpaid positions through which their personal satisfaction with life is heightened. Often, assisting others or refining one's own personal skills in a chosen area, as long as it makes a meaningful contribution to self or society, is enough of a justification to participate! The reward is in the "doing," not in being paid!

WHAT YOU MIGHT DO

EMPLOYMENT
1–I cannot work like this . . . what's going on in this arena?
2–I hope I can still return to work someday!

1–2 KEEPING EMPLOYMENT'S DOOR OPEN

Although returning to work is unlikely, it may be that keeping the door open to possible work-related endeavors is important and therapeutic. Work is often a major source of reward, personal value, and how people define themselves. If it seems desirable to the injured party, keep that option open!

1–2 WHAT TO DO

- See if a decision about returning to work can be postponed until after rehab concludes. Often the best tactic is to maintain that

**PERSON
WITH
APHASIA**

your loved one's true potential won't be known until then.

- If the employer is hesitant to postpone a decision about returning to work, and you suspect your loved one would value returning: see if he or she has sufficient sick leave to cover a postponement, either in part or full. You may want to investigate the option of leave-without-pay.

- If employment cannot be kept open for that length of time:
  ask if the employer might be willing to explore a mutually agreeable "work-related option" later. This endeavor would be totally voluntary, but if it should work out to everyone's benefit, then perhaps minimal compensation might be arranged down the road.

RECOVERY

*1–Treatment is finally beginning . . .
  now we can turn this thing around!*
*2–What should I expect from rehab
  and recovery?*
*3–What can I do to help this
  process?*

CAREGIVER

WHAT TO KNOW

1 To the caregiver, rehabilitation (rehab) is often viewed with great anticipation and high expectations! After days or weeks of chaos and uncertainty, finally there's something *positive* to look forward to, a rebuilding of functions that somehow went unexpectedly awry weeks ago. With this hope of forthcoming restoration, there often is a silent wish to *recapture* the preinjured person, to get back that individual you so desperately miss and still need!

1 Keeping a positive outlook about rehab is absolutely essential. These feelings over time, though, need to be realistic in order for the process ahead to work to its full advantage. You know by now, at least at a rational level of thinking, that aphasia is not another affliction that simply goes away. Even with the best care and the best of effort on your loved one's part, some form and degree of disability is apt to remain. Maybe in the future, modern medicine will devise better ways of stopping or reversing the effects of "brain attacks" (see Chapter 13, Medical Treatments of Stroke). However, for now, a part of your loved one's injury is likely irreversible. Try to erase any notions that this is not the case.

1 This fact does not diminish the role, importance, or value of rehab. It only ensures that you, as a "carer," or caregiver, stay grounded as to what

these restorative efforts may yield; they are intended to *enhance current*
levels of function, but not *eliminate dysfunction!* To keep the experience
of rehab positive, one needs to align one's expectation with what will follow.

1–2 Rehab's course is a brief, concentrated push to see if impaired skills
might be made more functional. In other words, it is an effort to see
whether their use in everyday life might be quickly and significantly
"jump started." In today's health care environment, though, rehab is no
longer a commitment to facilitate such use to its maximal level of performance. Instead, it is only a commitment to see if such function is possible within a narrow window of time. As a result, your loved one's use
of impaired skills *may have only begun* by the time rehab is ending!
Don't be confused by this! It is *not* a statement of what might be! Try not
to be dismayed. With ingenuity and effort, you can use this incomplete
treatment package to your benefit.

2 Expanding on the momentum of rehab is something we've chosen to
call **recovery.** As such, recovery is not synonymous with rehab, either in
form or mission. Rehab is a brief and important interim in this journey
to try to get basic skills in daily life up and running again. Recovery, on
the other hand, is a self-driven and self-realized continuation of what
trained rehab professionals help to establish and set into motion. Recovery typically involves a multitude of "real-life factors," that is, people, events, and settings, and, when properly "nudged" along, it may
continue to yield change and improvement for years to come.

3 Rehab helps set a direction and a way to allow functional skills to
return. It teaches your loved one *how* to resume use of impaired skills at
current levels of function, but as well, it teaches him or her how to slowly add on. How you can best assist at this time is to keep these rehab
"swings" of use engaged and moving in ever-increasing arcs. For example, his or her "talking swing" may require a number of potential nudges
on your part from time to time. Maybe that nudge is to simply wait, and
allow more time to process information. Maybe instead, it is to rephrase
what your loved one just said, or provide spoken options for him or her
to choose from. Shortly, each rehab specialist should be able to provide
you with a list of their own nudges to keep a particular skill or function
"in motion." Your role is simply to learn these well enough to permit
your loved one to actively "pump" these swings. **Even when pumping
is much harder for him or her than pushing is for you, you want to**

CAREGIVER resist the urge to do more! To the degree possible and safe, recovery means letting your loved take full responsibility for him- or herself.

3 Helping out, or caring for your loved one, then, means constantly providing a nudge only when your effort permits function and independence that otherwise would not occur. What nudges shouldn't do, though, is become a replacement for what your loved one can already do. As highlighted in later journey chapters, optimal recovery means giving people with aphasia every opportunity to venture forth on their own behalf. It is something that you want to carefully pay attention to from the very beginning. Making life better for you both begins right now by "caring for" instead of "doing for" your loved one. Suggestions follow for what to be aware of and how to act to promote these ends.

3 You can help as well by *starting now to get ready to cope with life after rehab,* rather than waiting until it is before you . . . as it soon will be! You've already been told that rehab's window is terribly brief; it will slam closed far more quickly than you ever imagined! **Certainly, starting to get "broken" functions working again is an important outcome of rehab. But recall that aphasia is not going to go away and its enduring deficits** *will impact you* **as much as your loved one. Because of this, your loved one's disorder is** *yours, too!* **For this reason, you need as much help in getting ready to shoulder the problems that remain, as your loved one needs in trying to get fixed what is broken.**

3 Finally, you can help by remembering there is *no single way* of dealing with rehab or recovery. Any system suggested for getting skills up and functional must feel comfortable to both of you. Recovering and reclaiming life is a *very personal experience*! Try not to push or be pushed into a course of action that doesn't feel right for you, your loved one, or you as a couple.

WHAT YOU MIGHT DO

1–2 SETTING THE STAGE FOR RECOVERY

Take out a sheet of paper. Copy the following text in large block letters:

CAREGIVER

REHAB

it's **NOT A CURE!**

it's simply **A BEGINNING STEP FORWARD** . . .

a **CONCENTRATED PUSH** to make things work again!

FOCUS ON the **THINGS THAT WORK**, not on the things that don't!

MORE IMPROVEMENT will come after rehab ends!

RECOVERY LASTS AS LONG AS PEOPLE ELECT TO TRY!

Put this message to yourself in a highly visible spot throughout the entire rehab process . . . like on the door of the refrigerator . . . see it . . . read it . . . and try to internalize it daily! Keep the last line of this message firmly in mind! In a couple of months, when rehab is over, you'll replace this list with another . . . about recovery (see Caregiver—Recovery, Chapter 6)! Getting better is just *starting*!

3 HELPING YOUR LOVED ONE

Keep your acts of caring and support within a framework that will ultimately foster your loved one's personal growth, self-esteem, and independence. The more of life you give back to your loved one, the more of life that will return to you. The more of life each of you are able to access independently, the more it will serve you jointly.

3 HOW TO FOSTER "CARING FOR"

• Encourage and maintain your loved one using as much residual skill as possible.

CAREGIVER
- Remember that inability and lack of use are two different things.
- If unsure whether a function or a portion of it is possible, confer with the professional directly responsible for managing such skills, e.g.,

  dressing, personal hygiene, hand-eye coordination—occupational therapist (OT).

  balancing, sitting, standing, and walking—physical therapist (PT).

  eating and communication—speech-language pathologist (SLP).
- Deny your loved one's request for help only when residual skills are *sufficient* to perform a task alone.
- Ensure that any refusals to help are portrayed as acts of "empowering your loved one" to do more, not as rule-enforcement or statements of your power.

3 HOW TO ENCOURAGE YOUR LOVED ONE'S PARTICIPATION

- Exhibit interest, caring, and confidence in your loved one's abilities, not your ability to act for him or her.
- Start where you know his or her skill levels are.
- Be present at first in case he or she should need your help.
- Reinforce function regardless of its proficiency or efficiency.

3 HOW "CARING FOR" SOUNDS IN WORDS

- "I love you and I'm right here."
- "You can do some or all of this."
- "Let's give it a try . . ."
- "If you can't . . . I *promise* to help!"
- "Come on . . . give it a try!"

3 USING A METAPHOR OF A SWING TO HELP YOUR LOVED ONE

- Your loved one is sitting in a swing.
- You know from talking to knowledgeable "swinging experts" that it is safe to try swinging.
- You position yourself behind him or her.
- Pumping is easier if the swing is already moving.
- So you give the swing just enough of a push to set it in motion.
- You encourage your loved one to try to keep that movement going.

- You push only when, and to the degree, needed.   **CAREGIVER**
- Inconspicuously, you give a slight push from behind on every third pump.
- Conspicuously, you emphasize your loved one's success in keeping the swing going.
- Weeks later, he or she is swinging alone.

3 WHERE "CARING FOR" LEADS

- To as much independence as your loved one's desires and residual skills permit.

3 BUILDING WORKING RELATIONSHIPS WITH REHAB STAFF

Whether rehab involves days, weeks, or months, keeping a good working relationship with the professional staff is vital. These individuals and their roles were overviewed earlier (see Chapter 4, Caregiver—Recovery). If rehab involves the same personnel from the hospital, then you are likely well on the way in knowing and feeling some comfort with rehab staff. If a different team of specialists is now overseeing treatment, you'll want to repeat the process of familiarizing yourself with them, and their emphases and preferences. Meet with each person who plays an active role in your loved one's treatment plan. Realize that their time is likely very limited; as urged before, come prepared and have an agenda in mind.

3 WHAT TO ADDRESS WITH REHAB STAFF

- Ask them to overview treatment from their perspectives:
    when it will begin or continue.
    where it is apt to lead over time, asking for "a range" within which expected change might fall.
    when it is apt to end, again asking for a range.
- Ask them what they would like or expect from you:
    now.
    throughout the duration of treatment.
    by its end.
- Ask them how they might prefer interacting and working with you.
    For example, some staff members prefer brief weekly meetings while others may urge you to drop in at the end of scheduled ses-

CAREGIVER

sions at your convenience. Some may encourage your attendance at treatment sessions while others may not. In any case, you'll want to establish a brief block of time weekly to meet and obtain their overview and express your concerns.

(minimally ask for 15 minutes weekly with each staff member).

3 HOW TO MAXIMIZE YOUR TIME WITH THEM

- *Listen* hard!
- Don't worry about talking at first. Let each specialist explain matters separately and collectively.
- Don't hesitate to ask for clarification of terms or concepts. Be sure you've gotten the message correct.
- At first, try not to be too optimistic, or pessimistic, about rehab's potential. Give yourself some time to truly grasp the significance of rehab's role in helping your loved one.

3 HOW TO BEGIN PREPARING NOW FOR LIFE AFTER REHAB

The brevity of rehab is a fairly new phenomenon in health care, and, unfortunately, no one has as yet constructed an effective bridge from it to daily life. You need to build your own road over this abyss, and Tables 5–1 and 5–2 outline what you will need to know and do to accomplish this. **You are apt to be the prime interactant with your loved one without the benefit of a speech-language pathologist in the near future. As such, you need to know how you can communicate effectively and comfortably right now before you forfeit access to this professional's assistance (see Caregiver—Communication in this chapter for more details). Don't view this "joint need" as anything less important than your loved one's restorative rehab.** Achieving some communicative connectedness as a couple is not usually automatic. You will need professional assistance in accomplishing this. Be aware that your joint needs have not always been a standard component of rehabilitative care, but, with the current threats to rehab services, your involvement in your loved one's subsequent recovery is more critical than ever. Get yourselves ready to deal with this right now!

- Tables 5–1 and 5–2 address what you may wish to consider in terms of getting the most out of rehab.

Table 5–1. Subjects relating to rehab, their prime concerns, related questions, references within book, and prime sources for answers.

SUBJECT	PRIME CONCERN	RELATED QUESTIONS	REFERENCE	PRIME SOURCES
Health Care System	How will it affect delivery of services?	Where will therapy occur? With whom? For how long? What options exist?	Chapter 3 Chapter 4: Caregiver—Recovery	Physician Rehab social worker Rehab staff
Health Care Insurance	What rehab services does your health care policy cover?	What types of services? What restrictions apply? For how long? Who determines when treatment ends? What is that decision based on? Are there any provisions for follow-up evaluations?	Chapter 3 Chapter 4: Caregiver—Recovery	Health care provider Physician Rehab social worker Rehab staff
Injury	How favorable is rehab for the type and degree of injury involved?	Is treatment an option? If so, how favorable does it appear? If not, why not? What other options exist?	Chapters 11 and 13 Chapter 4: Caregiver—Recovery	Physician Rehab staff
Functional Consequences	What functional consequences has the injury caused and how responsive are these to rehab?	What functions are impaired? How severe are these? Which can be improved? To what degree? What other options exist?	Chapters 9–13	Physician Rehab staff
You	What rehab services and methods might help now when rehab has concluded?	How might you relate to your loved one better? What skills would best prepare you to do this? How do you acquire these? What other options exist?	Chapters 5 and 6: Caregiver—Recovery	Rehab staff Physician

Table 5–2. Skills that may subsequently aid you if acquired in rehab.

SKILL	FOCUS	HOW TO PROCEED	SOURCE
Appraisal	To help you feel comfortable that your loved one is receiving the rehab services that may aid him or her and you the most.	Ask yourself upon finding out your loved one's rehab potential whether planned treatments address areas of dysfunction which stand to influence daily life the most; not just his or hers but yours together. Ask whether the type of therapy and its duration and intensity of treatment compares with what your health care insurance provides.	Rehab staff; physician and individual specialists; health care provider
Interactive	To help you re-establish, maintain, and hopefully promote past ties and comfort with your loved one in spite of impaired skills.	Ask rehab therapists to specify ways that you might *attain your former comfort level with your* loved one in spite of currently impaired skills. Ask if each therapist might *demonstrate these* for you. Ask if you can try these ways while *they monitor and comment.* Ask to continue to *refine them throughout rehab.*	Rehab staff; physician and individual specialists
Preparatory	To help you expand and enlarge your loved one's skills to act in his or her own behalf in daily life in spite of impaired functions.	Ask rehab therapists to specify ways, that if emphasized over time, might increase your loved one's ability and confidence to act in his or her own behalf in spite of impaired skills. Ask if they might demonstrate these for you now, as well as list a series of likely steps that might follow over time if targeted skills are expanded. Ask if there is a way to return periodically following rehab and have these adaptive skills reassessed and refined.	Rehab staff; physician and individual specialists

- Table 5–1 details common rehab-related concerns and how to procure additional information about them.

    These concerns are identified by subject, for example, health care system, insurer, or injury, and then by question, that is, what caregivers commonly need to know about each subject. Finally, there is a list of resources where additional information might be found.
- Table 5–2 details the acquisition of certain skills that may be beneficial later after rehab ends.

    Coming to the end of rehab requires *more* than simply reactivating some function in the impaired adult. It requires developing skills and ways that permit you, as a couple, to resume daily life. Ideally, rehab is not just about "the how to's," but also about feeling and remaining bonded as a couple in the process.

3 WHAT TO KNOW ABOUT TABLE 5–2

- These skills are most likely unfamiliar to you:

    They will require some time and patience to learn.

    They are not outwardly complicated.

    Their success, though, is more challenging than is apt to be apparent at first.

    They require a *subtle awareness* on your part of when, how, and how much to do.
- The aim is not to become an expert before rehab ends but simply to get oriented to these skills.
- Realize that some rehab personnel may not know of or endorse this type of therapy:

    Such skills are not typically a part of traditional rehab practices. Standard care has focused on restoring or circumventing impaired functions *in the patient*. Teaching caregivers ways of maintaining a personal connectedness with their loved one while dealing with the functional consequences of head injury and aphasia, may *not* be.
- Remember, though, to keep rehab comfortable and workable *for all*.

    You need to keep the rehab process moving forward in a positive direction. If you should encounter a rehab team member who is not inclined to assist with in such matters, carefully consider your next step. You do *not* want to disrupt the entire rehab process. The preferred option may be to begin looking for a rehab specialist who *would* assist you after the current treatment ends. It is never

CAREGIVER

too late to address such matters . . . even if it has been years since the injury!

3 WHAT YOU NEED TO DO BEFORE REHAB ENDS

- Rather than hoping to find permanent solutions, work toward feeling "enabled" to proceed independently.

  Your goal needs to be feeling "able" when rehab ends rather than find "solutions." Most of the *real* solutions, those of any true importance, are months and years away. You need simply to get oriented to, and partially skilled in, traversing the road ahead. If you have done that by rehab's end, you have more than done your job!

- Keep a daily or weekly log of change and the details of meetings with rehab personnel.

  Writing down key points along the way often helps sort out matters in your own mind. Also, written logs are extremely beneficial as a referral source, not just to document when certain changes occurred but to note their degree and consistency over time. For that reason, get in the habit of writing down what transpired, when, why, and their outcomes. Whether events seemed small or significant, a journal of key points along the road will prove invaluable later. Remember that change is often gradual and comes in small increments, but added up over time these small gains become large. A journal offers hard evidence of this fact.

> **ABOUT YOUR LOVED ONE**
> *1–He or she looks and acts so different. Is this change temporary or permanent?*

WHAT TO KNOW

1 People with aphasia are apt to "look" and "act" different in the beginning months after injury. There may be less movement of an arm or leg, more droop on one side to the face, more drooling, more food on or around the mouth, and possibly less control over bowel or bladder functions. As well, there may be other less apparent changes, like taking more time to think and react, focusing their thoughts and actions more personally than on others, and more sadness or crying. When such a lengthy and dramatic list of changes suddenly appears in life, it may seem to you that your loved one is "radically different." What do these differences signify? Are they brief changes or are they here to stay? **CAREGIVER**

1 First, recall from Chapter 2 that the "core person" is still present and well. Yes, some of the outward manifestations are different, and yes, some of these will remain so for months or indefinitely. However, many of the physical and behavioral changes will gradually evolve toward more normal and socially acceptable levels. In addition, the differences that do remain are apt to mean less and to stand out less vividly as time goes on. You are likely to grow more accustomed to, understanding of, and accepting of these changes over time.

1 At times, the extent of physical or behavioral change may seem simply too much to allow you to recapture a sense of the person of old. It may seem that the person of today is no longer remotely related. If differences in outward function were the *only* criteria . . . you may be right at times! You have *lost* someone who ran, joked, hosted incredible dinner parties, played the piano with ease, or played a competitive game of Trivial Pursuit! Recall, though, getting off that plane in a foreign country (Chapter 2). You were outwardly unable to exchange information and insecure over what to do next, but inwardly your core self was no different. Chances are, neither is your loved one's; the person from before is well and present. It is more that the outer wrapping on the package is different and perhaps a bit tarnished or seemingly unkempt. That wrapping will not look or seem quite so different once you are given some time to adjust.

WHAT YOU MIGHT DO

1 COPING WITH OUTWARD CHANGE

> **ABOUT YOUR LOVED ONE**
> *1–He or she looks and acts so differently.*
> *Is this change temporary or permanent?*

Visible differences in your loved one are apt to be most pronounced at this time. Rest assured that their form and severity should lessen. You are *not* likely to "get back" the person of before, but you are apt to see and feel the intactness of the inner person or soul. For many caregivers, it is this quality they knew best, admired most, and loved most dearly.

CAREGIVER

1 WHAT TO DO

- If you *are struggling* with current differences, begin by giving yourself permission to do so:

    It is not strange or wrong to feel personally ajar in the face of such physical or behavioral change.

    It takes time to put these changes into a different and more comfortable perspective.

    It may take time to see that the person from old is still present and well.

- If months later, you are still struggling to adapt to these differences:

    Specify what aspects of his or her changed self are most disturbing or disruptive to you and why.

    Consult with rehab specialists in those areas of dysfunction for their advice and assistance.

    Search out peer group forums that include people with whom to interact.

    Look to family, friends, and/or clergy for support or advice.

    Keep addressing any protracted feelings of personal rejection or withdrawal.

    Do not "give in" to accepting a "lesser existence."

    Keep pursuing ways of strengthening what is possible.

> **COMMUNICATION**
>
> 1–What can be done to improve his or her talking?
> 2–How can we make our own communication better?

WHAT TO KNOW

1 By now, you likely know the severity of your loved one's communication difficulties and whether or not treatment might help. Since disruption to talking is often the most obvious obstacle to communicating, it is often the prime concern of most caregivers. They often ask first, "What can be done to make my loved one's speech return?"

1 Talking may or may not be the first focus of therapy. If it is, it usually is because some speaking function remains and it can be easily accessed and stimulated. That is, there is a clear and easy way of giving that "talking swing" a push. If giving it a push, though, is not easy or possible, the speech-language pathologist is apt to look to other realms of language or communication to treat. Should this happen, be assured that it does *not* mean that talking isn't important or that it won't be addressed later on. It will! **People with aphasia need time to stabilize whole brain functions. As a result, nonspeaking tasks, like pointing to pictures or words when named or described may be far easier and more accessible in the early going. Over time, the speech-language pathologist will fashion a diverse treatment package that likely will stimulate all modalities of language use, depending on their current levels of function and how they might be expanded.**

CAREGIVER

1   As "whole brain" functions improve, more use of communication usually follows. For some, this improvement includes the emergence of some usable speech. When this is the case, talking is apt not to return abruptly, but instead in small, gradual portions over a period of weeks or months. For other sufferers, the return of "whole brain" functions may produce little or no change in talking. Recall that roughly half of the people who incur aphasia regain functional use of their ability to talk, that is, an ability to express their basic needs and wants through speech. Should your loved one fall in the "have not" category here, do know that there are other means of conversing without spoken words. Your loved one's speech-language pathologist should be able to advise you on which combination of these might be most appropriate in his or her case. You will want to keep close, ongoing contact with an experienced speech-language pathologist, not just about fostering better use of speech, but about how therapy might address other aspects of his or her impaired language and communication.

2   Improving your own communication with your loved one is likely a slightly different matter from trying to "fix" his or her disordered system. It means finding and developing ways of keeping the two of you socially bonded as a couple or pair. As noted in Caregiver-Recovery, the speech-language pathologist may tend to stress your loved one's remediation and be less concerned about remediating your communication as a couple. However, both areas of dysfunction require careful attention and intervention before rehab ends.

COMMUNICATION
1–What can be done to improve his or her talking?
2–How can we make our own communication better?

CAREGIVER

WHAT YOU MIGHT DO

1 IMPROVING HIS OR HER ABILITY TO TALK

If you haven't done so already, talk with the speech-language pathologist about your loved one's potential to resume communicating through speech. Don't be discouraged if speech has not been a prime focus initially. This does *not* mean that talking won't be a focus later, or that it won't return as time goes on.

1 HOW TO APPROACH TALKING AT FIRST

- Stay positive. You are likely some time way from knowing whether his or her talking will support any form of normal conversation.
- Keep your expectations within a "restorative" framework, not a curative one.

  Few people can claim to "cure" aphasia, but many lives and relationships of persons with aphasia and their loved ones have been restored.

- Resist the initial urge *to correct* your loved one, much as you would a child first learning to talk.

  Remember that people with aphasia still *have* and know the words they want to say. It is not beneficial to revert to "teaching" them how to talk again. As time goes on, there usually are specific ways of "facilitating" talking, but you need to review these first with the speech-language pathologist.

- Work at judging change *since* the injury, not comparing current skills with those before the injury.
- Stay informed and interested in the treatment process.
- Provide steady doses of encouragement regardless of the amount of change.
- Keep in mind that one's inability to talk in the early going does not preclude later use.

  Many people with aphasia are *speechless* in the beginning days and weeks. Give your loved one some time, and treatment a chance to work, before starting to "conclude" anything about what might evolve.

- Even if talking is nonexistent, both in the short and long term, the inner person you knew before remains.

2 HOW TO APPROACH YOUR JOINT COMMUNICATION NEEDS　　**CAREGIVER**

- Approach the speech-language pathologist about learning ways of comfortably interacting as a couple or pair.

    The aim here is not just to share information better but to allow the two of you to remain personally bonded in real life.

- Ask if this professional would make out a list of ways that might enhance your communication together.

    Each couple's communicative list will differ depending on their inherent strengths and challenges. For this reason, you need the speech-language pathologist's assistance in detailing how best to "input" and "output" information.

- Ask if you might watch how these supplemental "inputting" and "outputting" methods for communicating are used.

    You need to know precisely *the best way(s)* and *best order of steps* to follow to make your communication work ideally.

    Supplemental ways for *inputting information* to your loved one might include having you:

      talk slower, use fewer words, write out key words in big block letters, draw simplified sketches, gesture or pantomime, or use maps and pictures.

    Supplemental ways for helping your loved one in *outputting information* might include having him or her:

      write, draw, point to printed words or pictures, gesture or pantomime, or change vocal tone or stress.

    Because some working combination of these ways is probably what you most need, you cannot do this alone! You need an experienced speech-language pathologist to guide you through this process.

- Ask next whether you might practice these ways as a portion of treatment.

- If so, strive to perfect these methods with the speech-language pathologist's guidance.

- Make it a point to leave rehab with a "working knowledge" of how to communicate with your loved one.

    Journey Chapters 6, 7, and 8 continue to expand on the foundation established here. As highlighted in Chapter 8, your communication success as a couple actually sets the foundation for relational and societal well-being later. Skip ahead and read the tennis metaphor in the section entitled, "The Quality of Your Communication." You may benefit from a glimpse of where you

CAREGIVER   want to be years from now. At the moment, you need only get a
                     sense of where and how to begin.
                   • Start working on interaction at the beginning of rehab, not at the
                     end!

HEALTH
1–How much can my loved one do physically?
2–What else do I need to know at this time?
3–Is there any chance that this injury might reoccur? If so, how do we prevent it?

WHAT TO KNOW

1 Depending on the severity of your loved one's injury, physical activity may need to be curtailed at first. **However, staying physically active is an important part of recovery, not just during rehab but long afterward. Your loved one's physician and physical and occupational therapists can advise you about the proper amount, type, and frequency of physical exercise.** Occasionally, there may be other medical or physical restrictions that limit your loved one's freedom to take part in exercise, such as prior heart or lung disease. However, even when such restrictions exist, it is likely that this team of specialists will recommend some safe form of exercising rather than none. You do not want, though, to proceed into any physical exercise plan without their consultation and approval.

1 Often exercise plans to strengthen and expand compromised physical skills are begun in rehab, but abruptly halt when the patient returns home. Some of this failure is due to an unclear picture of what to do and how to do it once outside of the rehab setting. To avoid this, you can find out the types of activities that might be sustainable later outside this setting and ways to pursue them. It is important that midway through rehab's projected tenure you obtain a working knowledge of the type of exercises that are possible and prescribed. Scheduling and maintaining regular ongoing meetings with your loved one's physician and physical and occupational therapists should help assure that you know and can maintain these levels of activity.

2–3 By now, you likely know what caused your loved one's injury. It is not uncommon, though, that certain health-related details remain unclear. The realms often requiring further exploration are: what ongoing medical treatment, if any, will be needed; what are the purposes of these treatments; what health-related consequences may follow this

type and severity of injury; how might its recurrence be avoided. You
need to get understandable and clear answers to all of these questions
before rehab ends. A "side trip" into Chapter 13 will familiarize you
with basic information and terms commonly associated with answers to
these questions.

CAREGIVER

WHAT YOU MIGHT DO

1–3 ADDRESSING HEALTH CARE IN GENERAL

Keep a strong working relationship with the team
of health care professionals attending to your
loved one. If you have questions about how to do
this, you may wish to review previous considerations from Chapter 4: Caregiver—Health.

1 WHAT TO DO

- Ask your loved one's physician and physical and occupational therapists what physical activities are and are not possible at this time.
- Ask if there are any "special instructions" regarding their
implementation:
    how
    when
    where
    for how long.
- Keep a written record of their recommendations for review.
- Acquaint yourself with what to expect in the weeks and months
ahead.

2–3 WHAT TO DO

- Scan Chapters 12 and 13 for any "particulars" that relate to your
loved one's condition.
    Chapter 12: What else may accompany aphasia
    Chapter 13: What can be done to minimize further injury.

HEALTH

1–How much can my loved one do physically?
2–What else do I need to know at this time?
3–Is there any chance that this injury might reoccur? If so, how do we prevent it?

CAREGIVER

- Construct a list of questions about any of these features that remain unclear in your mind.
- Ask your loved one's physician to review your list of questions:
  clarify which of these issues pertain to your loved one.
  determine how they will be managed over time:
    in the short-run
    in the long-run.
- Monitor the progress of these issues as rehab evolves by keeping notes in your daily or weekly log.
- Midway through rehab start working on a plan as to how you might manage these alone.

EMOTIONS

1–He or she looks so unhappy . . . I just wish I could "fix it!"
2–My inability to do more totally drains me emotionally.

WHAT TO KNOW

1 For caregivers, agonizing over their loved ones' suffering is often one of the most difficult parts of coping. The intensity of wanting to fix the broken parts and extinguish this pain is understandable and a part of caring for one's loved one. However, as with physical support of a partially immobile arm or hand, it is not in your best interest or that of the injured party to extend help beyond what is needed to allow that person to assume full ownership and responsibility for him or herself. In other words, you want to avoid "doing for" your loved one in realms where it is not necessary. So to state the obvious, you cannot remove his or her agony; you cannot "fix" his or her broken parts; you cannot take responsibility for something that isn't yours. On the other hand, you can: acknowledge his or her feelings and the challenges they present, express a willingness to "assist" him or her, provide constant "pushes" on his or her recovery swing, and offer an unqualified "endorsement" of him or her as he or she is right now. But that is *all* you can do. **Trying to assume your loved one's pain as *yours* may only prevent him or her from confronting and resolving the issue him- or herself. Coming to grips with what is not working or broken is a lengthy proposition. You can be a facilitator, but your loved one must do the work.**

2 Rationally *knowing* what might work best doesn't necessarily make acceptance of it automatic or easy. You likely will need to set aside special time to internalize a working plan. In that regard, it may be helpful to schedule half- or full-day trips away to remove yourself from the immediacy of these feelings. Such freedom to focus on *just* these matters often permits insights otherwise overlooked. Quite frequently, the emotional overload is bound to elements other than just your loved one's injury. For example, you may feel personal pain and suffering of your own that is contributing to this anguish. Possibly you feel guilty over not having acted sooner. Maybe there were some *telling signs* that your loved one's injury was about to occur, and you failed to act. Regardless of the parts, it is likely a necessary step to sort out what is contributing to your anguish and to systematically work toward their reduction or elimination.

CAREGIVER

WHAT YOU MIGHT DO

1–2 SETTING THE STAGE

The first step is to try to identify *your* source(s) of anguish. From there, it becomes a much easier task to move forward and fashion a workable plan.

EMOTIONS
1–He or she looks so unhappy . . . I just wish I could "fix it!"
2–My inability to do more totally drains me emotionally.

1–2 WHAT TO DO

- Ask yourself these questions:
  "Did I *cause* this problem?"
     "If so, in what way?"
  "Am I responsible for seeing that my loved one's aphasia goes away?"
     "If so, why?"
- If the answers to both of these questions are solid "No's":
     You are moving in the right direction, keep at it!
     Keep well in mind your role and responsibilities as your loved one's emotional burden mounts.
- If either answer is a weak "No" or possibly a "Yes":
     Diligently set time aside to address their "why's."
     These answers likely will reveal some insights into your own emotional anguish and where to move next.
  If they are too much to resolve alone, seek outside assistance: other people confronting aphasia, a support group.

CAREGIVER

> friends or family.
> clergy.
> social worker or family counselor.
> psychotherapist.

DAILY LIFE

1–I've managed to keep things together, but I don't know how long I can keep juggling demands at work, home, and the rehab center!

WHAT TO KNOW

1 In the beginning, you were so involved in life and death issues that multiple demands didn't seem to compute. Now, 2 or 3 weeks later, you are beginning to sense a different schema to life. Your loved one is likely no longer in danger of dying, however, his or her recovery is apt to extend over months and years. Also, the many demands on your time have not abated and, for the first time, you are beginning to question your own endurance. Your worries are not so much about the days immediately forthcoming, but rather how you are going to manage in the weeks and months to come.

1 In this changing scenario, it is not strange to detect some feelings of entrapment, that is, an inkling that this ongoing dilemma may have only begun, and worries over how personal freedoms and daily responsibilities might be different now. And, as strange as it may seem, the best and healthiest way to begin looking for relief from these concerns is to reduce the amount of time spent with your loved one at the rehab center.

1 Such an option may seem impossible to do. But rethink for a moment where you want to be months and years down the road. For most caregivers, it is not hard to recognize or say, "I want my loved one as recovered as possible, but, as well, I want us to be personally strong as a couple." For this to happen, it means relinquishing the natural tendency to "do for" your loved one (see Caregiver—Recovery in this chapter). "Caring for" him or her means consciously protecting without overprotecting and consciously giving back the responsibility for living daily life rather than taking on those responsibilities yourself. It means working constantly to empower your loved one, not yourself.

1 For a brief moment, reassess where you have come from and where you are. Initially your loved one's medical condition required your constant attention and vigilance. Now, matters have changed.

His or her immediate survival is no longer in question. Yes, many demands still exist with respect to his or her recovery but there are also others, a team of rehab specialists, to assist you. Now *is* the time to redefine your role and purpose in this process!

CAREGIVER

1 Redefining what might work best for you is often easier if separated into categories. For instance, you may need to establish time at and away from rehab. Also, while at the rehab center, you need to attend to some "quality time" with your loved one, but as well, to find time to learn about, advocate for, and acquire new skills (see Caregiver-Recovery).

1 By "quality time," we refer to daily periods within your busy schedule where you can meaningfully connect and relate to one another. Once in rehab, your loved one's time from early morning until late afternoon is likely quite obligated. Depending on his or her needs, reducing your visits to late afternoon or early evenings might work best. Even then, due to the rigors of therapy and his or her diminished endurance, you may wish to keep your visits short. Weekends may be more conducive to sharing and interacting, but even then, you want to guard against sliding into a protective posture, "hovering over" your loved one.

1 Besides lessening your time at the rehab center, you need to reproportion what you do there. Make it a priority to start gathering the information and skills in Tables 5–1 and 5–2. Rehab staff members' time during the day is limited to patient care. When meetings are prearranged and their purposes are well defined and agreed on, though, such interactions are possible. Getting information and learning "how" to manage disrupted functions as well as possible as a pair is critical, and does not "intrude" on these professionals; it is in many ways reinforcing some prime themes in therapy and simultaneously guaranteeing the two of you the best working basis from which to manage life after rehab ends.

1 Allow in this whole mix sufficient time, too, for keeping home and job together. In the very beginning, both of these arenas in life were apt to suffer, but by now, you need to find a more comfortable and enduring solution. As urged before, *you need not feel obligated* to be at the rehab center except for brief visits with your loved one and preparing for what lies ahead. Focus the rest of your time and energies on maintaining home and work.

CAREGIVER

WHAT YOU MIGHT DO

1 REARRANGING ONE'S PRIORITIES

Making the initial changes in priorities requires conscious thought and choice. There are many ways of proceeding. Carefully examine your options and preferences before selecting your own course.

1 WAYS OF ALTERING TIME WITH YOUR LOVED ONE

- Write out things *you* need to attend to that lie outside your loved one's needs or the rehab center:
  Visibly seeing what needs your attention often frees you from being constantly present.
- Slowly change the frequency and duration of visits:
  Emphasize your pledged devotion to your loved one but note that "other demands" in daily life are going to lessen your actual time with him or her. This reduction in time has nothing to do with your level of caring; it remains the same. You keep his or her needs and wants at the top of this list and you'll be present as much as your joint schedules permit. Let him or her know that much of his or her time will be spent "in therapy," and you need, at those times, to attend to matters at the rehab center, home, and work.
- If such a shift seems too dramatic to you or your loved one, slowly modify visits.
  Maybe you were present constantly before. Now, come for an hour or half-hour in the morning and afternoon, and slowly reduce it to an hour in the evenings. Eventually modify that to a visit every other day. Try not to think about what you are *not* doing; try to think about what you are doing to help both of you recover.
- If less time with your loved one bothers you:
  Consider getting updates the first several days via the phone.
  If possible, talk to your loved one over the phone . . . even if communication is poor . . . it simply allows you to stay and feel connected.
- Avoid accompanying your loved one to every rehab session:
  Don't promote dependency by escorting your loved one through

> his or her daily rehab routine.
> Schedule separate appointments with rehab staff for things you want help with.
> - If concerns about your work remain, see Caregiver-Employment in this chapter.

CAREGIVER

WHAT TO KNOW

1 As you come to feel more familiar with all that has happened, you may feel freer to begin interacting with the outside world. Depending on your personal style, making contacts with others may or may not be what you want. **However, just as constantly accompanying your loved one through daily life is not advisable or healthy for him or her, so too, constantly isolating yourself from friends or routines is not advisable or healthy for you! You may need, even when it does not feel natural, to briefly and frequently escape the current setting and its dilemmas. Getting out with personal friends is one effective way of doing this.** Yet, it somehow may feel disrespectful or empty doing so—joking with others about trivial matters compared to your loved one's current condition. Although the joking is trivial, it is essential in helping you restore some balance to life. It is not so much the content of the respites that matters as it is being able to momentarily escape and think about something else. So, if necessary, push yourself in the beginning to keep contact with past friends. *You need to* in order to better cope and serve in an effective supportive role for your loved one.

> **FAMILY/FRIENDS**
> *1–I appreciate their concern!*
> *2–What is the best way to respond to them?*

2 Inquiries from others are appropriate but likely still too much to cope with. Again, until matters get more stabilized, it is not wrong, impolite, or insensitive to acknowledge their thoughtfulness, provide a brief overview, explain that it may be several months before anything more substantive is known, and that visitation will be more comfortable at that time.

2 It is important to know, too, that aphasia tends to erode past relationships with others. The loss of old friends is not a simple issue; it is discussed in more detail in Chapter 6: Person with Aphasia and Caregiver—Family/Friends. For now, know that keeping close ties with family or friends is important. Know, too, that this injury is theirs as well . . . like-

CAREGIVER ly not to the degree it is yours, but it likely alters their lives as well. To the degree people are willing to adapt and change to what aphasia ushers in, past bonds or ties need not be sacrificed.

> **FAMILY/FRIENDS**
> *1–I appreciate their concern!*
> *2–What is the best way to respond to them?*

WHAT YOU MIGHT DO

1–2 INTERACTING WITH OTHERS

Work to keep important connections with close friends up and running. For those special few who naturally add to daily life, reach out and move toward them rather than retract. You needn't be perfect . . . you needn't be fully there as you would have been before. But you do need to go and participate. Your well-being, especially over the long haul, demands the nurturing of contacts beyond your loved one . . . be they friends, places, events, or activities of personal reward and pleasure. Start attending to these right now . . . even if it does not feel perfectly natural or desirable!

1–2 STAYING CONNECTED WITH THE OUTSIDE WORLD

- Force yourself to reconnect with someone or something weekly outside the rehab environment.
- Do it as a favor to yourself. It is not an act showing either neglect or disfavor to your loved one.
- Down the road, you are apt to need others with whom you can relate and interact . . . keep key friends present.
- Call such a friend . . . arrange to have lunch:
    You can set the agenda. Depending on your feelings, you may or may not wish to discuss what is happening with your loved one. It is perfectly acceptable to simply indicate: "I sort of need to sit and chat about anything except what's happening at the rehab center."

1–2 COPING WITH OTHER ONGOING INQUIRIES

- If you are not already doing so, you may wish to monitor phone calls by:
    Purchasing a telephone answering machine.
    Obtaining "caller identification."

- Know that it is perfectly acceptable to acknowledge others' kindness but to decline assistance at this time.
- You may wish to ask a close friend to:
    - screen calls.
    - contact concerned individuals and let them know:
        - how much their inquiry was appreciated.
        - a general overview of matters.
        - how they might be of assistance.
- You may wish to have others aid in certain ways:
    - feed pets.
    - minimal grocery shopping.
    - upkeep items, e.g., mowing the yard or shoveling a walk.

CAREGIVER

WHAT TO KNOW

> **EMPLOYMENT**
> 1–*How can he or she return to work . . . maybe I should tell his or her boss right now!*
> 2–*How am I going to work and attend to him or her?*

1 This concern was addressed earlier (see Person with Aphasia—Employment).

2 Keeping your own employment at this time is important for several reasons. First, your loved one likely will not be able to return to work and the financial burden of the family may rest solely on your income. Second, work often defines an essential part of who we are or what we might be in life. If your work is of high choice and personally rewarding, then sacrificing to support your loved one's needs is likely not in your or his or her best interests. Third, if you are not working in order to *be available* to attend to your loved one's needs, this likely hinders rather than aids his or her optimal recovery. For reasons addressed earlier, your loved one needs every opportunity to fashion a lifestyle of his or her own based on existing skills and interests. As caring as your intentions may be, being constantly with your loved one is apt to reduce rather than increase his or her self-confidence and independence. For your loved one to grow and resume as much independence in daily life as possible, you may need to physically remove yourself from that environment daily. For all these reasons, it is important not to change or jeopardize any long-term employment now. Wait until you know better what residual abilities he or she will have before making any irreversible decisions.

<table>
<tr><td>

EMPLOYMENT

*1–How can he or she return to work
. . . maybe I should tell his or her
boss right now!*

*2–How am I going to work and
attend to him or her?*

</td></tr>
</table>

WHAT YOU MIGHT DO

1–2 CONFRONTING JOB CHANGES

Move deliberately and slowly with all of these decisions.

CAREGIVER

1 WHAT TO DO

Review suggestions earlier in chapter, Person with Aphasia—Employment

2 WHAT TO DO

Consider these options first before deciding to leave or quit your job:

- Carefully look at what is so essential "to do" at home or with your loved one that would require your quitting.
- Look to other ways of getting these essential parts accomplished without quitting your job.
- Also, look to other ways of attending to unessential parts over the short term.
- Explain to your loved one how your work is a priority.
- Ask if he or she would support you in this endeavor.

2 WHAT TO SAY

- "I want you to know that I'm very much with you."
- "I want you to know I'll remain so."
- "But . . . I need to keep my job . . . "
- "That means . . . I'll need to be away during the day."
- "I need your help in being patient while we work out a solution to this."
- "We will find one that works for both of us."
- "Other people have faced this, so can we."

Facing rehab's conclusion

Before you know it, rehab will be ending! It's likely still months away, but these months will pass quickly. You'll look up one day and find yourself attending a conference of medical and rehab staff members to review your loved one's progress and discharge. In this meeting, rehab team members will voice their assessments of what has and has not changed, and specific recommendations for the future. If you have carefully attended to those aspects of recovery that we highlighted in Tables 5–1 and 5–2, then you and your loved one are likely prepared for, although not necessarily pleased about, leaving rehab.

Undoubtedly many parts to daily life remain "broken" or not fixed the way you had hoped they would be! But know that what still remains undone in rehab's wake will not doom the success of your journey. There are *always* ways around what didn't get fixed or accomplished in rehab. In fact, it is likely that only a "smidge" did get accomplished. This journey is not just about *quantity of change*. If it were, much of the road ahead would, indeed, be treacherous. Change from traveling these roads usually comes in gradual and small increments. **Thus, what is more important than quantity of change is constancy of change. Is change still occurring and if so, are you and your loved one in the best position possible for fostering its continuation?** If you have come to know about your loved one's diminished skills (Table 5–1), and if you know ways to work with these skills as they currently are (Table 5–2), you are where you need to be. Not all of your information need be complete, nor your skills perfectly honed, they simply need to have been gathered and prepared for the road ahead.

❖ CHAPTER 6

Leaving formal care. . . going home

The second major crossroads involves returning to everyday life. By its very nature, the next stretch of your journey contains some of the rock-iest, bumpiest terrain of the entire trip. It comes after weeks or months of specialized attention, support, and retraining to restore parts of life that went amiss months ago. Even though these restorative efforts have fallen short of what you or your loved had hoped for, they have pro-vided a plan and some constancy from which to work. Now, just when the impaired parts were beginning to show signs of improvement, treatment is ending! At this moment, travelers commonly feel depleted and cheated. You wonder, "What sense does this make?" and "Why can't we continue with therapy until more, or possibly *all*, function has returned?" As alarming as stopping therapy is, this fear is secondary to those about what will replace it.

Whether it was intended or not, you likely are feeling a not-too-subtle shift toward *having to* assume a new role in relationship to your loved one, one of responsibility for the duties of formal care. At the beginning of this journey, you worried whether your loved one would get better at all. Then you worried about him or her receiving proper treatment. Now you worry that getting better resides *solely with you*. The magnitude of this shift, along with the other new duties and burdens since injury, is enough to make you feel like the paths you'd like to take look further away, rather than closer to you.

In the last chapter, we offered suggestions aimed at preparing you for this precise moment; hopefully some of them have reduced whatever load and worry you have been feeling. In this chapter, we detail how to get the most out of your loved one's discharge plan and how to continue receiving consultation from rehab specialists. Even so, as treatment ends and access to professional support becomes more difficult, you are apt to worry over the challenges ahead. Suddenly the road has gone from having a somewhat smooth surface to something rocky, treacherous, and unknown. As emphasized previously, however, there is nothing that can't be faced and negotiated with time, persistence, and dedication. Consider what lies ahead as simply that: a rough section of road, nothing more! Other travelers have gone before you and made it through, and so will you!

In addition to noticing some looming dark clouds on the horizon, you will also learn that leaving formal care ushers in strong and varied emotions. For people with aphasia, they are *finally going home!* It has been some time since they were in this favored and familiar spot, and for many, it was the last place where they were free of injury. They may cling to a hope that returning might minimize, perhaps even "erase," their current impairments. Even when they realize that such notions are unrealistic, they cannot help leaving rehab with an inflated sense of hope and restored confidence.

For this reason, the beginning days at home for people with aphasia often soften their worries. Just being in one's own bed or favorite chair and having home-cooked meals is enough to "forget" momentarily the unmet needs from rehab. Unfortunately, this respite is usually brief. As the novelty of home subsides and the remaining presence of impaired skills increases, it becomes apparent that this setting has *not erased* chronic disability. Given this realization and a new shortage now of others to help, their spirits tend to head downward. Pulling out of these moments of despair is often not easy and requires a concerted effort on everyone's part.

The caregiver is not as apt to be "lulled" into false hopes related to bringing his or her loved one home. Yes, you are happy to have your loved one physically and emotionally closer, and to not have to juggle the complexities of rehab, but the enormity of what still remains impaired has probably dampened your personal enthusiasm, comfort level, and confidence. It was one thing when trained rehab specialists assumed responsibility for these dysfunctional aspects; it is an entirely different matter to feel that they are "yours" to deal with. With this shift, many caregivers are more aware of what *is not working* about their loved one than what is. Not surprisingly, they worry about *their ability* to manage single-handedly the parts that aren't working. And worse yet, they worry that their loved one's long-term care might suffer because of something they overlooked or didn't do.

Given all of this confusion, your first instinct may be to simply push the accelerator pedal to the floor and race ahead to the next smooth section of road. All guide books advise against this. Instead, consider just the opposite: Let off on that accelerator, slow down, and pull off on the next safe shoulder. Turn off the car's engine, grab your coats, and get out of the car! Take a few minutes to look around at this familiar setting, which now greets you under "new" circumstances. Be prepared to expect that the place of old is not apt to hold the beauty or appeal it once did. In fact, you may even need to force yourself to examine some of its old landmarks. In terms of getting where you want to go, you need to know that there is no escaping it: **These changes you see, at least in part, are here to stay. They will look formidable for only as long as it takes you to incorporate them into a new way of life, one that will become comfortable and, with time, familiar.** So . . . get out of that vehicle . . . and start exploring and smelling the air. Slip on your "tennies" and pull out the wheelchair if necessary. Take a short exploratory hike on a well-marked route . . . maybe around the backyard. It doesn't matter where or how far you go, just go!

While looking, think about *looking in a different way!* It probably won't work at first, but try, and keep trying until it does. That is, try to view these new circumstances not as your adversary or enemy, but as something you simply need to learn more about. Your challenge is to learn and personally grow and flourish in this new but familiar land, not to wither, withdraw, or die. It is not the lay of the land that will determine the outcome; it is you. So refrain from attributing more to these differences than they deserve. Yes, some of the landscape is different, but if you are cautious, perceptive, and willing to risk within reason, you can reside in this "new" country with minimal anguish and a fair share of pleasure and comfort.

Remember that there is no urgency to act. If you need time to readjust and gain a sense of composure and direction, do so; nothing will be lost! You can remain parked along the side of these bumpy dirt roads for weeks and months without doing any real harm. Most importantly, the two of you need to figure out *your own* solutions *together.* They will come gradually by selecting out what is or is not important to you. So, settle in . . . relax . . . and find your own natural pace. There are numerous places to rest, think, make choices, and replenish your reserves. We'll continue to show you possibilities for finding beauty in something that may feel raw and barren. Rapidly accelerating ahead, though, is not a solution. Remember, time is your best ally. It is on your side, not against you!

Profiles

PERSON WITH APHASIA

- continuing to show improvement in health and physical appearance but still notably different
- following a plan for sustaining self-cares, although the level of assistance may range from none to a lot
- wanting very much to be at home whether or not current physical or functional skills permit
- tending more toward a self-centered position in thought and actions . . . less able to step outside one's own personal doubts and worries
- still showing gains in the areas of dysfunction, but not as pronounced as at first

CAREGIVER

- feeling encouraged by improvements during rehab but equally concerned over the lack of major change
- feeling intensely panicked over treatment ending, just when some momentum was starting
- feeling torn between wanting loved one at home and worrying that his or her condition is too severe to manage alone
- worrying over the prospect of having to assume responsibility for loved one's care
- feeling the most overwhelmed since the initial days of injury
- asserting that there *must be* more to recovery, yet stymied as to how to pursue it

- increasing interest in partaking in life although lacking self-initiation and confidence
- realizing that functioning is *not* back to anything close to one's pre-injured level
- worrying about how he or she will manage without professional support
- increasing bouts of fear, anxiety, depression, and/or loneliness . . . even anger at times
- showing signs of reduced self-esteem and increased self-pity
- unconsciously trying to shift his or her burden of care onto caregiver
- shying away from being around others, including friends

- beginning to entertain the notion that a full recovery may not be possible
- trying to figure out what a partial recovery will mean now and in the future
- noticing that friends inquire less about loved one's condition
- feeling surprised and hurt by the reaction of many close friends to what's happened, i.e., you sense a growing distance and discomfort in them . . . but you are unsure why

Primary concerns

PERSON WITH APHASIA

Recovery
1–Treatment can't be ending! I was just starting to get better!
2–I'll continue to improve, right?
3–How will I ever manage this alone?

Feelings about self
1–I'm better . . . but far from where I was!
2–I can't see myself staying like *this*. I'm a mere shadow of the person I once was!

CAREGIVER

Recovery
1–Golly, we were just starting . . . how can treatment be ending?
2–How do we deal with all that remains?
3–Where do we go from here?

About your loved one
1–He or she still needs a lot of assistance!
2–I know I need to be more patient . . . but it is hard at times!
3–Slowly, I'm starting to see signs of his or her "old" self.

Daily Life

1–How well will I manage alone?

2–Being at home should help!

3–Why are some of the smallest tasks still so hard to do?

Emotions

1–This is a real mess . . . and I'm the source of the problem!

2–I feel clumsy and awkward a lot of the time!

3–I sure hope I can manage this alone.

Relationship

1–I'm no longer physically attractive . . . certainly not like this!

2–Will my significant other even want to be close to me again, I hope so!

Communication

1–How can treatment be stopping now?

(a) despair: How will I manage this alone?

(b) determination: I cannot stay like this . . . I must, and I *will* talk better!

2–I'm no good to others if I can't talk.

Family/Friends

1–What are my family and friends going to think of me?

2–It cannot be good . . . I'm embarrassed . . .

Daily Life

1–How well can he or she manage alone?

2–Am I asking or demanding too much?

3–Why doesn't he or she try harder? I would!

Emotions

1–Whew, I've got a lot on my shoulders!

2–I know we'll manage, but I'm hanging by a thread.

Employment (yours)

1–How are we going to manage?

. . . I can't give up my job!

. . . but he or she can't manage alone?

2-What options do we have?

Communication

1–If he or she could only *talk*, everything would be OK!

2–We're doing better with *our* communication!

. . . I understand his or her basic needs.

. . . Still it is *very hard* and *frustrating* at times!

. . . How can we get better?

3–What should I do when we're around other people?

Family/Friends

1–We cannot avoid seeing or being around others now!

2–What should I do?

3–How can I make this easier on
   my loved one?
      for them!
      for me!
3–I know I have to meet them
   sometime, but I'm not looking forward to this!

Employment

1–It's time to decide about
   working . . .
      What can I do?
      What do I want to do?
      What should I do?

Relationship

1–I still love him or her but I'm
   unsure how to express it.
      . . . is it physically or
      medically OK to be
      intimate again?
      . . . what can or can't he or
      she do?
2–How do we approach this
   realm?

Health

1–Why am I so tired all the time?

Health

1–Are there any other health
   issues that need explanation or
   attention?

WHAT TO KNOW

1 The ending of formal treatment serves as the
first indicator that aphasia is here to stay. Most
people with aphasia tend to enter rehab thinking
that disability will pass, if not in full at least to a
large extent, much like a variety of acute afflic-
tions have. But now treatment is over and many difficulties still persist.
Yes, there has been change, but compared to preinjured levels of function, they may seem insignificant. Because of this, it is the presence of
injury, not the benefit of therapy, that is apt to stand in the forefront of
your loved one's thoughts as he or she leaves formal care. *You* have
many questions, and these are amply addressed under Caregiver—
Recovery in this chapter.

> **RECOVERY**
> *1–Treatment can't be ending! I was
>   just starting to get better!*
> *2–I'll continue to improve, right?*
> *3–How will I ever manage this alone?*

**PERSON
WITH
APHASIA**

PERSON WITH APHASIA

1 Even though some awareness of permanent injury has taken hold, it is likely that any true appreciation of what this really means is still months away. The changed status of the person with aphasia is much *too new* to incorporate or accept that this altered state is lasting. What dominates instead is the image of the person prior to injury. All of one's lifetime, with the exception of the last 1, 2, or 3 months, has been spent injury-free. It is not surprising that this earlier image should prevail now! It is the *only form* of being that your loved one has ever known. Now this thing called "aphasia" stands between everything that once was and everything that now is. There has *not* been sufficient time to even start to revamp one's prior perspective of self or life. To do this, the injured party must actually come to see his or her injured state as *not* resolving. Accomplishing this transformation in full takes years! In fact, for a small number of aphasic sufferers, coming to grips with their changed selves never occurs, they continue to use their pre-injury status as the goal for recovery.

2 Aphasia's permanence does not imply that further improvement *is not possible.* In fact, most people with aphasia steadfastly believe they will get better with more time. What is most discouraging now, though, is the loss of trained professionals to assist them. Because both the person with aphasia and the caregiver have *only known* recovery through these specialists, it is perfectly understandable that both parties feel abandoned and terribly worried at the moment. For many aphasic sufferers, their sole consolation is knowing that their caregiver is still nearby to support their efforts.

3 Because common functions of daily life still remain difficult, and "help" is less extensive, issues of diminishing self-confidence and self-worth are apt to be even more apparent now. These declines naturally threaten the person's viability to take charge and actively do more with altered states, as he or she had hoped. Such periods of inner anguish are common: However, as a caregiver, be sure that you not misconstrue them as signs of *not wanting* to improve further, or *not possessing* the ability. They are more suggestive of the feeling when someone suddenly lets the air out of the tires. We may need to stop and to reinflate those tires before moving on. How much air is needed depends on how much air was taken out!

3 Whether brain-injured or not, all of us face periods of uncertainty when we feel disempowered, ineffective, and highly vulnerable. When

such periods are prominent and lasting, we begin to question our abilities to even cope or function in life. **People with aphasia are no different. They, like the rest of us, require steady doses of "proof" that
current functions do "truly" make a difference to someone. Their
continued willingness and courage to continue to try in life is
dependent on this simple, yet often elusive, fact: that how they are
today still matters and has value! Both are unquestionably true!**

**PERSON
WITH
APHASIA**

WHAT YOU MIGHT DO

RECOVERY
1–*Treatment can't be ending! I was just starting to get better!*
2–*I'll continue to improve, right?*
3–*How will I ever manage this alone?*

1 FRAMING REHAB'S ENDING

Your direction following rehab depends on your
loved one's needs. Most importantly, if any
doubt exists in his or her mind about the possibility for further recovery, it is important to emphasize that recovery has *only begun*. True, the
rules and means for achieving these ends are about to shift, but this is
no reason to despair. It simply means that you, your loved one, and others must be more creative and committed to making sure current
progress continues. The journey chapters ahead are filled with notions
for doing more! Right now, let your loved one know that you are
wholeheartedly behind this mutual endeavor and pursuit.

1 WHAT TO DO

- Acknowledge that treatment is about to end.
- Counter quickly that you will, together, find new ways of continu-
  ing what was begun in rehab.
- Emphasize that current gains are *only the beginning* of recovery.
- State that over time, more *will return*, and better skills will follow.
- Assure your loved one that current abilities are more than sufficient
  to work from.
- Acknowledge that the initial weeks and months may be the most
  difficult, but that you can, and will, forge a new plan for daily life
  together.

1 WHAT TO KEEP IN MIND

- Your loved one needs to develop some inner strength.

PERSON WITH APHASIA

Gaining back a sense of self comes from *participating in life*, not from being isolated and pitied for what is or isn't present or working.
- Building a working foundation from which he or she can *act* means:
    Encouraging participation in situations where current skills exist and are safe.
    Selecting activities that he or she chooses rather than prescribing them.
    Giving your loved one constant encouragement and reason to act.
    Making sure that chosen activities, are fun especially at first.
    Emphasizing the importance to you of your loved one's intact and valued *inner core.*

2 WHERE TO BEGIN

- Focus on what has improved, not what remains impaired or yet to be improved.
- Avoid arguing whether or not current skills are sufficient to participate.
- Urge use of the skills that currently exist (see Caregiver—Recovery in this chapter):
    You may need to ask rehab therapists to help translate current rehab skills into daily life functions: for example, helping with the laundry, meal preparation, or housecleaning.
- Resist doing for your loved one—overattending or doting on him or her.
- Make participation inviting by commenting on how beneficial his or her efforts really are.

2–3 WHAT TO SAY

- "Treatment is ending . . . but your ability to get better, though, is not!"
- "You can, and will, continue to improve as long as you try to!"
- "It all depends on your willingness."
- "If you choose to work at it, I'll help."
- "We need to explore new ways of making this happen."
- "It may take time to get these new ways up and working."
- "Others have done it, so will we!"

WHAT TO KNOW

ABOUT YOUR SELF
1–*I'm better . . . but far from where I was!*
2–*I can't see myself staying like **this**. I'm a mere shadow of the person I once was!*

PERSON WITH APHASIA

1 Even though the gains are probably small so far, most people with aphasia leave formal care knowing that they *are* better off now than they were before treatment started. Many see current gains, though, as minimal or even insignificant when compared to where they once were. Changing one's feelings about one's altered self entails finding legitimacy in something that doesn't seem to have much. It means coming to view daily life from a vantage point of "what is." It means having the courage to work with and expand upon current abilities, as poor as they may seem, rather than succumbing to the angst and despair of what seemingly is not.

1 We've told you . . . the person with aphasia is the *same person inside* in spite of outward differences. **As hard as it may be for your loved one to acknowledge this, now is a good time to begin commenting on your awareness that his or her "inner parts" are unchanged. You will need to say it over and over again in a variety of ways and contexts before your loved one is apt to begin to believe it. Providing this focus allows your loved one to give credence to a core from which to build more quickly than if he or she had to discover it alone.** Also, it tells him or her unequivocally that you are there—and that you do care!

2 Remaking one's diminished image of self is not a quick undertaking, nor is it the only readjustment necessary. In fact, setting the stage for continued recovery requires readjusting everyone's expectations. It starts by consistently showing and acknowledging that more is possible than the person with aphasia, the caregiver, and even society are apt to view as possible. As just noted, it means bringing current levels of function to the forefront, encouraging and rewarding their use, and promoting preferred ways of expanding them. Over time, what may have seemed so insignificant in the beginning, actually provides the leverage to develop something more tolerable to the person with aphasia, more acceptable and even more valued.

2 You cannot force your loved one to adopt this or any other plan for making life better! If he or she is so intractably "stuck" at the moment in the shortcomings of self and life, *exerting force* to make him or her act is *not* good either. Keep giving that swing a gentle and constant

PERSON WITH APHASIA

nudge; sooner or later your loved one is apt to start pumping of his or her own free will. You cannot demand that he or she pump; the impetus has got to come from him or her.

2 Within the range of what your loved one will allow, the most valued element at first is reestablishing some comfort in the use of everyday functions. It is better at this time, as you leave formal care, to work toward building a familiar and achievable repertoire of existing skills than trying to add on to them. Form a firm, known, and operative base, then slowly begin expanding in preferred directions . . . but not at first!

2 The seeming immensity of the task may discourage you at times. Know that the process ahead, though, is not like acquiring new functions in childhood. Instead, it is more like getting a snowball moving down a mountain slope. In the beginning, the process may be quite difficult: the snow must hold together and a constant pushing and prodding is necessary until it begins to accumulate some size and momentum. Once moving, though, your effort becomes minimal; the expanding mass and velocity of the snowball will ensure its continuation without your assistance. Like the snowball, your loved one's recovery of a sense of self is hardest at first. Once moving with sustained force, however, its momentum is often enough to provide recovery with a direction and course of its own.

FEELINGS ABOUT SELF

1–I'm better, but far from where I was!

2–I can't see myself staying like **this**. I'm a mere shadow of the person I once was!

WHAT YOU MIGHT DO

1–2 IMPROVING SELF

Improving your loved one's image of self is linked to establishing and building on rehab's roots. This process is detailed in this chapter in Caregiver—Recovery. Fundamentally, though, it rests with molding daily life around what is possible until time permits acceptance of what is not.

1–2 WHAT TO DO

- Start small, on solid footing, and build a reinforced base from which to expand.

- Target simple, basic functions and ways of assuring that they are more of your loved one's choice, and valued in everyday life.
- Seek assistance from rehab staff in how to do this (review Table 5–2 in Chapter 5 and See Caregiver—Recovery, Chapter 6):

  in telling you what they think is or isn't currently possible.

  in helping you learn ways to foster optimal use.

  in demonstrating full use of functions at this time.
- Work to keep the process fun, positive, and successful.
- Don't try to do too much too quickly.
- Don't expect a lot at first.

PERSON WITH APHASIA

1–2 WHAT TO SAY

- "I know I can't truly feel all of what you must."
- "I do know it must feel scary and discouraging at times."
- "But *I know* the person I've always cared for and loved is still here."
- "Yes, there are differences, but they mean little to me."
- "What matters is that you are here and still able to do a lot."
- "We'll work through the differences in our lives together."

WHAT TO KNOW

DAILY LIFE

1–How well will I manage alone?

2–Being at home should help!

3–Why are some of the smallest tasks still so hard to do?

1 Since "lots" of dysfunction is apt to remain at the time of discharge, your loved one cannot help but wonder how he or she will manage in daily life now without assistance. For some people with aphasia, these worries are outwardly expressed, while for others, they remain more hidden and concealed. In either case, they are likely present and prominent at the time of discharge.

1 Knowing precisely where to stand on this issue is often difficult for caregivers. **Too much support is apt to promote unwanted and unnecessary dependencies, but too little support is apt to create fear, uncertainty, and perceived inability. When in doubt, it is best to err toward giving too much in the beginning, that is, being too forgiving and protective.** Your loved one's sense of self is apt to be as "fragile" as it will be at any time throughout the entire journey. For this reason, slightly overextending yourself is important. This act does not mean, however, acquiescing to any or all demands or needs. It means support-

PERSON WITH APHASIA

ing existing functions as a "confidence builder" until your loved one can and will act more independently. **The key, here, is not doing the task in full, but supporting your loved one's effort to do so. Over time, it permits you to slowly withdraw your support and not jeopardize the continued recovery of his or her image of self or ability.**

2 As noted in the introduction, "being in one's own bed" at home usually is not enough to remove the stark reality of permanent injury. Although your loved one is apt to be more comfortable and relaxed in this setting, the consequences of injury are apt to become every bit as distinct again in a matter of days or weeks. In fact, in some ways, being at home may only accentuate your awareness of injury. After all, it was here that your loved one functioned normally for much of his or her adult years. Now, current skills interfere with the simplest of tasks! **Be ready, then, for a "mixed bag;" initial enthusiasm and relief on returning home, followed by alarm and disappointment over how matters are different.**

3 What is often the greatest frustration is that some of the simplest functions of daily life, tying one's shoes, putting on one's socks, or buttoning a button, remain so difficult. When this is the case, realize that these moments of despair are usually transitory. In the beginning, your loved one has a reduced reservoir of energy and resources from which to draw. Because of this, such moments of frustration are apt to loom larger in life than they warrant. With time, his or her tolerance for coping will improve: so too, will his or her skills in performing or circumventing these annoyances.

DAILY LIFE

1–How well will I manage alone?
2–Being at home should help!
3–Why are some of the smallest tasks still so hard to do?

WHAT YOU MIGHT DO

1 KEEPING THE REHAB MACHINERY UP AND RUNNING AT HOME

The key words here are "operational" and "pleasurable." Many adults with aphasia return home and their skills quickly regress from the levels achieved in treatment to something far less. There was a forward momentum in rehab, and to keep that momentum going, it is essential to keep that machinery up and running—and enjoyable.

1 WHAT TO DO

PERSON WITH APHASIA

• Again, look to Caregiver—Recovery in this chapter. This section details these principles:

to know your loved one's current levels of function from each rehab specialist before discharge.

to develop a plan for how you might "empower" your loved one to act more in his or her behalf.

to implement this plan from the beginning.

to be more forgiving at first.

to start slow, and build from what exists.

2 WHAT TO CONSIDER

• Diffuse any inflated or deflated assessments of what home might provide.
• Acknowledge, too, that, because of familiarity, being home is apt to make some adjustments easier.
• View each day separately, and try to do a little more in a manner that meets with your loved one's approval.
• Over time, constancy and persistence will pay off.

WHAT TO KNOW

EMOTIONS

*1–This is a real mess . . . and **I'm** the source of the problem!*
2–I feel clumsy and awkward a lot of the time!
3–I sure hope I can manage this alone.

1 About now, the many ramifications of having aphasia and its related disabilities are starting to appear. Yes, there has been visible dysfunction or disability from early on, but now these changes are beginning to show symptoms of their own in the form of reduced self-worth and self-esteem. These consequences of disability have been previewed earlier in Chapter 2 and in the Feelings About Self section. A more thorough explanation of factors appears in Chapter 12, Psychological and Emotional Aspects. They start surfacing about this time in recovery when the person with aphasia begins to entertain the likelihood of chronic dysfunction.

1 Initial brushes with *permanence of injury* are apt to be met with complete denial (feeling as if consequences of the injury will pass with just

PERSON WITH APHASIA more time), or some form of bargaining (feeling that, "If I can only get such and such back, then I'll be OK and able to function in life"). Although these ways of coping are understandable when having to face an unwanted and enduring reality, neither rejecting nor negotiating are long-term solutions. Within months, the person with aphasia is usually again having to confront the permanency of this injury. Quite likely, your loved one may be in the beginning stages of doing just this right now, and feeling terribly responsible for having created this mess.

1 As a result, be prepared for strong and varied emotions in this adjustment period: anger, despair, denial, frustration, persistence, determination, and fluctuating "highs" and "lows." Some mixture of these is apt to come with confronting permanent injury. **Once your loved one is able to "give in" to the possibility of the injury's permanence, you are apt to see periods of intermittent or sustained depression. These emotional consequences of the permanence of injury are as much a part of aphasia and its related disabilities as the more visible physical impairments to talking, walking, dressing, or eating.** As such, they deserve careful attention, but often they do not *mean* what these emotions might have prior to injury. Caregivers become confused when they begin to see and deal with them. **An effective strategy is trying to avoid riding your loved one's emotional roller coaster, but instead see these expressions as a necessary part of getting better.** We offer suggestions for working with them in the sections ahead.

2 Although some use of physical skills has returned, these skills may feel quite unrefined or awkward. Your loved one may be steadily withdrawing from participating in life, not because of the inability to perform, but because he or she feels so clumsy and inept with current skills. Tasks at the moment are apt to require much more effort and concentration than every before, but more worrisome to people with aphasia, they feel ungainly and *not under one's full control.* This constant need for maximal effort to achieve minimal results is enough to make many people with aphasia withdraw from trying at all. You are apt to see frustration and pain accompanying your loved one's efforts to try. If patience is not his or her "long-suit," then your helping to foster use may be a challenge. Backing away from participation, though, is usually not a good option, instead, we need to find and foster ways to help your loved one keep frustration low and skill use ongoing.

3 Inactivity that results from discouragement should not be confused with inability or incompetence. Adults with aphasia are quite

able to act . . . the difference rests in their levels of proficiency and efficiency. Certainly on a normative scale, it is understandable how your loved one may tend to degrade his or her efforts as "unworthy" or "unacceptable." However, most functions in daily life are retrievable, at least to a limited degree even when impairment is severe. Chapters 6 (Caregiver—Recovery), 7, and 8 detail numerous ways of crafting more out of existing levels of function while keeping expectations and frustrations to a minimum.

PERSON WITH APHASIA

YOU MIGHT DO

1–3 COPING WITH YOUR LOVED ONE'S EMOTIONS AND DIMINISHED SENSE OF SELF

EMOTIONS
1–This is a real mess . . . and *I'm the source of the problem!*
2–I feel clumsy and awkward a lot of the time!
3–I sure hope I can manage this alone.

One of the hardest tasks associated with aphasia's recovery is "truly" understanding and integrating the complexities of what this impairment and its related disabilities impose on your loved one's feelings about his or her person or self. Once caregivers and others are "truly" oriented to these complexities, recovery is usually much easier to manage.

1–3 REMEMBERING WHAT IS HAPPENING AT THE MOMENT

- Your loved one's difficulties with self-worth are not solely about inability, they are about "perceived" inability. Society tends to judge one's worth by one's skill in performing. However, there is far *more* to one's value as a person in life than his or her ability to perform any task. In fact, level of function may not reflect the ability, skill, or character of a person at all. For example, consider someone suddenly paralyzed below the waist who wishes to relearn how to ski. It is unlikely that in this paralyzed state, performance following injury will match or exceed prior capabilities. **Yet, it is *quite possible* that skiing down a slope on a modified ski-sled requires far *more* skill and courage than skiing ever did before. Thus, it is not "how well" one performs in life that matters; instead it is the willingness to challenge one's self within one's capabilities.**

PERSON WITH APHASIA

- It is a willingness to venture forth "in spite" of "perceived inability" that is needed.
- There is no short cut around it:

    It will take time, effort, and likely "some" anguish.

    but the entire process need not be anguishing . . . sections ahead speak to helping you with this.

RELATIONSHIP

*1–I'm no longer physically attractive . . . certainly **not** like this!*

2–Will my significant other even want to be close to me again . . . I sure hope so!

WHAT TO KNOW

1–2 Hopefully our suggestions in Chapter 5, Person with Aphasia—Relationship, have minimized the impact of these doubts now. The difference, though, is that your loved one likely imagined that much of his or her physical disfigurement from injury would have passed by now. But it has not! Now, the thought of going home with restricted use of a hand and arm, not being able to walk properly, and having changed facial movements and expressions looms large. Your loved one likely wonders, "Can you—and do you—still even find me physically attractive? If so, how can that be? I'm not sure I would!" And related to this are questions like: "Will he or she want to hold me?" "Kiss me?" "Or even be close again?"

1–2 When viewing what he or she has to "offer" as less, your loved one may not possess the courage to take the first step in affectionately extending to you. Rather, he or she may await your initiation as some measure or indication of your willingness or desire to be near him or her. Whether such overtures are even possible on your part at this time is a different matter, but your loved one's injury should not change the quality of your personal relationship. If you, as a couple, were prone to share physical affection with one another, this part of your relationship need not be sacrificed or changed now.

1–2 You may need to know what is possible, and how best to approach such moments now, given your loved one's physical limitations. These questions are addressed in a later section of this chapter (Caregiver—Relationship). Know, however, that staying personally and physically close is apt to require adjustments, just like with most realms of life. These modifications need *not* exclude or interfere with your previous choices about sharing your affection and love for one another.

WHAT YOU MIGHT DO

RELATIONSHIP
1–I'm no longer physically attractive . . . certainly **not** like this!
2–Will my significant other even want to be close to me again . . . I sure hope so!

1–2 KEEPING YOUR RELATIONSHIP STRONG AND SECURE

PERSON WITH APHASIA

Try to focus on your loved one's "inner self" at first and less on the outward manifestations of his or her injury. This does not mean ignoring physical differences; it means attempting to put them in the perspective they deserve. Often coming home poses striking contrasts in your loved one's physical appearance and behaviors. If you look at *just* these, it is apt to inhibit your actions and possibly skew your view of what is. For this reason, responding to your loved one's inner self (since that is typically unimpaired) may allow you to slowly incorporate and overlook his or her physical differences. In the entirety of sharing with one another, his or her physical limitations are typically less important than they seem at first.

1–2 WHAT TO DO

- Frequently move closer rather than away from your loved one. Just this act and posture is often enough at first to let your loved one know you are together rather than apart as a twosome.
- Sit close by, and physically reach out if possible.
- Strive to place minor significance on what is physically different or not working.

     Read Caregiver—Relationship in this chapter. You may need some time and assistance to do this. But it is a worthy goal and usually attainable.

- Stress how you are far more drawn to the person that's *still* there (inside) . . . and intact!
- Know that it usually takes some time to feel totally comfortable caressing and holding one another.

     Quite possibly, nothing is more familiar, or intimate than the touch and sharing you provided one another before injury. It is not strange that when the manner and form of this sharing "changes," so too, may your ease and level of comfort. Give it some time.

- Smile and reach out and invite him or her to come to you.
- If possible, *frequently tell* your loved one that you love him or her. If possible, tell him or her it is every bit as much *as you ever did.*

<table>
<tr><td>

COMMUNICATION

1–How can treatment be stopping now?

   (a) despair: How will I manage this alone?

   *(b) determination: I **cannot** stay like this . . . I must, and I **will** talk better!*

2–I'm no good to others if I can't talk.

</td></tr>
</table>

PERSON WITH APHASIA

WHAT TO KNOW

1 Of all rehab areas, communication often is the slowest to improve. For this reason, ending treatment now feels totally unreasonable. Quite likely, only the rudimentary parts of communicating have emerged, while skills in eating, toileting, dressing, sitting, and walking are much farther along. Your loved one's disordered speech and language have probably only begun to show signs of change. Even so, if you elected to follow our earlier suggestions at the beginning of rehab (Caregiver—Communication, Chapter 5), you should have some working basis for communicating with each other. **Although your loved one's minor speech-language gains and a communicative system of your own may feel totally inadequate, it is not substandard for people leaving rehab. It is more the rule than the exception!**

1 Recall that reimbursable rehab services in today's health care system require immediate, substantial, and functional improvement (see Chapter 3). The degree of return, much less full return, was never the criteria for rehab services. That treatment has ended, then, is not a statement of prognosis, because the possibility of a full return was never even addressed. Health care providers are simply looking for ways of reducing expenditures. Decisions about treatment are not dependent on whether further gains are possible, but on how quickly they can be enacted (cost effectiveness), and how influential will they be on later life, in terms of its quality and effect on overall health. Discharge is not based on whether your one loved might become a better communicator if treated. Don't be confused, then; the stopping of treatment does not signal an end to communicative gains.

1 Treatment's ending can trigger different reactions. For some sufferers, there is despair and diminished hope; for others, there is a staunch determination to push harder to find other ways to improve. Because the loss of communication, and especially talking, is so new and often life-altering, most people leave rehab wanting desperately to do more. The question then becomes: "What more can be done to promote my loved one's talking or communication? In Caregiver—Recovery in this chapter a section entitled: Keeping Rehab's Momentum Ongoing At Home offers suggestions and a plan for pursuing additional rehab services.

1 Briefly, extended treatment for communication likely depends on three factors: money, location, and need. Regarding money, know that any continued treatment is apt to be partially or completely out-of-pocket. It depends on how your health care insurer defines speech-language services and what medical or clinical criteria are necessary for reimbursement. Quite likely, though, this resource is nearly, if not completely, depleted. The private services of a certified speech-language pathologist will cost you between $50 and $100 per hour. Regarding location, know that where you live is apt to influence what services are possible. Generally speaking, the more rural your location, the fewer options there are available. Should you reside in or near a city, the likelihood of other "low-cost" alternatives, such as aphasia support or conversational groups, and university training programs increases (see Appendix C). Before seeking services, you may wish to know first whether further treatment would be advantageous. What further functional gains in communication might follow? Besides consulting with your loved one's speech-language pathologist, you may wish to ask the advice of other professionals who specialize in aphasia rehabilitation. The National Aphasia Association (NAA) provides a list of regional and area representatives whom you might contact. This information is available by phone (800–922–4622), or by consulting the NAA's website on the Internet at: http://www.aphasia.org/index.html.

PERSON WITH APHASIA

2 With rehab's ending, your loved one may worry about his or her communication skills with others in the outside world. He or she is likely fearing current communicative limitations, especially if his or her speech is severely restricted or absent. Since talking was so imperative and common to life and communication before, thinking of communicating without it now is apt to feel "impossible." To the degree the two of you have pursued *alternative means of communication* with each other (as suggested in Caregiver—Communication, Chapter 5), nontalking ways of interacting may or may not be familiar. Even if they are, your loved one may view these methods as possible with you, but as less socially acceptable or less likely to work with others. Both of these impressions are accurate to a degree, but as will be emphasized in Chapters 7 and 8, communication with others in the outside world likely will require special attention to become an effective and regular occurrence. Either your loved will need to become less sensitive to current speech limitations and supplement his or her communication with other forms of expression, or he or she will need to find environments where other people are familiar and adaptable to his or her communication needs. Most likely, a combination of these forms of modification will evolve with time.

COMMUNICATION

1–How can treatment be stopping now?

   (a) despair: How will I manage this alone?

   (b) determination: I **cannot** stay like this . . . I must, and I **will** talk better!

2–I'm no good to others if I can't talk.

PERSON WITH APHASIA

WHAT YOU MIGHT DO

1 KEEPING COMMUNICATION VIABLE

You need to treat seriously your loved one's worry and focus on wanting to talk better. Your basic options here are: more therapy, a different form of therapy, or "your" therapy. Sorting through these decisions is not always easy. Don't rush them. Be sure your route fits your needs. Often "less" is not necessarily worse; it depends on your needs and means. Communication "repair" is typically a *slow process*. Seldom after an intense period of several months of speech-language therapy are you apt to find "night and day" changes from more therapy. In special cases, it may make a significant difference, but even then progress is apt to come gradually rather than all at once. Basically your choice here depends on personal choice and motivation, potential return, cost, and the availability of you or others to assist.

1 WHAT ABOUT FURTHER THERAPY?

- Ask your loved one's speech-language pathologist whether additional intensive, one-on-one, therapy might produce further functional gains in communication.
- If so, ask where such gains would likely occur and how they might impact daily life.
- If the areas of communication that could improve do not include the areas you are most concerned about, ask specifically about these.
- If substantial or meaningful change might follow, ask who, how, and where such treatment might be offered.
- As suggested above, you may wish to obtain one or more options about such matters.

  The NAA and other stroke or aphasia agencies in your region of the country are good referral sources.

  Contacts in other countries are listed in Appendix C.
- Next, check suggested agencies for continuing services.

  You are going to want to know their charges, whether your insurance may cover any of these costs, and specifically what their services include. You need to find "a match" here, that is, treatment that addresses your needs within your means. As alluded to above, more options are apt to exist in urban than in rural areas.

PERSON WITH APHASIA

- Go visit any treatment option or facility a couple of times with your loved one before making a decision.

  Speaking to others in your community who have experienced treatment from these referral sources may be helpful too.

- **If your loved one's motivation to do more is intense and if further outside treatment is not an option, either due to potential return, resources, or cost, then ask the rehab speech-language pathologist about fashioning a home program tailored to your loved one's needs.**

  For instance, your loved one may want to work specifically on talking. It may be that the collective opinion of the specialists consulted is that further usable speech is apt to return only slowly or not at all. What is important to you, however, is that "something" be done to address this unmet need. Quite likely, a specialized set of speech exercises at current skill levels can be prepared for home practice. Some time may be needed on your or someone else's part for this practice. On the other hand, it is important to keep exercises as self-sustaining as possible, that is, within a realm your loved one can practice at his or her discretion. His or her speech-language pathologist should be able to help with suggestions here.

- Sometimes more therapy is not the answer. Rather you and your loved one may simply need more time to adjust and adapt to "what is."

  What is crucial is that the two of you currently have a way to remain as connected and "interactive" as possible. We've been stressing this point from rehab's beginning. Now it is absolutely *crucial* as you attempt to confront daily matters alone.

2 ADDRESSING YOUR LOVED ONE'S WORTH IF TALKING ISN'T POSSIBLE

By now, you know that your loved one's inner worth is unrelated to his or her ability to talk. It is likely, though, he or she may not see or feel this way, especially this early on. We've given you suggestions for furthering talking, if this should be his or her strong desire. Additionally, you may need to keep pointing out how alternative communicative methods are

PERSON WITH APHASIA

helping, too. Making your communication the best it can be is apt to rely on a combination of speaking and nonspeaking methods. In Caregiver— Communication, we reemphasize the importance of having some sense of just what this combination may entail before rehab ends. Also, this section provides simple options for helping your loved one communicate with others when talking is limited or not possible. These will apply to both familiar and unfamiliar interactants.

2 WHAT TO SAY

- "I know you are discouraged about communicating because of the difficulty talking."
- "We are going to continue to work on making your talking better, I promise!"
- **"But you need to understand, too, that talking and communicating *are not the same thing*."**
- **"*We can communicate* even though your talking doesn't work."**
- "Yes, it takes longer; it's harder; it's not as complete—but is it possible? . . . *it is*!"
- "Until talking does get better, we need to remember this and keep using these other methods, too."
- "Getting better means staying together, and staying together means communicating even if all the parts don't get said."
- "Who you are is not tied *solely* to what you say, even though it may feel that way to you now!"
- "I know you well, and you'll never be any less to me simply because you can't tell me something."
- "We'll work this out together, I promise!"

WHAT TO KNOW

1–2 Your loved one will soon have to confront interacting with friends. In some respects, both of you had hoped to avoid this by having the more visible aspects of injury "fixed" before rehab ended. Since this has not occurred, these interactions may pose some concern over how others may react. For this reason, many people with aphasia attempt to conceal their changed identities from others for as long as they possible can. Most people with aphasia are extremely aware of, and sensitive to, what the outside world might think. Since they do not find their current status "worthy," it is not surprising that they would assume others will not either.

PERSON WITH APHASIA

1–2 Therapeutically it might have been in your loved one's best interest to not have many visitors in the beginning months of injury. Now, though, this scale begins to tip in the opposite direction. Staying completely isolated from others in the outside world is likely not a good or healthy long-term solution. Instead, it is important to *start* exposing your loved one to others soon after leaving formal care. This exposure need not be long or frequent in the beginning, but allowing him or her to remain isolated only tends to magnify those feelings that he or she is unworthy of other attention. Often brief visits from a friend or family member are beneficial. Be aware that moving out again into everyday society is one of the hardest tasks people with aphasia face. Successful experience often begins here through interactions with close friends. As you'll see in Chapters 7 and 8, it involves many other steps before your loved one is apt to feel some comfort and ease being outside the home alone.

3 You need to know that a certain number of friends will simply "disappear" out of your lives in the months ahead. Unfortunately, this percentage is apt to be higher than you expected. However, there often is a core of people who remain present and interactive, although many of the relationships with these people are apt to be different. If you cherish these people and your relationships with them, you likely need to understand their perspective in coping with your loved one's injury. A later section in this chapter, Caregiver—Family or Friends, describes common issues confronting close friends and family members as they come together with you and your loved one.

PERSON WITH APHASIA

WHAT YOU MIGHT DO

1–3 KEEPING OLD FRIENDSHIPS FUNCTIONING

At first, putting friends at ease by showing them "how to" interact may help a lot. However, this aid alone is likely not enough. You will need to redefine your togetherness with friends much as you did with each other. Some friends may be more vested in this process than others. Those individuals who are vested are apt to remain good friends for life. Unfortunately, this number is often limited. It does not mean, though, that you are destined to be without friends. It means that, with time, you and your loved one are apt to select and foster new friendships, people who *only* know you as you are. You may certainly influence the likelihood that old friendships remain, but you cannot ensure their long-term quality or resilience.

1–3 WHAT TO DO

- Look for compatible visitors or interactants for your loved one:
  You want to encourage your loved one's contact with people who are less apt to retract from or focus on your loved one's current communicative or physical restrictions. Those people are ones who had previously valued him or her as a "person" rather than solely as a participant in some mutually shared interest or activity, like playing golf or cards together. A long-term friend may be someone who has enough of a history with your loved one to be light, personable, and warm. In the beginning, you may want to keep all visits brief. It helps both parties gradually learn and adjust to each other's changed status, style, and skills. Trying to cope with the whole gambit of dysfunction at first may simply be too overwhelming. **Visitors need to be led along at first and not given too much too quickly. You likely need to provide a simple model for sharing and interacting. Try to reinforce the visitor's communicative attempts by rephrasing and aiding their interactiveness with your loved one.**

- Orient the visitor to your loved one.
  In Chapter 5, Person with Aphasia—Family or Friends, you will find a list of ways for making an initial visit and interaction from

a friend more natural and comfortable. The most crucial component is finding a way that permits a natural, relaxed, casual, exchange within existing communication skills rather than embarrassed silence or confused "over-communicating." In the sectio, Caregiver—Family/Friends, at the end of this chapter, you will find ways of explaining this objective to a potential visitor.

PERSON WITH APHASIA

- Orient your loved one to visitors, too:

  It is important to let him or her know:

  > that communicating is *not* going to be perfect . . . but that *does not matter.*

  > **the purpose now is not to do** *a lot of communicating,* **but** *just some sharing* **with one another.**

  > that it took the two of you time to learn how to communicate.

  > it is apt to take "others" a little time, too.

  > You will work at it together.

WHAT TO KNOW

> **EMPLOYMENT**
>
> 1–It's time to decide about working.
> What can I do . . . ?
> What do I want to do . . . ?
> What should I do . . . ?

1 Rendering a final decision about employment is likely easier now. The restorative efforts of rehab have either moved your loved one closer to an employable status or provided the opportunity to access this possibility and then to eliminate it from consideration. As noted earlier, it is the latter outcome that usually occurs; most individuals with aphasia either agree to or are forced to "retire" from their former jobs. The exception may be adults who are relatively young (in their 30s or 40s), possess mild impairments, and are highly motivated to work again. Even for this group, the free-enterprise system often works against rather than for their retention. Any enduring solution that allows for employment usually takes years to resolve.

1 There are many barriers facing people with aphasia who want to stay employed. Most involve finding a conducive setting, and an employer who values the person's residual skills and the person enough to modify the job to match his or her skills. As a result, it is far easier for an employer to look to a non-head-injured employee with lesser knowledge or experience than to change existing operations to include a person who cannot communicate or use language normally. Thus, people with aphasia may be dismissed from prior employment, not because they *lack the*

PERSON WITH APHASIA

knowledge to do the job, but because they lack fundamental skills. Because spoken and written communiqués are so intrinsic to most jobs, people who cannot produce them are denied reentry.

1 Not all employers or work settings reject people with aphasia. It is possible that if the person with aphasia is willing to "accept" a lesser position, duties, and salary, and if his or her injury is mild, some form of paid employment might follow. Should your loved one fall into this category, it may be especially important not to close the employer's door immediately following rehab. Even if returning to that setting is not possible perhaps "other" settings within the organization might be workable over time. However, you will likely need the support of the rehab staff to help you, your loved one, and the potential employer match current skills with possible job related tasks. This assistance is not confined to simply where to begin, but he or she, you, and the employer are apt to require ongoing consultations to make employment an enduring reality.

1 If returning to work is not possible or of your loved one's choice, you may wish to determine if your loved one qualifies for disability compensation. Usually such monies originate with the employer or government social programs, such as Social Security Disability. Often compensation depends on a physician's written declaration that your loved one's injury will preclude any further employment in the years ahead. Before compensation begins, there is usually a short interim (6–9 months) to verify the chronic nature of his or her injury. The other stipulation about such programs is that any subsequent employment can only provide a small fraction of one's previous earnings. As a result, most people with aphasia who do return to work often work in a limited capacity to protect their disability benefits and livelihoods.

EMPLOYMENT

1–It's time to decide about working.
What can I do?
What do I want to do?
What must I do?

WHAT YOU MIGHT DO

1 ADDRESSING WORK-RELATED ISSUES

Keep available as many options as possible. Rather than having the decision imposed, strive to let the person with aphasia make his or her own decision about whether or not he or she would like to pursue returning to work.

1 WHAT TO DO

- If your loved one is unable or does not want to return to work, it is time to inform his or her former employer of this decision.
- If he or she does wish to return to work, then you need to obtain the rehab team's opinion on these questions:

    Is *any* form of employment still possible?

    If so, *what type* of endeavor might be possible and *where* might such an endeavor begin?

- **If the rehab team's recommendation is against his or her returning to work, yet he or she strongly opposes this option, it is prudent not to deny your loved one the *opportunity to try*.**

    You certainly do not want to promote "false hope," but even more important, you do not want to extinguish or discourage your loved one's desire to act in his or her own behalf. Chapter 7, Person with Aphasia—Recovery details the dynamics of how you might slowly and reasonably progress toward locating a work environment where current skills match the desired outcome. To the degree possible, allow and support your loved one's right to make his or her *own* personal choices in life!

WHAT TO KNOW

HEALTH
1–Why am I so tired all the time?

1 Injury to any part of the brain often disrupts total efficiency. What typically would have taken little or no effort before now requires considerable effort. In fact, if your loved one does not make a concerted effort at this moment, even small tasks may go undone. For this reason, his or her mental and physical reservoirs may never fill to capacity. Furthermore, once called upon, they are apt to deplete much more quickly. Tasks that would have taken minutes before now take two or three times as long. Once completed, there is little residual strength from which to draw.

1 Diminished mental and physical reserves are common for people with aphasia whose injury occurred just months before. However, after a year's duration, your loved one should be in a better position to gauge his or her own energy level on a daily basis. Careful attendance to exercise, diet, and medications is apt to restore these functions to near capacity in the months and years ahead. However, many sufferers still notice that their physical or mental reservoirs may diminish more quickly than before.

HEALTH

1–Why am I so tired all the time?

WHAT YOU MIGHT DO

1 BUILDING ENDURANCE OVER TIME

PERSON WITH APHASIA

It is important to separate chronic fatigue from being unhealthy. In the early going of aphasia, fatigue is a reality, but it does not signal other health concerns. Counteracting its effects, though, requires more than simply recognizing it exists. It requires pressing one's system daily and weekly in order to stay active and to try to do more and more over time. If extended slowly and consistently, it is likely that your loved one's levels of energy will continue to increase in the months and years ahead.

1 WHAT TO DO

- Chapter 13 describes the importance of diet, exercise, and medications in minimizing further injury.
- Ask the physical therapist for suggestions about an exercise program to follow before leaving formal care.
- Contact the National Stroke and American Heart Associations, which distribute exercise videos for people who have incurred stroke or heart injuries (see Appendix C).

RECOVERY

*1–Golly, we were just starting . . .
how can treatment be ending?*
*2–How do we deal with all that
remains?*
3–Where do we go from here?

WHAT TO KNOW

1 Caregivers are apt to panic when rehab ends, no matter how much was done in preparation for it. It came too quickly and life is still too chaotic to imagine trying to function without it. All you know for sure is that your loved one can't function as independently as he or she once did, and that your future remains cloaked in uncertainty. You likely are being forced to confront a number of dilemmas and their built-in complexities: not enough improvement so far, yet a favorable impression that more may come; not sufficient function to expect normal performance, yet feeling unable to concede that it might not evolve with more time; not enough experience in working with or minimizing current dysfunction, yet feel-

ing that continued improvement is now *your responsibility*. All of this is   **CAREGIVER**
apt to leave you feeling overwhelmed, and wondering how we live in a
society where so little help exists.

1 You are fully justified in these feelings. However, the problems before
you are not going to disappear, or halt the process of your loved one's
discharge from rehab. If you haven't already followed the suggestions in
Chapter 5: Caregiver—Recovery, go back and review them right now.
Even if some of them were too much to cope with during rehab, and they
weren't considered until now, their value is no less at this time. In fact,
needing this knowledge and skill now may make this action easier to
confront.

1 Remember rehab was *never* intended *to fix* your loved one's aphasia
or its associated disabilities. That grand goal was only partially possible
at best, and even the possible part was too broad and time-consuming to
accomplish in these brief weeks or months. **The objective of rehab was
to establish *a working foundation* from which to expand and build.
You need to garner as much information as possible about this foundation before it ends.**

1 Try not to get lost in the many details of going from a highly controlled and regulated setting governed by others (rehab), to a more loose-
ly structured environment of your own making (home). As you did with
the chaos you faced and successfully endured when aphasia was new and
unknown, so too you will sort through these transitional details. Right
now, the task is to *identify* the important parts that need attending to and
start arranging them into a workable plan.

2–3 Actually, a starting point already exists! As formal care comes to an
end, a plan is prepared to assure that your loved one's current medical
and rehab needs match the extent of outside care. The formal name for
this process is a ***rehabilitation discharge plan***. For your loved one to be
released to an outside setting, there must be adequate environmental and
professional support to permit a safe and sustainable form of daily life.
If your loved one's medical or physical condition remains severely in
question, it is likely that a more restrictive living environment, like a
skilled nursing home, may be recommended (see Figures 3–1 and 3–2 in
Chapter 3). If such an option does not correspond with your own desires,
it may be possible to provide such health care services at home. The lim-

CAREGIVER   itation on this option, though, is money. Such expenditures are not typically covered by most health care providers past a period of 2 to 3 months following discharge. If your loved one's condition requires long-term care, a skilled nursing home may be the only option. There are signs, though, of an increasing trend in today's health practices to provide health care services in the home at a cost lower than in traditional institutionalized settings.

2–3 Chapter 3, and most likely Figure 3–2, Road Under Construction, spelled out discharge options that you are likely facing at the moment. It is just the options at the bottom of Figure 3–2, those dealing with discharge from the rehab center, that apply now. Typically, rehab staff members begin pointing out options weeks in advance of discharge. Thus, it is likely you know now how and where this team thinks your loved one's needs might be served best after rehab, and these options are displayed in Figure 3–2. You want to listen carefully to these recommendations, even though they may not coincide with your own wishes. You want to be cautious about abruptly rejecting or overruling the team's input. **These professionals** *have you and your loved one's needs and best interests in mind.* **As well, they have years of knowledge and experience in making such decisions, and somewhat of a "sixth sense" about what may or may not work outside a rehab setting on a sustained basis. Listen to their plan and their reasons for the route or routes they have in mind.** If you still "object," and have the physical and financial means to secure the requisites they feel must be met, it is likely that your preferred course will be approved. However, you need to know well the pros and cons of each option.

2–3 Leaving formal care magnifies two concerns: (1) how to make daily life work and (2) how to keep rehab's momentum ongoing. The extent to which these questions may be addressed by rehab specialists varies considerably. However, it is crucial to your well-being that they be sorted out as completely as possible before you walk out the door. Table 5–2 (Chapter 5), facilitative and preparatory skills, spoke to the issue of preparing for discharge. **Hopefully, you began the process of learning to interact effectively as a couple months ago. But if you haven't, do so** *now!* **Even if there is not sufficient time to practice or refine these skills, make every effort to acquire them. They will prove invaluable as you travel over the road ahead.**

2-3 *Making daily life work again* is not so difficult conceptually, but is often much more difficult to enact! A cornerstone to getting life working again is keeping its main parts as *interactive* and *mutually shared* as possible. What this means is forging a workable means of *staying together* in spite of many impaired functions. At the top of the list of impairments are one's concerns over disordered communication. Although these problems *are* hindrances in the exchanging of information, you will, if you haven't already, come to modify and bridge them with more time. **What is far more important in the early stages of living with aphasia is acknowledging and interacting with the person behind those communicative problems. Staying connected means de-emphasizing the need or importance of exchanging information perfectly. You want to let the "telling" of messages be secondary to the "sharing" of messages. The core person you knew before this injury is still there. If you concentrate on staying in touch with the *person*, and not just the adequacy of his or her message, your journey ahead will be considerably easier.**

CAREGIVER

2–3 At first, you need to find ways of making your shared parts of daily life work better. Finding these routes takes time, not days or weeks . . . but months and years. Initially, you need to simply get "the knack" of what they are and how to deal with them. And with lots of practice, you will gradually become skilled and proficient in their use. Keep remembering, though, that time is not your enemy, it is always working in your behalf. Nothing must get done at once; usually it cannot! It takes time, probing, trying, revamping, and trying again, to find a solution that works for the two of you. Carefully making your way along in a thoughtful manner is far better than trying to race ahead.

2–3 Next, you need to give yourself permission and the leniency to work from *where you are*, not fretting over where you *aren't* or where you *wish you might be*. If you can stay focused on the realities of the moment and judge progress from there, not according to what once was, you are ideally situated for moving ahead. The bends in this road do not always take you forward. There are apt to be numerous ups and downs, switchbacks, and even periods where you need to back up. But through some constancy and interaction with each other, life's inherent reinforcements will help guide the two of you down the preferred route.

CAREGIVER **2–3** *Keeping rehab's momentum ongoing:* The key here is to understand that your loved one's disabilities run far deeper than their superfi-
cial manifestations might suggest. Very likely, he or she is feeling *disempowered,* that is, simply *unable* to act in his or her own behalf, given
the enormity of perceived dysfunction around him or her. As a part of
this, your loved one is apt to feel unworthy as a person. Both of these
internal (mis)perceptions of self stand in direct opposition to maintaining or expanding rehab's momentum.

2–3 The first step toward counteracting feelings of disempowerment or
devaluation is to establish a core of real-life activities that are possible at
existing skill levels (see Person with Aphasia—Recovery earlier in this
chapter). At first, it may seem to you, and your loved one, that such tasks,
like sorting or folding laundry, setting the table, or vacuuming and dust-
ing the living room are simply "fillers," menial tasks to give him or her
something to do. Such a view is accentuated by the fact that these tasks
often were done quickly and secondarily to the more important functions
in life, like working or recreating. At this moment in recovery, though,
these tasks are neither menial, nor secondary: They often represent the
very framework your loved one most needs in life! **Coming to feel
"enabled" starts with his or her participating in life at whatever
level of function is possible. Even when one's participation may be a
painful reminder of what is *not* possible, if properly elicited, nur-
tured, and acknowledged, doing *something* does more to ensure
rehab's momentum than any other single act. Nothing aids subsequent growth more than establishing success with what is possible
and safe. It is from this foundation that an expanded participation
in life takes root and slowly emerges.**

2–3 Besides providing real-life situations where your loved one might
participate, it is crucial to keep his or her destiny more in his or her
hands rather than yours. Every time your loved one acts in his or her
own behalf to assume more responsibility for self, the more it empow-
ers him or her to do more. The act itself, like performing simple everyday household chores, may seem insignificant and even cruel to suggest. But objections, from your loved one or yourself are bound to what
such actions may have meant prior to injury. Now, though, it is important to reorient, and redefine, and reaccept what these actions mean
now! It is not in your loved one's interest or yours to simply "while
away" the day because there is nothing within his or her abilities.

Having "nothing to do" is a scenario that is no more vaild than the ear- **CAREGIVER**
lier one that found household tasks degrading. The scenes come simply from the perspective taken. The more your loved one is willing to
act today, in whatever form he or she chooses, the more of a basis he
or she has established for doing something tomorrow, whether returning to this task or trying a different one. Thus, the more you can
encourage and support your loved one to participate in life, regardless
of its form, the better off he or she is apt to be in the weeks and months
ahead.

2–3 Remember, too, you cannot force something on your loved one that
is not of his or her choice. Meaningful participation in life *requires* that
whatever action occurs be taken on willingly. Thus, people with aphasia
cannot be conscripted to act if they refuse your offers to assist them.
Such early refusals to act can represent some of the most trying moments
in the journey. Once outside rehab, and after becoming more aware of
his or her seemingly limited capabilities, your loved one may simply
decline to make any effort on his or her behalf. If this should be the case,
you most certainly need to urge, in a caring and complimentary manner,
that he or she reconsider and try participating with your assistance at
first. But if it is clear that such encouragement detracts rather than adds
to the desired outcome, then you need to respect and accept your loved
one's decision. Empowering someone fundamentally means letting the
person decide for him- or herself.

2–3 Although you are obligated to "honor" your loved one's wishes, it
may be important to understand why he or she might elect not to act. For
a disempowered person, it is often the fear of failure and rejection that
prompts such a decision. Rather than try, and appear to be even more
unworthy than people thought, it is far safer and simpler to refuse to participate at all. That your loved one might judge his or her actions as looking foolish is apt to be quite different from how you might judge those
same actions. **Nevertheless, any action that is deemed socially ques-
tionable or of minimal worth on a normative scale is likely to be seen
by the person with aphasia as unworthy or foolish. It will take time
and some concerted effort to convince your loved one that you view
such efforts differently. The legitimacy of your loved one's efforts,
though, cannot be mandated. With sincerity and great care, you
must slowly and consistently demonstrate in everyday life that such
efforts of his or hers *matter* to you.**

CAREGIVER   **2–3** If your loved one elects not to act in his or her own behalf, how can you demonstrate that such actions do matter? **One option, alluded to earlier, is to take any intended task to your loved one and *to do it together*. In fact, do not ask for or emphasize his or her participation Instead, ask him or her to help you!** If your loved one is reticent to try, you do not want to provide an open window through which he or she might escape. Instead, bring the task to him or her and have a set function in mind that is within his or her existing skills. At first, keep your attention focused on doing the task together and not on his or her separate role. Keep bringing the task to him or her until your loved one chooses to come to you to assist. By this time, you can begin to emphasize how important his or her role is. Once you can get your loved one's foot in a door of his or her own choosing, it typically is easier.

2–3 Realize, too, that working together isn't just about getting a job done, it's about *doing things together*. The more you promote this type of interaction in the months ahead, the more recovery you are apt to experience. You likely have complemented one another's efforts through much of life and you need to foster this partnership again. Yes, some of the roles and tasks have likely changed but that fact has not lessened the importance of who does what now. Everything must get done. And as long as you attribute legitimacy to all the actions and reinforce your loved one's equality in the partnership, so too, over time, will your loved one.

2–3 If bringing the task to your loved one and suggesting doing it together is not enough to enlist his or her participation, then do not insist. But, as emphasized earlier, his or her refusal to act in life should not fall on your side of the ledger. A partnership requires both parties to act within their means, and with caring for each other. Letting his or her clothes sit unsorted and unwashed in the basement until a time when he or she needs some clean underwear may prompt a different action. Such an action, though, needs to be clearly dissociated from any form of "punishment." If he or she wishes to go without clean clothes, you will honor that wish. If he or she does want clean clothes, you are willing to work with him or her to achieve that outcome. His or her sorting and doing laundry would help tremendously. If that task is simply unacceptable to your loved one, then you are more than willing to find something else that would be more acceptable and within his or her capabilities. You can do that together!

2–3 When an unwillingness to participate in life involves basic functions, like eating, standing, walking, personal hygiene, or exercising, it may be advisable at first to extend your assistance beyond what is likely necessary. Once again, the purpose in doing so is just to establish a baseline from which the two of you can begin slowly shifting the burden of function onto your loved one. If he or she still refuses to assume greater responsibility, seek guidance from a rehab or health care professional at follow-up reevaluations on how to further your loved one's participation. It may even be possible for a professional to make a home visit and to demonstrate such methods there. Regardless of what happens over the long haul, letting your loved one's refusal to act become your burden only breeds feelings of entrapment, discontent, and ultimately anger.

2–3 Finally, do not let personal stagnation and despair reign over you or your loved one's well-being for any extended period in the early going. If you loved one remains immobilized for weeks at a time, seek professional assistance (see suggestions ahead). The first 6 to 12 months following rehab are terribly influential in establishing what will or will not occur in the years ahead. It is a time to make sure that *hope and promise for the future* are both fostered and set into motion. Forward momentum only adds to the equation. You need to come to the first year's juncture with the snowball moving on its own, not resting at the top of the mountain's slope.

CAREGIVER

WHAT YOU MIGHT DO

1 KEEPING RECOVERY ONGOING

You began rehab by posting a list of reminders for daily viewing. Now it is time to replace that list with a different one:

RECOVERY . . .

We're at the **BEGINNING OF GETTING BETTER** . . . NOT the end!

RECOVERY
1–Golly, we were just starting. how can treatment be ending?
2–How do we deal with all that remains?
3–Where does we go from here?

CAREGIVER

this is **NOT A RACE**!

SLOWLY ADD to what works.

SUPPORT . . . do not demand!

PROMOTE HIS OR HER PERSISTENCE AT GETTING BETTER!

THE MORE DONE, THE MORE THAT RETURNS.

GETTING BETTER NEVER ENDS . . . unless people stop trying!

STOPPING IS OK . . . as long as it is out of informed choice!

when living with aphasia feels more **COMFORTABLE** than changing something about it . . .

YOUR JOURNEY IS OVER!

The time to get there may be a matter of months, years, or an entire lifetime!

The **TRIP'S LENGTH IS UNIMPORTANT**.

It is **WHAT YOU LEARN ALONG THE WAY**!

2–3 ESTABLISHING A WORKING FOUNDATION OUTSIDE FORMAL CARE

- Suggestions for establishing a working foundation in the real world were offered in Tables 5–1 and 5–2.

  Table 5–1 emphasized the gathering of information that you need to proceed.

  Table 5–2 emphasized the skills that will help you the most.
- You need to ensure that this information and skill acquisition occurs before leaving rehab.
- Also, you will need full updates from each rehab specialist before discharge regarding:

      what is and is not functional at this time.

      what else might make these areas of current dysfunction work better.

      how this might be accomplished.

- If these suggestions are not familiar to you or you have never tried using them:

      ask each rehab specialist to observe any suggested ways that may aid you in:

         staying connected as a couple.

         helping or circumventing functional impairments at the moment.

      if possible, ask if you might try out these methods yourself while the therapist observes.

      get as much "hands on" direction and experience as possible before discharge.

2–3 MAKING DAILY LIFE WORK AGAIN AT HOME

- There are multiple parts to this such as:

      knowing that what lies ahead is something that requires a lot of "trial and error."

      knowing that you can, and need to, get some consistent help along the way (see next paragraph).

      starting to develop small expectations from what is possible and gradually adding to them.

      providing support, help . . . a push of the swing, but not pumping for your loved one.

         See Chapter 5: Caregiver—Recovery.

      encouraging activities and pursuits of your loved one's choice.

      finding opportunities for expanding current levels of function:

         See Person with Aphasia—Recovery in this chapter and Table 5–2.

      maintaining a weekly log of where matters stand, and what has and hasn't worked.

         These entries need not be long or complicated, a small paragraph is plenty. Note your general impressions over time. Sometimes these may involve change; many times they do not. Simply record whatever stood out in your mind over the past week. **Get in the habit of making these entries now. You will need these logs later as a reference to judge change. They are invaluable. Don't skimp here, do them and keep them up!**

CAREGIVER 2–3 ARRANGING FOR PERIODIC REASSESSMENTS ALONG THE WAY

- **Try *not* to leave formal care without an established plan to revisit rehab personnel down the road.**

  It is crucial to keep ties with these or other rehab personnel in the months ahead. The purpose of these return visits is not to simply to assess whether further change has occurred or to ask for more therapy, but to determine where you stand in getting your daily lives operational, comfortable, and harmonious.

- If the professionals who saw you throughout rehab cannot provide such services now, ask who might.

  There are many home-based care agencies coming into existence in America. That trend is apt to continue in the years ahead.

- **Try to arrange for the first follow-up meeting in the first 2 to 3 weeks after discharge.**

  The most challenging period of adjustment at home is *in the beginning*. You likely will need the most assistance then. If at all possible, plan for monthly follow-ups over the first 3 months and then depending on your needs and the rehab staff's impressions, modify your schedule to every other month or once every 3 months up to a year postonset.

- Often costs of such follow-up assessments are reimbursable, but they may not be.

  You'll want to check into these matters ahead of time.

- Even if matters are progressing well at home, *meet anyway*—at least at first.

- Minimally, you'll want to have convened at least three times before the first year's anniversary of injury to:

  Provide copies of your journal or log notes in advance of these meetings.

  Make clear to the rehab professional you visit that your objective is to confirm whether you are on the right path and to add to what currently is functional.

  Ask for a reassessment of what is or is not working.

  Ask for help in refining your efforts to push life's "swing" at just the right time and place.

Rather than meeting each rehab staff member separately, it
may be preferable to meet them together and ask them to share
ideas.

It's likely that the PT and OT can address specific functions
and activities around the house or in daily life that might be
fostered or enlarged on. The speech-language pathologist
may offer suggestions within that context about how to
approach such matters communicatively. Together they may
fuse a package of notions for keeping your loved one's participation in daily life more active and personally rewarding.

2–3 KEEPING REHAB'S MOMENTUM ONGOING AT HOME

Because not enough return has occurred, keeping rehab's themes ongoing is often a prime concern for both your loved one and yourself. The
most likely possibilities are either to take as much of rehab's exercises
home with you or to consider more therapy as an outpatient. The latter
option was detailed earlier for communication (See Person with Aphasia—Communication). Many of the concerns overviewed earlier for
continuing communication therapy are apt to apply equally to physical
and occupational therapies.

2–3 WHAT TO DO

- Ask each rehab specialist:
    Would more formal therapy be beneficial in his or her opinion?
      In what way?
    Who might we turn to for such options?
    How long might additional treatment be beneficial?
    What would their costs be?
    What portion of these costs would be ours versus our insurer's?
    In lieu of more therapy or in conjunction with it, how might we
    best continue with rehab exercises at home right now?
- If you know you want to seek out additional support, here are
  common community resources to explore:
    visiting nurse services or other home-based providers in your
    community.
    local aging coalitions or senior centers.
    local, state, regional, or national aphasia or stroke support
    groups or clubs (see Appendix C).

CAREGIVER

other known residents in your community who have suffered from aphasia or stroke.

graduate student training clinics at nearby universities.

long-term rehab centers, devoted to the treatment of aphasia.

ABOUT YOUR LOVED ONE

1–He or she still needs a lot of assistance!

2–I know I need to be more patient . . . but it is hard at times!

3–Slowly, I'm starting to see signs of his or her "old" self.

WHAT TO KNOW

1 Quite likely, basic daily life skills are less than totally functional. Often, "broken" or disabled parts are seen as needing assistance in order to function, and to some extent, this is true. However, the kind of assistance is often different from what one would describe as "broken." Remember how the circuitry in people with aphasia often goes awry (Chapter 5: Person with Aphasia—Communication). Because of this, their abilities typically get *blocked*, rather than lost. That is, people with aphasia usually *know* what it is they would like to accomplish, but their poorly wired nervous systems won't allow it to transmit as it once did. **Thus, the assistance that your loved one needs is apt to be more in unblocking or circumventing the blockage than in relearning tasks. Because of this, teaching, as you might think of this term, is often not a useful strategy or concept for you.** Rather, your loved one needs a lot of support, encouragement, urging, and *facilitating* . . . giving the swing a push at just the right time and in the right direction.

1 Remember, too, you need not be your loved one's sole supporter. Even prior to injury, you likely were not all things at all times to your loved one. Don't fault yourself for what you cannot do now. Much is offered in the chapters ahead for finding other people, who of their choosing, would elect to spend time to assist your loved one. Looking outside yourself for contact with others is not simply a benefit for you, but for your loved one as well. He or she needs many other contacts for life to work as it should or could. Some of what you do not naturally possess within your personality and resources will likely exist freely in somebody else. Instead of seeing yourself as a problem if certain functions are not possible for *you*, look for resources outside yourself that might supplement what you naturally provide.

2 Your desire to be more patient is admirable. Your patience, though, is apt to be taxed repeatedly throughout this journey. If being calm and consistent is difficult at times, it doesn't mean that you are an unworthy companion or that you cannot help in other ways. In fact, patience alone is not what your loved one needs. True, allowing more time for him or her to process and react is likely high on the list of things that would help, but this is less about patience than about the timing. You can help the most by coming to learn where and how to apply brief "pushes" to your loved one's swing (see Caregiver—Recovery, Chapter 5). It is apt to take you awhile to learn just how your loved one's system works and how you might best complement its operation.

CAREGIVER

3 It is probable that some signs of the person you knew before the injury are starting to re-emerge. Perhaps, he or she had a tendency to kid you at times. It would not be surprising for him or her to laugh or show some recognition of that trait again, something that he or she had not done since the time of injury. Old habits and preferences may start to resurface. Possibly he or she was meticulous, keeping everything in a set location or being sure clothing was properly arranged and worn. You may begin to see signs of these tendencies once again.

3 What may seem directly contrary to this pattern is that some new or previously unseen personality characteristics may emerge as well. These differences often fall across a broad spectrum of categories: likes and dislikes regarding foods or how they are prepared, preferred activities during the day, sleep patterns, or personal hygiene. On the whole, though, there are usually fewer *new additions* than there are old tendencies that have re-emerged.

WHAT YOU MIGHT DO

1 PROVIDING ASSISTANCE

As a general rule, try to regard and treat "the person" with aphasia no differently than you did before the injury. Obviously, your means and manner of interacting require some adjusting. But

ABOUT YOUR LOVED ONE
1–He or she still needs a lot of assistance!
2–I know I need to be more patient . . . but it is hard at times!
3–Slowly, I'm starting to see signs of his or her "old" self!

CAREGIVER your intent does not. Keep it as before, that is, one caring adult to another caring adult.

1–2 WHAT TO DO

- Resist *teaching* or *telling* him or her how to do things!
- Instead:
  see if your loved one will attempt some or all of a task alone.
  give whatever he or she *can do* slight, encouraging nudges in the right direction.
  as much as possible, encourage your loved one's participation, or do it together.
  try not to take over the task.
  instead, *share* and *demonstrate* how to do the task.
- Try to get in synchrony with your loved one's need for a gentle push of that swing.
- Pay attention to his or her signals, they indicate when the push should come.
- If he or she stops participating, so should you:
  back up to an easier, do-able, step.
  again, provide just enough of a push now to get him or her participating again.
  resist assuming *full responsibility*—even if it is easier to do so.

3 HOW TO USE THE PAST TO AID THE FUTURE

- Yes, performance is different, but your loved one's likes and dislikes are apt to remain much the same.
- Give thought to ways that might recapture *pleasurable* aspects of the past.
- Try not to accentuate *how well* he or she accomplished these things, but *how fun* they were.
- Try to highlight recapturing some of that pleasure by matching challenge and current skills.
- To do this, you need to be ready to sacrifice performance and to think more about the "doing of it."
  for example: you may have frequently joked or kidded with one another.
  your loved one *may not* be able to carry the speaking load now as he or she did before.

instead, now you may need to support the actual *telling*, i.e.,

Play with a fun story or a joke.

If your loved one responds, probe areas he or she may be reacting to.

Keep a smile and stay upbeat . . . that was what was important before.

Don't expect a lot at first. Persist. Keep it positive and fun.

Over time, your loved one may well begin to joke in this new way.

CAREGIVER

WHAT TO KNOW

1-2 These questions are not new. They've been asked and answered from your loved one's perspective already. In terms of daily life, though, the prime issue is how to get day-to-day routines up and running when so much appears impaired. The prior section provided some basic notions: look for parts of life that are "of choice," acknowledge your loved one's participation in them, and slowly add to existing skills. In the section involving recovery, we outlined a number of ways of getting functional skills started at home. Making daily life more operational, though, requires more. It requires re-establishing the legitimacy of your loved one as an *equal* partner in all aspects of daily life.

DAILY LIFE
1–How well can he or she manage alone?
2–Am I asking or demanding too much?
3–Why doesn't he or she try harder? I would!

1–2 Caregivers commonly report that the functional skills they witnessed in a clinical setting are not in full use at home. Why people with aphasia would revert to lower levels of use or function in daily life is often a concerning issue. One obvious reason is that rehab personnel know a lot more than you about your loved one's disordered machinery and how to make it work efficiently. They know *when* and *how* to give your loved one's different rehab swings a "proper" push. Also, rehab is highly structured so that treatments occur regularly and at designated times, something not likely to continue at home. But neither of these reasons is apt to influence restricted use at home as much as the perceived inequality surrounding functional abilities. For this reason, it is important to guard against this inequality from the outset.

CAREGIVER **1–2** Before your loved one's injury, your daily lives included two self-sufficient routines of your and your loved one's own choosing. Yes, you interacted and shared regularly, but you did so from your own perspectives and personal strengths. Also, it was probably common for one or both of you to elect to work independently for a period of time before resuming a joint activity again. Now, with your loved one's injuries, it may seem like the rules for sharing in daily life have changed. It may seem that you are the "abled," "dominant" force in the partnership and that your loved one has become the "disabled," "dependent" party. Unquestionably, if activities in daily life were judged solely on a normative scale of skill, then you *are* the more able adult. However, it is this misperception in daily life that often causes the inequality cited above.

1–2 Simply because you are the more able person in the relationship does not mean that you should be the more dominant force. **The very reason rehab specialists often succeed in getting maximal effort from their patients is not simply because they know how to facilitate function; it is because they strive to treat each person as an equal in their treatment environments. Far more important than always nudging the swing in motion at the right time, is letting the person with aphasia know he or she is valued and retains equal status in the relationship with you.** Experienced clinicians know that the level of disability has *no bearing* on their feelings about the person whom they are treating. It is from this foundation of respect that many people with aphasia are encouraged to try even harder. As a result, it is important early on to distinguish level of dysfunction from level of status in the relationship.

1–2 The best way to achieve equality is to afford your loved one equal footing as a self-governing person from the time he or she arrives home. Just as prior to injury, this means mutually consulting on daily matters rather than deciding for him or her or for yourselves; it means not feeling any sense of devaluation toward your loved one because of diminished communication or physical skills; it means revising life's activities so your loved one can share in them, regardless of what his or her level of participation might be. Keeping a sense of equality within your home is essential to building a stronger relationship and making daily life more effective. Chapter 8 elaborates on this specific principle. Make sure you begin setting the proper foundation for daily life right now!

3 In the beginning months of recovery, your loved one's endurance is apt to suffer. Getting the machinery up and working involves a concerted effort, but keeping it running for any extended period of time is often wearing and unsustainable. As a result, your loved one's physical and mental stamina is apt to lag and it will continue to lag for months to come. You do not want to interpret this lower ability to sustain effort as a sign of not wanting to take part in life, but as a continuing state of fatigue. It takes more effort and energy to "set things into motion!" His or her ability to start or initiate actions is apt to be slower and more hesitant. With time and actual participation, though, this hesitancy is apt to fade. Up until 24 months postinjury, afford him or her the benefit of the doubt and assume he or she is giving you his or her full effort!

CAREGIVER

WHAT YOU MIGHT DO

1 ESTABLISHING FUNCTION AT HOME

DAILY LIFE
1–How well can he or she manage alone?
2–Am I asking or demanding too much?
3–Why doesn't he or she try harder? I would!

The section of road ahead is seldom easy. Even if you are gifted at dealing with crises in life, the transition ahead is apt to be taxing at times. Start with the expectation that it is going to take months, or years, to get daily life functioning properly again. Keep in mind that the roughness of this section of road, though, is nothing to fear. You have plenty of time to negotiate it. Persist. It is very much worth the effort.

1–2 WHAT TO DO

- Ask each rehab specialist to detail current levels of function and how they may specifically translate into use at home.
- Ask how they manage to afford your loved one every opportunity to be an equal participant in such activities.
- As recommended earlier, ask for a demonstration of these methods. Besides allowing you to see what your loved one can do, it establishes *you* as a knowing "insider" in the eyes of your loved one.
- Some rehab specialist are willing to make home visits before discharge occurs; request this.
   It allows you to see firsthand, within your home environment, how certain functions might work.

CAREGIVER

It allows you to ask how to modify your environment to help you and your loved one.

It allows you to ask how you might expand existing functions over time in this setting.

- If possible, consider videotaping the therapist working with your loved one because:

  It allows you to view their manner over and over at home in a more relaxed environment for learning.

  It allows you to share these activities with your loved one as proof that such functions are possible.

- If videotaping isn't possible, try to observe each therapist's work, and note all of what seems important:

  later share this list with them and ask how they might modify or add to it.

- Keep a simplified, visible list on "do-able" functions prominently displayed at home:

  It provides a nice, documented statement of what *is* possible.

  It allows you to *add* to it over time.

  It serves as another means of documenting progress.

  It helps identify what likely needs further work when you return to follow-up rehab sessions.

- Ask rehab specialists if you might call them during the first several weeks should questions arise.

- Videotape your own efforts at home:

  This allows documentation of what you've done and what has or has not worked.

  It may allow rehab specialists to better aid you in establishing the desired function:

    drop the tape off for the therapist a week prior to your follow-up conference.

    provide current questions, concerns, and desires.

    ask the therapist if he or she might demonstrate how to improve on these efforts.

    videotape the therapist as "a model" to take home and study and learn from.

3 WHAT TO DO

- Understand that short durations of activity in the beginning do not signify "lack of effort."

CAREGIVER

> Remember that continuing a function is infinitely harder than simply doing it once.
> - You may need to provide a gentle nudge to get an activity restarted. Ask him or her *to help you!*
> - Slowly increase the length and frequency of chosen activities.

WHAT TO KNOW

EMOTIONS
1–Whew, I've got a lot on my shoulders!
2–I know we'll manage, but I'm hanging by a thread.

1–2 For good reason, the ending of treatment heightens anxiety over how unmet needs might be resolved. In this shifting of who is responsible for what, caregivers commonly feel overwhelmed, entrapped, and victimized. Not only is your loved one seemingly in need of more attention than when he or she was in rehab, but much of what he or she was providing in daily life around the home before is now yours to deal with as well. Maybe it was his or her responsibility to pay the bills, make home repairs, and clean the house, or take care of the yard or garden. The thought of continuously adding these tasks to your side of the ledger is simply too much. You realize this predicament is not your loved one's fault or doing, but you may have difficulty not feeling "caught" in something that is beyond your means to deal with. As difficult as it is to imagine that these added duties are *not your responsibility*, at least in the manner you are envisioning, they are *not!*

1–2 The truth is, people with aphasia *can* and *should* be given every opportunity to *care for themselves*. Not only does this help the caregiver, but it is essential to restoring worth and value to the injured person's sense of self. Furthermore, it is *not wrong* to look to others for support and help in this pursuit. Such help can be tailored to you and your loved one's needs and personal style. Remember throughout this journey that it is *not incumbent on you alone* to be the sole supporter! You are not alone in this struggle, although it may feel that way at the moment. There are other ways to live life besides one that requires your constant participation or supervision. We begin detailing these in the sections ahead. However, if these concerns are at the top of your list of concerns, you may wish to scan sections of Chapter 7 (Caregiver—Recovery) and Chapter 8 (Daily Life) that speak to this issue in more detail.

EMOTIONS
1–*Whew, I've got a lot on my shoulders!*
2–*I know we'll manage, but I'm hanging by a thread.*

CAREGIVER

WHAT YOU MIGHT DO

1–2 ESTABLISHING SOME BALANCE TO DAILY LIFE

Time, once again, *is* your greatest ally! With it, you and your loved one *will* establish ways of dividing the duties of daily life more equitably. Chapter 7, Caregiver—Recovery, discusses a method for putting these aspects of daily life into a more workable framework. If you are struggling to find a long-term perspective, you may wish to review this section now. In the next 6 to 12 months, though, you need to work toward a more equitable sharing of duties at home. Caregiver—Recovery in this chapter addresses this issue. **Above all, do know that while you can facilitate matters in life for your loved one, you need not and should not accept responsibility—that must be his or her role.**

1–2 WHAT TO DO

- Identify the most worrisome and overpowering concerns at the moment.
- Make sure that you ask the appropriate rehab specialists how they might manage these concerns.
- Work to develop plans that serve both of your best interests.
For example: A caregiver, who had never managed the family finances before, was faced with having to find a workable plan. Through meetings with the injured person's speech-language pathologist, she learned that her loved one could still do simple arithmetic but not check writing or bookkeeping. Her loved one's inability to write checks was not because of writing but because he could no longer recall the proper spelling of key words. However, by introducing computer software containing an easily managed bookkeeping program, a printed list of service pro-viders, and a self-styled aid for converting dollar amounts into their written equivalents, the injured adult was able to resume most of his past functions. For a while, the caregiver carefully monitored his entries and checks to be sure they were adequate. Within several months, all of the financial matters were back in his hands. Not only did it help the caregiver, but it helped tremen-

dously to restore some direction and purpose in the injured person's life.

CAREGIVER

- Resist the temptation to make it your *sole responsibility* to account for what your loved one cannot.

  Look for ways of sharing that load with your loved one and others.

- Allow yourself some free time in any equation . . . just for yourself!

  If necessary, look for alternative ways that would allow you to feel comfortable *not* being present or responsible. You need and deserve regular respites where your own needs can be met. If this is not possible within your home, look for ways of comfortably stepping away from this environment from time to time, even if it means occasionally finding a place for your loved one outside the home. For instance, look into activities or functions at adult daycare or senior centers in your community. Also, seek out others who have already faced this dilemma in your community and ask how they have coped with such issues (see Appendix C).

WHAT TO KNOW

1 As a couple, you likely need the income from your job, but may feel anguish about leaving your loved one unattended at home. The emotional trauma of not being there may be greater than the sadness of having to stop working. However, as

> **EMPLOYMENT (YOURS)**
> 1–How are we going to manage?
> . . . I can't give up my job!
> . . . but he or she can't manage alone?
> 2–What options do we have?

difficult as this may be, sacrificing your employment is likely a poor choice, at least in the beginning months of moving from rehab to home. Besides the loss of income, it is important not to succumb to the strong nurturing impulse to rush to your loved one's side. As emphasized earlier, being present constantly to support and attend to your loved one is apt to do more harm than good. To recover, he or she needs to gradually assume more responsibility for his or her life, even in its currently tenuous and seemingly fractured state; you need to do as much as possible to promote this desired outcome, and his or her independence. Additionally, it is quite likely that your employment is a prime reward and motivation in your life. Losing this opportunity for self-satisfaction

CAREGIVER should not be discarded or sacrificed quickly or lightly. It deserves careful consideration!

2 The first step is to place the current situation in the perspective it deserves. That is, your loved one's recovery is going to *take time.* None of the essential parts of this equation is apt to transpire in a matter of days or weeks; instead they will require months or years. Your immediate availability or presence in daily life is not likely to alter the eventual outcome that dramatically. Yes, some of the initial stages of transition might be more comfortable and operational if you were present at certain times. But being present at these moments does not justify *your continuous presence.* It is not so much your constancy at every moment in daily life that is needed; it is your constancy in periodically nudging the living of daily life in a direction that would benefit everyone. This latter objective is a slow and cooperative undertaking, but not something that requires your continual presence.

2 For this reason, look into other options that might provide several months' leeway to evaluate your needs before considering any long-term change in your employment. Reducing your work hours temporarily from full-time to part-time, or taking leave without pay may afford the time you need at home to reach a mutually agreeable solution. Should being away from work simply be impossible, the rehab social worker might assist you in locating social resources in the community that would support and satisfy your loved one's needs in your absence. You do not, though, want to jeopardize your work environment now if it represents a vital part of your daily life! Consider, too, that resigning work, unless it is truly your informed choice, is not a good solution for managing your loved one's perceived needs!

EMPLOYMENT (YOURS)
1–*How are we going to manage?*
   . . . I can't give up my job!
   . . . but he or she can't manage alone?
2–*What options do we have?*

WHAT YOU MIGHT DO

1–2 ATTENDING TO WORK

You need to ensure that your well-being is factored into any decision that is apt to affect daily life over the long haul, such as your employment. Keeping yourself engaged and rewarded in life in a manner of your per-

---

sonal choice is as essential to any long-term solution as meeting your loved one's needs now or down the road! You may need to give yourself permission to attend to your own needs as well.

1–2 WHAT TO DO

- Before leaving rehab, discuss your work-related issues with the rehab social worker:

    ask about community-based options to support both your working and attending to your loved one.

- Ask rehab specialists what safety factors would preclude your loved one staying at home alone:

    Ask them how they might be minimized or overcome:

    For example, you may worry that your loved one might fall and not be able to get up.

    The physical therapist can demonstrate how your loved one should cope with such a situation. You may need to learn the prescribed routine in rehab and practice it later at home. It may take several successful occurrences before you and he or she feels comfortable that falling is not a concern.

- You want to develop a plan that all parties can agree on.

    Do not expect that any new plan will work perfectly, it is apt to take some time and effort before it becomes comfortably established. As before, keep in mind that *you* are not the sole resource for making sure it does work. Look to your loved one and others to accept ownership, too.

- You don't want to endorse any solution where your needs are ignored or sacrificed.

    Even if such a plan is sustainable, it is *not* a healthy choice for *either* of you!

COMMUNICATION

1–If he or she could only **talk**, everything would be OK!

2–We're doing better with **our** communication!

   . . . I understand his or her basic needs.

   . . . Still it is **very hard** and **frustrating** at times!

   . . . How can we get better?

3–What should I do when we're around other people?

CAREGIVER

WHAT TO KNOW

1 Continuing communication breakdowns are now seriously impacting daily life, especially if they involve difficulties talking. Caregivers typically feel that *if only my loved one could talk,* then everything would be all right! They deeply miss and *mourn* the loss of being able to readily connect with the person they so freely shared with before. Besides sharing, talking was the prime vehicle for resolving everyday conflicts and dilemmas. Now, its restricted form feels cumbersome and unnatural. Because of this, caregivers often find themselves longing—more likely obsessing over—ways of making communication better.

1 Your desire for your loved one to talk is perfectly understandable as long as it remains a desire and *not* an expectation. It may be that the immediate urgency comes from knowing that real-life challenges are about to occur. It didn't matter so much that communication was restricted in the hospital or rehab center where little conversing was essential to living of daily life. Now, though, the rules are changing, and you and your loved one are about to face daily issues together, and alone. How will you manage like this?

2 If you've followed through with the earlier suggestions about communication (see Chapter 5, Caregiver—Communication), you should have some operative ways of interacting at the moment. If you don't, it is highly advisable to seek these out right now. The path ahead requires ways of comfortably exchanging simple content, but just as important, of maintaining ways that allow the two of you to stay personally connected. Even if that communication is incomplete or inaccurate, it will be acceptable as long as you remain bonded as people who care for one another. Communicating will improve over time. Now, however, you need to simply connect. As you leave formal care, you desperately need to have some way to relate as a couple in spite of your loved one's significant language impairments.

2 If you have your own communication system up and running, you need to know that going home is apt to tax it. It was one thing to *prac-*

tice ways of communicating with a speech-language pathologist present **CAREGIVER** at the rehab center, but maintaining these strategies alone and in real-life situations is often a different matter. If the strategies seem less helpful at first, simply back away from focusing on the content of the message. Such a move may seem counter to what you most need, but before you can exchange freely you often need to de-emphasize the importance of getting every aspect of your loved one's message. Staying connected with your loved one communicatively often means interactively sharing in a "back and forth" or "give and take" manner. Chapter 8 introduces hitting a tennis ball back and forth as a visual metaphor for what you and your loved one now need to strive for communicatively. If you are struggling with this notion, you may wish to skip ahead to "Quality of Your Communication" in that chapter.

3 Heading out into everyday life with minimal use of speech is often a real heart stopper! It will require time to establish the best ways of coping. People with aphasia vary considerably in which routes they choose, often depending on their perceptions of their impairments, their prior communicative styles, and personalities. Severity of injury and severity of the handicap do not always align. For instance, some people with mild aphasia, who can readily express themselves with speech, see their lives as dramatically changed. Perhaps they were dependent on the use of superb speaking or writing skills in vocations, such as an attorney, salesperson, or author. Talking now is far beneath what they view as tolerable. Other people with aphasia, who have no functional means of talking, may remain highly conversant with others in spite of their communication difficulties. Usually these individuals were "outgoing" and unaffected by the negative opinions of others. Even though their speech may suffer, they exuberantly continue interacting as if it was not impaired.

3 Your goal in the months ahead needs to be fostering more interaction between your loved one and others. To do so, means *not* speaking or communicating for him or her, but instead looking for effective and desirable ways of making exchanges work simultaneously or with minimal nudging on your part. You certainly do not want to leave your loved one unsupported in social situations where he or she is unable to function. In the same sense, though, you do not want to intervene constantly when he or she may develop ways of managing alone.

3 The most detrimental tactic is to turn all communiqués into miniature "treatment sessions." For instance, interrupting your loved one's attempt

CAREGIVER   to say something like: "Now I know you can say that word, you did it this morning. It starts with a 'BEEE!'" or "Remember the fruit you slice up and put on your cereal? . . . it's yellow . . . you peel it back . . . it's a . . . .???" Such stimulation tasks, if properly laid out and explained to you may facilitate talking at home, but when prompted, in public, they more resemble a dog trick than a helping hand. Avoid doing this to your loved one—*ever!* In everyday life, you constantly want to search for ways of communicating which your loved one can control and use rather than you. More about these methods follows.

COMMUNICATION

*1–If he or she could only **talk**, everything would be OK!*
*2–We're doing better with **our** communication!*
*   I understand his or her basic needs.*
*   Still it is **very hard** and **frustrating** at times!*
*   How can we get better?*
3–What should I do when we're around other people?

WHAT YOU MIGHT DO

1 PUTTING TALKING WHERE IT BELONGS

Keep remembering that your loved one's worth or value is *not* bound to his or her ability to communicate. Who he or she is extends far beyond his or her talking or even his or her communicating. If these terms remain confusing in your mind, Chapter 9 describes the difference between them. Your loved one remains internally intact. Ease and access to symbols for communicating is no longer the same, but the underlying person is. Try not to fixate on what isn't working, concentrate instead on making the most of out what is. Also, if talking remains a key concern of his or hers, refer to Person with Aphasia—Communication earlier in this chapter for suggestions on how to further this skill.

2 IMPROVING YOUR OWN COMMUNICATION

What is important is to keep that snowball moving down the hill. Certainly, the more you've done so far to set this in motion, the more comfortable you should be right now. But if you are just beginning to move in this direction, your late start need not prevent putting together a working system right now. You need *your own communication system* up and running before worrying about how best to communicate with others.

2 WHAT TO DO   CAREGIVER

- If you have any confusion about what is "talking" versus what is "communicating," refer to Chapter 9.
- Get a clear understanding of what might aid *your own* communication at home:

  review the questions and issues in Chapter 5, Caregiver—Communication.

  review them with the speech-language pathologist before discharge.

  Minimally, you need from the speech-language pathologist a defined set of ways of exchanging ideas and feelings back and forth with each other. If your loved one is not talking, you need a prescriptive list of what to do, how to do it, and in what order, to augment talking or deal with other communication barriers. Have these ways and their proper use spelled out in a written or videotaped form. Ideally, you should have attempted them yourselves with the speech-language pathologist observing their use.

- Establish a plan for consultative help as you try to implement these ways of communicating at home:

  Attempt to schedule follow-up consultations monthly over the first 3 months, and then at 3-month intervals through the first year postonset.

  You need an effective way of interacting at home. You need some help, especially in the beginning stages. For that reason, return monthly for the first several months and review what has and hasn't been working, and how you might improve on what isn't.

  Do not attempt to do this alone.

3 AIDING COMMUNICATION WITH OTHERS

Because interacting with others in the real world typically takes on a variety of forms, you likely will need a variety of forms of communicating. If talking is not viable, then other augmentative ways are important. What these are and how they are used differs according to the interactant and the situation. We address several common possibilities below: communicating with complete strangers, with familiar people in specific situations, and with family and friends.

CAREGIVER **3** COMMUNICATING WITH COMPLETE STRANGERS

In that communication is apt to brief, tied to a specific topic, and unlikely to recur, the best alternative options are to quickly orient the normal interactant to what is happening and how best to determine whatever the communiqué may be about. A simple, laminated card of introduction may prove beneficial.

- If some talking is possible and yet not sufficient to quickly communicate, the person with aphasia may wish to provide a general printed statement like:

  I'm . . . John Doe.
  I've suffered a stroke.
  Talking is difficult but my mind works well.
  I can understand your spoken message.
  Give me a moment, I usually can get my point across.
  Thanks.

- If talking is not possible at all, but understanding is good . . . change the latter portion of the card to:

  I can't talk but my mind works well.
  I can understand your spoken message, if you talk slowly.
  Please ask me some "yes or no" questions, I can answer these.
  It may take a few minutes, but we'll figure things out, OK?
  Thanks.

- If talking is not possible and you wish to request a specific task, change the card to reflect that desire:

  I'm John Doe.
  I live at 220 S. Monroe St.
  I've suffered a stroke and cannot talk.
  Would you mind calling a taxi for me?
  The number for Union Cab is 777–2678.
  Thanks.

3 WAYS OF COMMUNICATING WITH FAMILIAR PEOPLE IN SPECIFIC SITUATIONS

There are many aids commercially available that might assist people with aphasia in these situations (see Appendix D). What is far more important than the aid's use is whether it fits with your loved one's communicative needs. The speech-language pathologist should be able to assist you in determining their appropriateness for your loved one.

CAREGIVER

For example:

perhaps your loved one likes to visit a farmer's market on the weekends.

he or she is unable to state basic desires.

many of the vendors personally know him or her.

he or she may want to carry a pocket notebook with a listing of:

items commonly purchased by categories, e.g., vegetables, fruits, flowers.

quantities of items desired, e.g., dozen, half-dozen.

price scale, e.g., in dollars and cents.

3 WAYS OF COMMUNICATING WITH FAMILY AND FRIENDS

Most normal interactants, even if they are caring and interested in the person with aphasia, find it difficult to constantly alter their *own* communication to meet the needs of others. This is especially true if communicating with a person having aphasia requires a lot of time and methods with which they are only vaguely familiar. It does not hurt to explain *how to communicate* in more depth if they are highly interested and vested in that process. However, it is usually best to keep suggestions and aids to a minimum when involving others, and focus more on easy ways to exchange common everyday information in a simple and familiar manner. Again, the speech-language pathologist may help you with such suggestions.

WHAT TO KNOW

1–2 Going home ensures more contact with the outside world. The preferred strategy is to slowly ease into visits and to attempt to keep these encounters brief and as positive as possible. **The difficulty in getting together with friends or family members may not be simply yours, but, as alluded to earlier, these meetings may be equally challenging for them. Before venturing forth, it may help to familiarize yourself *with their perspective* as well.**

> **FAMILY/FRIENDS**
> *1–We cannot avoid seeing or being around others now!*
> *2–What should I do?*
> *3–How can I make this easier on him or her?*

2 Seeing a friend or relative with aphasia often stops people dead in their tracks. They are speechless, stunned by the physical differences that

CAREGIVER brain injury may bring, but even more overwhelmed by the apparent absence of communication. Within minutes, they are often in a state of panic over what to do or say. Above all, they do not want to do anything wrong, yet they are unclear about what is right. As a result, they often sit startled, and awkwardly search for signs of what to do next. Frequently, the person with aphasia senses their alarm and discomfort, and immediately assumes that it is his or her changed status that is responsible. Although to an extent this is true, their discomfort is apt not to be *as personal* as your loved one might imagine. Friends and family simply do not know how to act or what to say!

2 In addition, close friends or family members cannot help wondering how they would feel if they were in your loved one's position. Would they want others around if they couldn't talk? Would they wish to cope with life like this? It may be terribly painful to see someone they care for in such an altered state of being. For someone of approximately the same age, it may be a vivid reminder of one's own mortality or vulnerability to lasting injury. Although they know that aphasia is not contagious, they cannot help wondering how they would be reacting if it had happened to them. All of these thoughts serve to dissociate them from the injured adult. But collectively, these tendencies to withdraw are *not* because they no longer care for the injured party, they typically do! Rather your loved one's injury is too "threatening" to their own mortality and way of life!

2 Finally, close friends may have chosen your company in the past to share in a particular activity or agenda. Maybe you, as a foursome, enjoyed playing cards, eating out, or dancing together. Without this common theme, and with the awkwardness imposed on communication by your loved one's aphasia, such relationships often tend to slip away. Occasionally, though, there may be a couple who is able and willing to adapt to a different format and a different way of relating.

2–3 For all of the above reasons, it is may be easiest on everyone if you select friends or family who were more tied to your loved one as a "person" than through a mutually shared activity that is no longer possible. Additionally, it is important to let visitors, whoever they are, know what they should expect communicatively, how best to cope with it, and the importance of their remaining as natural and unchanged as possible. Keep letting them know that your loved one is no different; there is simply a communication problem!

WHAT YOU MIGHT DO

FAMILY/FRIENDS
1—We cannot avoid seeing or being around others now!
2—What should I do?
3—How can I make this easier on him or her?

1–3 SETTING THE STAGE FOR VISITS

Carefully consider the time, place, and individuals who visit. Often the tenor of these initial encounters with other friends and family plays an important role in shaping your loved one's sense of self and his or her relationship to the outside world.

CAREGIVER

1–3 WHAT TO DO

- Review the suggestions in Chapter 5: Person with Aphasia—Family or Friends about how to orient visitors.
- Strive to place the visitor at ease from the beginning:
  have close friends and family read Chapter 2 on what aphasia is and is not.
  - Depending on the likelihood of their extended contact with your loved one, you may want to give them the entire book to scan on their own time and in their own manner.
  - Before they visit, talk briefly about what they might expect.
  - De-emphasize the need to exchange a lot of information.
  - Let them know that it is the social connecting that really matters.
  - Reassure them that, with a little time, they'll each "catch on" to each others' communicative attempts.
- Close friends need to know that you recognize that this process is difficult for them too:
  - It was for you . . . it has got to be for them as well.
  - However, the worst time was in the beginning before you understood what aphasia was.
  - Now that you know, it's much easier.
  - It takes some time, it takes some reaching out, but, there are rewards in doing so.
- Think of ways of staying connected that do *not* involve a lot of talking:
  - Watch videos or favorite TV programs together.
  - Take brief rides in a car.
  - Play simple board or card games together.
- Focus more on the quality of personal "sharing," and less on the completeness or adequacy of communication.

CAREGIVER   **1–3** WHAT TO SAY TO VISITORS

- "Aphasia is *nothing* to fear."
- "It is a *communication problem*."
- "Over time, it *can* be compensated for."
- "It will take some time, though, to learn how to do that."
- "Interacting with our loved one is apt to feel awkward at first."
- "You cannot do anything terribly bad or wrong."
- "Simply try at first to be your "old self" and remain natural and upbeat."
- "Focus on extending, and being *with* him or her rather than exchanging a lot of information."

RELATIONSHIP

1–I still love him or her but I'm
   unsure how to express it!
    . . . is it physically and medically
   OK to be intimate again?
    . . . what can or can't he or she
   do?
2–How do we approach this realm?

WHAT TO KNOW

1 Society favors normalcy and rewards one's physical appearance and vitality. Many people define themselves by how they look and what they can do. Aphasia frequently plays havoc with one or both of these realms. Few sufferers escape injury without visible or subtle characteristics that society might classify as undesirable or unattractive. As a result, it is not strange that individuals with aphasia and their caregivers may struggle at first to recapture the physical attraction they once held for one another. Such disconnected feelings, or thoughts are not bad or wrong. In fact, they are quite understandable within the context of all that has happened.

1 Such feelings are likely associated with standards outside your own. The strongest evidence for this is the steadfast devotion and commitment you've already provided. **Your constancy and your caring for your loved one from the moment of injury until now speaks strongly to your loving or caring for him or her. What may prove problematic at the moment is that injury-related changes in his or her physical appearance and behaviors have possibly detracted from what society judges *as desirable*.** And if so, these changes now do make a difference in how readily you accept or feel a willingness to be physically close to your partner.

1 None of this sense of personal alienation need worry you unless it persists, or feels as if it is no longer a reflection of a societal standard but of *yours alone*. If you fear this may be the case in the beginning, give yourself a little time "to adjust" internally to *seeing* and *being around* these new physical features and behaviors of your loved one. Remember what these outward manifestations *really are,* outward manifestations! They are the *consequences of injury* to the brain, not a lessening of the person inside! Allow time to redefine these changes in your *own terms and feelings.*

2 Some caregivers are not dramatically affected by physical change in their partner. Even so, they may worry about what is or is not possible or safe sexually. Because such matters are highly personal and intimate, many people prefer *to read about* such topics rather than to openly discuss them with trained professionals or other sufferers. If that should be true for you, then you may want to start by examining "Sexuality" in Chapter 12. However, if your questions and concerns are not addressed in Chapter 12 or here, it is advisable to seek answers to your specific questions from trained professionals. To do this, you may wish to request a private meeting with your loved one's physician, physical therapist, and/or rehab social worker. One of these individuals should be able to advise you on such matters and how to proceed given your loved one's physical restrictions at the moment.

2 Reuniting as a couple requires more than readjusting one's feelings and knowledge of what needs to be done. Sharing intimately with one another is often a foremost manifestation of couplehood. As such, it represents an act and process that molds and fuses the personal preferences of two individuals participating in a highly mutual activity. You have likely watched couples from afar on a dance floor and noticed how they express themselves. As a group, they share some features of movement and rhythm, but separately each couple manifests their own personalized style and flair.

2 In light of all that has happened, your loved one is apt to return home feeling that dancing may be a thing of the past. As the other in this twosome, you may feel that the old tango is a thing of the past, too. It may even concern you that *attempting to dance* may be more painful than simply going without! Well . . . do know that there are thousands of ways of dancing, none of which is inherently *more acceptable* than another. It

CAREGIVER

CAREGIVER   is not so much the manner as it is the mutual sharing and personal close-ness that counts. Although it may be difficult to think of stepping out on the dance floor without moving with that old familiar style and flair, it is likely that simply recapturing the beat of the music and the pleasure of being physically near one another is the first order of business. Do know: chances are that many forms of movement and dancing are still possible, even including some form of the old tango.

RELATIONSHIP

1–*I still love him or her but I'm unsure how to express it!*
Is it physically and medically OK to be intimate again?
What can or can't he or she do?
2–*How do we approach this realm?*

WHAT YOU MIGHT DO

1 RECONNECTING WITH YOUR LOVED ONE

If this part of living life was important prior to injury, chances are that with a little time and patience, it can be again. Depending on the importance of these concerns, you may wish to address specific questions of your own prior to discharge. Be prepared for this realm to take some time to return to its former form.

1 MAKING AN INITIAL PLAN

- Read the earlier suggested material on this topic, Chapter 12, "Sexuality."
- If additional questions exist:
  arrange a private meeting with your loved one's doctor and physical therapist before discharge.
  you may wish to advise them of your topic and quickly preview your concerns:
  Are there any physical or medical reasons to preclude sexual activity now?
  Are there any physical or emotional reasons that my loved one may not be able or wish to take part in such activity?
  If so, what are the best ways of minimizing or overcoming these difficulties?
  How might I make physical contact positive and pleasant at first?

Is there any other literature that might help explain the nature of restoring physical intimacy with someone after stroke with aphasia?

CAREGIVER

2 WHAT TO CONSIDER IN THE BEGINNING

- Strive to maintain the potential for as much physical intimacy as prior to injury:

   If you slept in the same bed before, continue this practice unless his or her medical or physical condition precludes.

   At first, you may wish to simply snuggle with one another without a further sexual intent.

- Do not think about "dancing" as you once did, just think about getting back out on the dance floor:

   See if you can hear and feel the beat of the music—that's a meaningful beginning!

   Simplify everything in the beginning, both in action and expectation.

   Plan to help and support in ways you never needed to previously.

   Keep movement functional, safe, and pleasurable.

   Give yourself some time to make the "new ways" of dancing feel right.

- Do not let this sphere of life stay unaddressed, especially if it was important before:

   Actively pursue whatever it takes:

   Talk about it with your loved one.

   Experiment.

   If it does not feel right, it is always modifiable.

   But if you do nothing at all, over time, the potential for modification becomes less viable.

- If you've seriously worked at this, and it has not felt right or comfortable over time, seek further professional guidance, possibly a marriage counselor or a rehab psychologist.

WHAT TO KNOW

1 There are a number of health-related issues that require careful tracking as you prepare to leave

> **HEALTH**
> *1–Are there any other health issues that need explanation or attention?*

CAREGIVER formal care. Many of these issues were identified in Chapter 5: Caregiver—Health. Review these again to determine which, if any, need addressing now before discharge. High on that list needs to be any medical issues that pertain to current, ongoing medical treatments. For example, your loved one may require the use of blood thinning or blood pressure medications, or he or she may need a special oral diet. Such matters need to be completely clear in your mind prior to discharge.

1 It is a good idea, as well, to discuss the likelihood of *seizures* down the road. Your loved one's physician should be able to address their likelihood and potential management. You do not want to leave formal care without a basic orientation to what these are and what they mean, should they occur. Suddenly and unexpectedly, this complication of head injury may appear! For many caregivers not aware of what they are, they fear *another stroke* is occurring! Do not put yourself through such an ordeal! Find out *right now* . . . what are seizures and what can be done about them. As a prelude to the topic, you may want to scan the section in Chapter 12 on this topic entitled, "Seizures."

HEALTH

1–Are there any other health issues that need explanation or attention?

WHAT YOU MIGHT DO

1 ESTABLISHING A PLAN OF ACTION

Keep yourself pointed forward and in control of what medical issues remain before you. There are often unexpected bumps along the road ahead until all these health-related concerns get stabilized. Be careful and diligent in attending to them before discharge.

1 WHAT TO DO

- Review potential health-related issues from Chapter 5: Caregiver—Health.
- Take any unresolved concerns to your loved one's physician before discharge.
  Make sure that a discussion of seizures is included in this.
- Also, it is a good time to try to network with others:
  Besides peer support groups, there are all kinds of information about all aspects of health care issues on the Internet. You may wish to scan this resource or ask someone who knows how.

The journey ahead

What may have looked like a brief light at the end of the tunnel, that is, seeing some initial improvement through rehab, may suddenly appear dark and gloomy. It is as if someone has just blocked the tunnel's exit. Shortly, you and your loved one will need to put together your own solutions for coping with diminished functions that previously were managed by the rehab staff. Because of this, you are about to experience one of the more challenging phases of this journey. **But, do know: there is much, much more to this trip that stands on the positive side of the ledger. There is more growth, more improvement, and more meaning to be derived from what exists at the moment.** In fact, for most people who look back at all the change that accrues over the years, this point in time is marked *with little significance*. For most, leaving formal care *was traumatic*, but it was not the end of recovery—no, not by a long shot!

The accomplishments from rehab are not the end of recovery's tunnel. The light that you thought was there still *is*, and the darkness now is not because that light is gone. It is because the tunnel is much longer than you or your loved ever expected! Don't despair with the surrounding darkness at the moment. The tunnel's end is ahead and it is still well lit. And as you continue your way along, there will be more light emanating forth. Reaching the end over time has much more to do with realizing you and your loved one's potential in your much-changed world. There is plenty of room for progress, and much more light still to come. Just keep moving forward, you'll get there!

❖   CHAPTER 7

One year later . . . finding "your stride!"

The anniversary of aphasia's onset is an important landmark in this journey. It was a year ago today that this all began. In some ways, it feels like it was just yesterday, and in other ways it feels like 10 years of living and effort have gone into these last 365 days! Quite likely, this striking contrast between what once was, and now is, best characterizes life at the moment. There is still a sharp, almost biting, remembrance of life prior to injury, but as well, there is the vivid reality of the last year's struggles and accomplishments. And it is from this blending of old and new that a *different* reality in life is beginning to emerge.

This new view has come from steadily confronting functional differences over a sustained period of time. Yes, you were told that aphasia and its associated disabilities would come and likely stay, but you had no idea what this really meant. Now, after 365 days of having confronted these changes daily, you do! Some lost skills have returned, but many still remain impaired. Some skills are present in a restricted form that at least works well enough to live with. There are other skills, though, that haven't returned at all, and it is their absence that likely stands in the way of resuming a lifestyle you once knew.

Even so, such absences have not stopped your living of daily life. The two of you have molded together a routine that is *at least tolerable.* By "tolerable," we don't mean that every part is perfect or of choice, but rather that what life does transpire now is a life with a minimal degree of dissonance or pain. It is this process of replacing the workings of before with the workings of today that allows the door to open to something entirely new. For the first time, travelers can begin to *choose* a new direction, one that promises to add pleasure to life, not simply another way *to cope* with injury.

Some travelers, however, aren't ready or able to accept this new identity before them and its inherent choices and responsibilities. To them, the old way of life still seems *like the only way* to view life, even now. Current skills may seem totally unacceptable and unlikely to improve over time. Instead of accepting the permanence of injury and choosing to take the next road ahead, these travelers see their journey as over! To them, it appears as if there are no viable routes to choose from, but rather that living life has turned into an inescapable "life sentence." Until travelers can accept the permanence of aphasia, and transform the concept of *having aphasia* into *living life with aphasia*, the routes ahead are inaccessible. Should you be such a traveler, these routes ahead *are not washed out*; they are only temporarily blocked. You should know that your survival on this journey is assured whether you elect to take these routes or not. What is sacrificed if you choose not to, though, is quite significant—the road ahead can take you to places that put more pleasure, meaning, and comfort back into daily life. Do know that these routes await your travel at any time in the months or years ahead. You need to be ready to confront life *as it is* in order to proceed down this byway, but take your time and proceed *at your own natural pace!*

You will need something more than a workable way of confronting daily life to move forward from here. You and your loved one need to feel some mutual comfort in sliding behind the wheel of your vehicle; you need to feel that driving ahead is not only of choice, but that it is highly desirable and essential for finding out who you may be. Chances are that the past 365 days have more than prepared you to drive these routes. If starting up the engine, sorting through the road maps, and setting out on a preferred course is enticing, then you are ready. You may not know precisely how or when you'll get to your next destination, but that does not matter. The road ahead will help point you in the direction you need to go.

What is apt to be most absent in life now is a sense of pleasure or well-being, at least compared to what you once knew. If more than 20% of your shared time together qualifies as enjoyable or of personal choice, then you are doing exceedingly well. Most travelers fall well short of this percentage after a year; although life may be working, it is not resonating like it once did. In this realm, the biggest gains are still ahead of you. What this chapter provides, then, are routes for increasing your personal satisfaction. These routes depend primarily on adding to what you've already set in motion at home, and then starting to explore meaningful additions in the community-at-large. It is this latter realm, interacting with the outside world, that is apt to take the longest period to figure out. Chapter 8 concentrates on just that, building better and stronger ties with the outside world. For now, though, keep in mind that all routes from here on out are solely of choice. You and your loved one can elect to take them or not! Not only that, you can take some while avoiding others, or you can opt to find *other people* who, of their own choosing, would elect to accompany one or both of you at times. In other words, there are many ways of negotiating the roads ahead.

So, strap on your seat belts, and don't worry if you still feel a little scared. We all do when we truly take life's choices into our *own hands*. Proceed cautiously and you can, and will, find your way safely to the next juncture. Keep on going!

Profiles

PERSON WITH APHASIA

- appearing more fit and healthy, although long-term deficits are now becoming apparent
- still improving in all realms, i.e., communication, standing, walking, and self-care

CAREGIVER

- often feeling discouraged that rehab gains have not fully blossomed
- trying to cope with the reality that many aspects of daily life are permanently different

PERSON WITH APHASIA

- noting smaller increments of change than in first 6 months, but gains are still evident, especially to those closely involved
- becoming aware that aphasia and related disabilities are not going to resolve over time
- starting to incorporate the concept of *permanent change* into self-image and daily life
- struggling with feelings of diminished self-worth, yet striving to move forward with more participation in daily life
- starting to gauge some changes with reference to months ago rather than with pre-injured status
- experiencing intermittent bouts of depression and anger over current disabilities and the lack of progress
- resisting giving up in spite of moments of discouragement and diminished self-worth
- feeling uncertain about the future but clinging to the belief that more gains can and will follow
- acquiescing to others who are "normal," and presumably more able, more often than relying on one's own abilities
- losing contact with past friends and business associates . . . likely feeling abandoned by many people

CAREGIVER

- if loved one is at home, likely delighted that a workable solution is evolving, but anguishing over the absence of certain aspects of daily life from before
- feeling particularly troubled over:

  restricted access and use of conversation

  increased responsibility in realms of life that previously were shared or handled by loved one

  diminished access to the same person who served as a prime confidante in life

  awkwardness in matters of intimacy, closeness, and sex

  diminished nurturing of your needs, i.e., aphasic partner too entrapped in his or her own misfortunes to see or attend to your needs

- possibly struggling with redefining ties with and commitments to loved one
- still hoping for ways of improving the complicated mix of issues in daily life at the moment
- starting to broaden your base of support, i.e., confiding in others, attending support groups, or looking for activities outside the home
- coming to realize that many past friendships were based on your being a "normal" couple

Primary concerns

PERSON WITH APHASIA

Recovery

1–I'm getting by—but it is *not* where I was or want to be!

2–How can I get more function back?

Emotions—Feelings About Self—Daily Life

One of several scenarios is likely evolving:

1–DEPRESSED—*self-deprecation*: I can't do anything. What's the use of even trying!

2–CHALLENGED—*self-doubt*: I'm doing some basic things. But I'm unsure whether I can do more!

3–EMPOWERED—*self-confident*: I'm slowly getting better. But I know I can do more and I *will* with time!

Relationship

1–I know you love the person I was, but do you respect the person I currently am?

2–For me, I need to be *more* my own person. Please allow me, and help me, to do more on my own—that's what I need the most!

Communication

1–I still want to talk!

2–How can I increase my progress?

CAREGIVER

Recovery

1–How can we make things better . . .they seem "stuck" to me!

2–I cannot accept that our lives may not get any better than this!

3–There has got to be *more* possible, but *what* and *how*?

Emotions—Feelings About Your Loved One—Daily Life

One of several scenarios is likely evolving:

1–DISCOURAGED—*He or she has given up*: What kind of existence is this? The good life is *over*!

2–STYMIED—He or she is still trying but little is changing: There's got to be more, but *where* and *how?*

3–DETERMINED—He or she isn't giving up and neither am I. We've always managed before, we'll manage this too!

Relationship

1–I *still* sense I'm not allowing my loved one to do all he or she might. How can I "let go" further?

2–How can we make *us* better?

Communication

1–We figure out almost everything now at home; however, occasionally we still get stuck!

PERSON WITH APHASIA

2–Is there anything more we might
do that we haven't already?

Family/Friends
1–What happened to our
"supposed" friends?
2–How will we ever gain new
ones when I cannot talk?

Employment
1–I couldn't go back to my old
job, but I sure would like to
have something meaningful to
fill that void!
2–What might that be?

CAREGIVER

Family/Friends
1–What, if anything, might
make past friendships better?
2–How might we add new ones?

Employment (yours)
1–Thank goodness, I still have
my work!

Health
1–This all happened a year ago.
Are we doing everything we
can to ensure it doesn't recur?

> **RECOVERY**
> 1–*I'm getting by—but it is **not** where
> I was or want to be!*
> 2–*How can I get more function
> back?*

WHAT TO KNOW

1 You and your loved one have now experienced
6 to 9 months away from formal care and its services. In that interim, you have had enough time to
explore earlier suggestions for recovery (see
Chapter 6; Person with Aphasia/Caregiver—Re-
covery). The core theme of these recommendations was: (1) to make
daily life work as well as possible and (2) to sustain the momentum
begun in rehab. To help daily life along, you were advised to target as
much self-determination, self-involvement, and self-independence as
your loved one's rehab status would permit. You were given ideas to
facilitate current skills. Your suggested role was to continue to be supportive but to turn over the task of performing to your loved one whenever safe and possible. Finally, you were encouraged to look for activities that were of choice, and pleasurable.

1 Quite likely, these efforts over the past 6 months have met with varying degrees of success. Their therapeutic value, though, is not in the

number of independent tasks currently occurring at home, or in how well they may be running. What is more telling is whether a solid basis for interacting and conducting daily life has begun to evolve *between the two of you*. People with aphasia return home with depleted feelings about themselves and their abilities. Nothing is more important to recovery than establishing a foundation from which you and your loved one can begin to judge life's possibilities in your own terms and thinking.

PERSON WITH APHASIA

1 The first 6 to 9 months at home provide an essential and often invisible ingredient for making life better. This hidden ingredient is time. It takes weeks and months of living with differences before you can begin to understand and accept them for what they are. People with aphasia need to experience their changed states of being and function day after day in order to truly come to understand what they mean personally. Skill levels are no longer apt to change quickly. However, participating in life can only help that process along, and even if the level of activity is less than desired, it is better than not doing anything at all! Coming to this point in the journey requires *time*, a year's duration is often minimal to *see* the situation and to *set* this process in motion.

1 After 12 months, people with aphasia often *start* to reframe life according to what *is* rather than what once *was*. They begin judging the path of their recovery differently. They begin to notice and respond to changes in relation to where they were weeks or months ago instead of to their preinjured selves. Viewing change since injury does not mean they have forgotten their "normal" beings. It means only that they are starting to accrue sufficient time with their disabilities to look at them as part of their changed selves. In the beginning days and weeks, no other referent existed except one's noninjured self. Now, gains in talking, walking, dressing, and so forth, are emerging, and although they may be less than desired, your loved one is likely recognizing them as improvements. Tying change to differences since injury is a tremendously important step in moving recovery forward.

1 It is common that people with aphasia first view small gains as insignificant. They acknowledge that they are better off than before, but quickly revert to a normal scale of comparison. If seen only that way, these gains constantly fall short of the mark. Yet, because they usually permit more participation in life, the recovery process is advanced. On occasion, though, certain travelers may refuse to acknowledge the value of these gains. If they elect, instead, to withdraw from participating in

PERSON WITH APHASIA

life, they are apt to slide toward states of depression and self-deprecation. On the other hand, there is a group of individuals who strongly summon their inner strengths to press forward and do more. The next section of this chapter, Person with Aphasia—Emotions—Feelings About Self—Daily Life addresses various ways that people with aphasia may elect to cope at this point in time. What is *most important* to recognize, though, is that recovery's true form *is only beginning to take shape.*

1 Therapeutic efforts in the early stages of recovery were devoted to fixing or repairing disrupted functions in the injured party. It is possible that your loved one is still practicing some of the specific treatment tasks begun in rehab. If your loved one wishes to continue specific exercises to improve speech, reading, writing, or arm and leg movement, it is important that such stimulation continue. However, *keeping the momentum of rehab moving ahead* no longer is just about striving to make impaired skills work better; it is contingent as well on refining processes in life that permit you and your loved one to work together freely and honestly, at existing levels of function, while maintaining your *own* identities and pursuits. Keeping rehab alive means refusing to let aphasia and its associated disabilities dominate life now or in the future. **Until living life with aphasia is a stronger force than not living life because of aphasia or its associated disabilities, there is much recovering left to do.**

2 The simple answer to this question is that people with aphasia will get back more function when they realize that they need to work with, rather than against, what they currently have. Existing levels of function are not inherently bad, even though they may seem that way at times. Yet the more people with aphasia are willing to nurture current skills, and persist in making them even better, the more daily life will begin to take on renewed meaning and purpose. Such an approach to recovery involves not only bolstering impaired skills but restoring a person's often diminished views of self. You may need, repeatedly, to provide a positive and caring reminder to your loved one about the nature of this process, without "demanding" his or her incorporation of your view. You need, with time, to allow him or her to adopt *his or her own version* of "taking charge" of life.

2 If seeing the permanence in dysfunction only pushes your loved one further away from wanting to take charge of life, there is likely a "fixation" on just seeing only the worst of things. Years ago I treated a gentleman with aphasia and a severe right hemiplegia (loss of movement of the right arm, hand, and leg) who suggested by his manner and limited speech: "Heck, this dumb arm doesn't work . . . what good is it! I can't use it! I can't pick anything up or write! It's a nuisance . . . why not cut it off!" The truth was, this gentleman's right arm and hand functions were significantly different than before injury, **but** they were useful in a number of ways! He could stabilize himself while using a walker, he could swim short distances, an activity he highly valued, and he could hold a fishing pole while reeling with his left arm! Were his skills like they were prior to injury? Not at all! But were impaired skills beyond *any* value? Not at all! Often, in cases like this gentleman's, there is confusion between what permanent injury and what permanent inability mean. However, these concepts are *not* the same, and it may be necessary in the months ahead to keep this distinction clear. We'll keep helping you with this task!

PERSON WITH APHASIA

WHAT YOU MIGHT DO

1–2 KEEPING RECOVERY MOVING AHEAD

RECOVERY
1–I'm getting by—but it is not where I was or want to be! 2–How can I get more function back?

Keeping recovery moving forward depends on your loved one's *willingness to try and to risk further change*. If this is lacking, however, recovery's path is apt to become temporarily blocked. Such blockages commonly occur throughout the first years after injury. Most people with aphasia move forward in bursts or spurts, that is, wanting and willing to do more and then retracting and resting or questioning what they want. Somewhere in this interaction of trying and retreating, these individuals come to adopt and hopefully accept, a different style of life and being. On the other hand, blockages are often due to fear, devaluation of one's self or skills, or uncertainty over one's ability to change further. In cases like this, it makes sense to have an arsenal of ways for getting life moving again. In general, the process is one of assessing why the perceived challenge was too great or the perceived skill too limited. Increasing participation in life is often tied to merging the perceived challenge one envisions with the actual skill level one possesses. **This is a process we discuss in depth in the next section.**

**PERSON
WITH
APHASIA**

1–2 DETERMINING YOUR LOVED ONE'S STATUS AT THE MOMENT

You were urged at the time of discharge to maintain contact with rehab personnel through follow-up reevaluation meetings and to keep weekly logs of change since then (see Chapter 6, Caregiver—Recovery). If you have done your version of these two suggestions, you and your loved one likely have a working means of approaching further recovery. This system may not function perfectly in all respects. That is well expected. The important thing is that you have been *building onto a framework*. More suggestions for adding to it follow in the next section. However, if you have reached this juncture in the road without any sense of direction, and your forward momentum has totally stalled, it is crucial to regroup and get matters heading along a preferred course. Each moment you delay takes you farther away from where you ultimately want to go. When accumulated over time, these moments can threaten the ultimate success of this journey.

1–2 GETTING MATTERS MOVING IN THE RIGHT DIRECTION

- Carefully reread Person with Aphasia and Caregiver—Recovery sections in Chapters 5 and 6.
- Sit down and write up a general summary of what has transpired since discharge:

  what you have tried to do to promote recovery, both individually and as a couple.

  which aspects have worked and which have not.

  what stands in the way of further progess at this time.
- Organize your summary by time and, if possible, according to rehab domains (see Table 4–1).
- **Schedule a reevaluation with a team of rehab staff members right now:**

  it may be helpful to return to the professionals who saw your loved one before.

    These professionals have a familiarity with your loved one's injury which may increase their ability to assist you.

    If these professionals are not available, look for recommendations for others who are.

    Again, you likely will need to be explicit about your needs during this reevaluation:

PERSON WITH APHASIA

That is, you want their collective assistance in specifying where and how current skills might be best utilized and expanded in daily life now and in the future. **You are *not* requesting *more therapy* . . . rather, functional ways of making life better given your loved one's residual skills and capabilities** *at this time.*

- Provide rehab personnel with copies of your written summary before convening.

  Remember that moving ahead with recovery means promoting the good in what has worked, while eliminating the bad from what has not. So if you have been asking your loved one to participate in as many realms of life as he or she can and wants to, you will have many observations to share with the rehab staff.

- Be sure you come away from these meetings with rehab personnel with a plan of what and where you and your loved one might begin, or continue, participating in life with what is possible.

- It may be best, if you have any questions about their recommendations, to ask them to demonstrate proper ways or methods of prompting activity or participation.

- You want this demonstration to be as specific to your living environment and circumstances as possible.

- **Don't leave without some clear sense of *what*, *how*, and *where* you might do more!**

WHAT TO KNOW

1–3 Depending on coping options chosen earlier in the journey, a variety of emotions, and feelings about self and performance in daily life are apt to exist now. It would be impossible to explain them fully here. For example, the emotions of people with aphasia often span the gamut from pervasive depression to strong feelings to act further in their own behalf. In between, though, most sufferers feel a steady push or internal pressure to do more, but with considerable worry about how to accomplish this. Feelings about self can be anywhere on a continuum from a complete denunciation of self to a sense of growing strength and confidence.

EMOTIONS—FEELINGS ABOUT SELF—DAILY LIFE
One of several scenarios is likely evolving:

1–***DEPRESSED***—*self-deprecation: I can't do anything. What's the use of even trying!*

2–***CHALLENGED***—*self-doubt: I'm doing some basic things. But I'm unsure whether I can do more!*

3–***EMPOWERED***—*self-confident: I'm slowly getting better. But I know I can do more and I **will** with time!*

PERSON WITH APHASIA Most commonly, though, there is considerable self-doubt, wondering whether the skills that remain are sufficient for living life. Performance in daily life varies from a near inability or unwillingness to act to a dedicated pledge to do much more. Interspersed between these two extremes are waxing and waning attempts, mustering the strength to act for a time and then needing to rest before trying again.

1–3 Often there are predictable ties between emotions, feelings about self, and performance in daily life. For instance, individuals who are deeply depressed over their altered states are more likely to tend more toward self-deprecation and feeling unable to act. The individuals who have grown stronger and more confident of their skills in the past months are now most likely to push even harder for greater and sustained improvement. Most individuals with aphasia, though, fall in a middle range of these characteristics, that is, feeling quite challenged, wanting to do more, and yet uncertain how to progress from here. In truth, *all* of the characteristics here probably apply at times to most adults with aphasia. That is, most are depressed at times, most question their abilities to do more at times, most are strongly inspired do more at times. But, to simplify matters, we have purposefully "clumped" this complex array of characteristics into the three profiles you see above.

1–3 Where, precisely, your loved one rests within these artificially created profiles is of less importance than whether there has been continuing change since leaving formal care. It is still quite early in the recovery process, and because of this, upward or downward shifts among these profiles is apt to occur. However, some of this variation should be starting to level off now. If earlier suggestions were followed, the forward momentum now ought to move toward empowering your loved one to take part in a more self-determined and active form of daily life. although this trend is important, it is even more critical by the end of the second year to have these positive forces highly visible and dominant in daily life.

1 *Depressed and unable to act.* When these descriptors dominate after a year's duration of aphasia, it is common to find that the sufferer is likely a passive observer instead of an active participant in daily life. People with pervasive depression remain intractably stuck in the mire and muck they perceive around them. What matters the most, should this be the case for your loved one, is whether such a state has been there for an extended period of time or whether it is part of a progressive downward trend. While the preferred direction in recovery is ultimately in the opposite direction, away from despondency and toward a willingness to act, *it is common* to find individuals with aphasia experiencing temporary bouts of depression as they confront the realities of lasting disability.

1 If your loved one's depression fits the latter form of temporary withdrawal from life, it may represent an essential step toward later recovery. That is, progressively sliding downward may be necessary for your loved one to relinquish his or her unrealistic expectations of a full recovery and finally muster the strength required to sustain an upward drive to cope with life as it is. Even if this is the case, you do not want to leave your loved one in a diminished state for any protracted period of time. Should depression reign at this time, it is imperative to monitor it closely and to get "the swing" of daily life back and moving again.

1 Successfully giving that swing a push probably involves refocusing the attention of the person with aphasia, providing steady doses of something positive, and taking smaller "do-able" steps forward. Indirectly, it means getting the depressed adult away from thoughts of either the past or future, or the seeming enormity of the task ahead. It is the sufferer's natural tendency to gravitate toward this gloomy scenario rather than take any action whatsoever. It may take some creativity and cleverness to break the pattern of old and get your loved one moving in the preferred direction, but most people with aphasia eventually choose to relent.

1 Finally, it may be a case that biochemical changes within the injured brain are contributing to your loved one's ongoing despair (see Chapter 12, Depression). If this is the case, no matter how much you try to give his or her swing a nudge, it is apt to quickly resettle to a motionless state. The best management under these conditions is to pursue a combination of treatments: drug and behavioral. An antidepressant medication may be necessary to get matters moving in the right direction. Your loved one's doctor, neurologist, physiatrist, or rehab psychologist are likely contacts about such matters.

2 *Challenged and tenuously moving forward.* It is within this profile that most people with aphasia find themselves at 1-year postonset. Quite likely, they have already experienced the downward slide into a period

PERSON WITH APHASIA

of depression, and have begun working themselves slowly upward. It has not been a completely predictable path. For every three steps forward, there have been one or two of slipping backward or sideways. But by continuing to try, they have continued to learn more about their changed selves and the new terrain around them. Even if such mixed results seem only minimally positive, these individuals are usually making sizable gains internally toward learning how to negotiate the roads ahead. By gradually building on existing ways of participating in life, as urged months ago, they have probably *begun to see some value* in what does exist, rather than succumbing to the belief that none exists and nothing is possible.

2 However, in this realm of actively living life, much more remains to be done. Prompting your loved one to help you around the house or in other fun or self-chosen activities was only a starting point. We need to significantly expand on this notion now and in the months ahead. To do so, you need to understand a phenomenon recently popularized in a series of self-help books by M. Csikszentmihalyi, called *flow*. **The fundamental principle of flow is that all people need frequent and predictable periods in their lives when the actual act of participating in life dominates self-awareness, self-consciousness, and even awareness of reward! It is, in fact, the captivating nature of simply "doing" the activity that causes its initiator to forget entirely about self, time, or outcome.** At the moment of "doing," a person in flow is outside his or her own needs, and it is *solely* the involvement in the act itself that matters, and governs the rest of consciousness.

2 For people with aphasia, there is a constant stranglehold on life's possibilities because of their altered perception of themselves and their many unmet needs and unsatisfactory skills. Often they find it very difficult to step out of their own injury-induced scenarios and begin any process "of choice" again. Part of this heightened self-awareness and introspection comes from knowing that current abilities do not fit into the normal range of performance. In addition, brain injury diminishes one's ability to abstract and maintain a clear perception of one's needs in relation to the rest of the world. As a result, suggestions for increasing involvement in life are often met with a bevy of reasons for *not being* able. And yet, you need to know that most people with aphasia are capable of doing at least the same type of most of the activities they did prior to injury. What is different now is that the proficiency, efficiency, or accuracy of their performance is likely to be less!

2 I once knew a gentleman with aphasia who, before his injury, dearly loved to play golf. He shot a score in the mid-80s for 18 holes and consistently drove the ball 250+ yards off the tee. Following his injury, and with restricted use of the right side of his body, his best effort was a drive 50 yards straight down the fairway and a typical occurrence was a ball that might travel 20 to 30 yards in nearly any direction. He saw these latter efforts as *unworthy* and *unrewarding*, and he was sure others would view them the same way. Because of this, he rejected *any* further association with golf, a position that is quite understandable. Yet when asked, Did he still enjoy the process of hitting a golf ball? He quickly responded, "You bet!" From this, a more accurate picture emerged: It was *not* that he couldn't hit a golf ball—*he could*—and it was not even because he didn't like the process—*he did*. His nonparticipation was due, instead, to *his* perception of what that performance meant to himself and others!

PERSON WITH APHASIA

2 In approaching this dilemma, I asked this gentleman which was more difficult: To hit the golf ball 250 yards with his full physical capabilities, or to hit it 50 yards now and keep it straight with his hemiparesis? Again, his answer was instantaneous: It was much harder and *more skillful* on his part to hit the ball 50 yards straight now. Yet, the inherent pleasure from doing this activity was far less than his past joy in hitting longer drives. Next, I asked him, "If no one ever *saw* how far your ball went, and if you were left alone to work at your own pace, would golf be more inviting?" His answer, somewhat delayed, was, "I'm not sure, but I think so."

2 As a result, I began reinforcing some of what he had told me. He obviously *could hit a ball* and he *liked doing that*. It was the interference of a diminished value attached to this effort that really stood in the way of his participation. That value was small because his drives now needed to compare with the drives of old and that expectation was much too challenging. However, if his current abilities and their potentials could be matched, pleasure in the activity might return. So instead of asking him if he wanted to go participate (hit a bucket of balls), I kept putting a more reasonable expectation before him to consider. "Why don't we see whether you can hit a ball 50 yards straight down the fairway, say, 50% of the time by the end of next summer? We can go at nonpeak times when nobody is around. And remember, this task *was not the easier* of the two. You've already told me that, and *I agree*, hitting a ball 50 yards now and keeping it straight is much harder than hitting 250 yards before your injury! Give some thought to that: I'm more than willing to come along and assist if you choose to try." By reframing his perception of

PERSON WITH APHASIA what was expected and adding an endorsement for its legitimacy, he elected to pick up the golf club and try again, but from a different focus and with a different outcome in mind.

2 Through this action, this gentleman defined a different type of pleasure in playing golf. It did not happen overnight, but it did after weeks and months of going to the driving range. While involved in the activity, he came to forget his injury! Would his golf balls ever go 250 yards again? No! Did this seemingly matter? After a period of adjustment, it did *not!* **Over time and with support, this gentleman managed to blend what once *was* with what *now is*, and what he *perceived* as possible with what actually was possible. In doing so, he was able to redefine himself in relation to this process and to recapture a state of flow while hitting golf balls in a much diminished physical capacity.**

2 This story points out that it is not so much how skilled one needs to be to enter a state of flow. Forgetting oneself and becoming absorbed in the task relies instead on equating challenge with skill. If natural skill was the sole determiner of optimal participation in life, then only the very best performers in the world, whether musicians, athletes, authors, teachers, and so on, would ever have access to it. In truth, we *all* enter states of flow on a regular basis; we need to, according to M. Csikszentmihalyi, in order to live life to its fullest! But to have any chance of becoming a true participant, we must be willing to push or expand our current skills to the next higher level of function, regardless of where they were to begin with. It is through responding to this challenge that one unconsciously escapes a preoccupation with one's self.

2 It is this, the pursuit of flow, that is the next step for you and your loved one in the months and years ahead. Being aphasic, being brain-injured, and being less able does not preclude your loved one from entering it. It is only through actively interacting with life's challenges in chosen realms of participation that the person with aphasia is apt to be able to forget that he or she is aphasic and to begin building a restored sense of self and life. Adding flow to life makes aphasia a secondary factor or influence. **To reiterate, it is when participating in life with aphasia outweighs the living life because of aphasia, that your loved one's journey is nearing completion.**

2 The next section of suggestions introduces specific ways for caregivers to help their loved ones establish and promote flow in their lives.

They depend foremost on a cooperative and honest interaction about what is and is not possible for both of you. Resuming a meaningful life requires careful study, patience, effort, persistence, adaptation, and more persistence. If these ingredients naturally fit into your make-up or nervous system as a person and caregiver, then the suggestions that follow should help you. If, on the other hand, patience, desire, or the ability to persist do not fit, then it is likely that you need to look to other sources or individuals to aid you and your loved one. These, too, are discussed. You cannot constantly try to be more than you are and feel comfortable with. Finding an enduring solution requires your honesty and steadfast dedication.

PERSON WITH APHASIA

3 *Empowered and confident.* There is another, much smaller group of people with aphasia who reach the first year of coping with an overwhelming urge or desire to do more. Such individuals usually are not timid about trying; they possess a burning desire to do whatever it takes to remake themselves and their lives. Quite frequently, these people were "street fighters" before their injury. Whereas this interruption in life was certainly not of their choice, it is not going to dictate their existence now. In the totality of what life was or how it might be, there is no other option for them except to throw *every ounce of energy* into getting better. These individuals look at their diminished functions as a specific reason to get out bed and try harder every day!

3 Most of these individuals will improve simply because of their dedication and persistence. If something doesn't work, they quickly shift to something that will. Their personal drive and energy to do more propels them forward in spite of what isn't working or other obstacles along the way. However, if one wishes to get the most out of their directed energies, it makes sense to do everything possible to permit these individuals "to pump" their respective "swings" as fully and as hard as possible. What complicates the process, though, is that conventional wisdom (the considered opinions of trained professionals) often challenges or even blocks many of their chosen paths.

3 It is very difficult to condone a pursuit if it might threaten your loved one's safety or lead to a unsatisfactory conclusion. Whether your loved one's most sought-after desire is to talk, walk, run, swim, ride a bike, play a piano, go back to work, or drive a car, it is not uncommon to find informed sources who may announce that such a goal is either not possible or unreasonable to pursue. It may well be that their considered opinions *are right*, that is, your loved one may not be able to attain such an end. However, it is frequently more detrimental to prevent your loved one from trying, than for such an effort to fall short of its intended target. **In fact, as long as the criteria for participation are well known and agreed on in advance, it is *most therapeutic* to allow your loved one to determine his or her own path. Such a courtesy is not irresponsible or uncaring: it is actually just the opposite; it is what we afford any other person who we hold in honor or respect.**

3 As an example, let us consider the desire of many people with aphasia to resume driving an automobile. It may well be that your desire and the opinions of medical or rehab personnel are that such a feat is not possible. Perhaps there are concerns over your loved one's vision, reaction time, physical capabilities, or knowledge of the rules of the road. No matter what the blocking concerns may be, prohibiting your loved one from any chosen pursuit, especially if higher thinking and reasoning are sound, needs to be considered with extreme caution and forethought. If your normally endowed son or daughter announces one day, "I think I'll become an astronaut," you may immediately caution him or her about what this may entail, but you likely would *not prohibit* his or her attempts. It is his or her life to live as he or she would choose! It is not *you* who is responsible for this potential failure, and you are apt to let the process of pursuing the goal dictate its own outcome. So, too, you need to let the process of living life determine what your loved one does.

3 Some ground rules for such participation in many pursuits are likely needed. For instance, it is not wrong to state, "The rehab staff questions whether you can pass a driving test. I must admit to having grave worries about your safety and the safety of others, should you drive. But if that is what you want, let's talk about how we can make this endeavor comfortable for both of us. For me to help you, we need your doctor's medical approval, procurement of a driver's permit, completion of a certified driving school program, and a satisfactory score on a written and an on-road driving test. If you're willing to do these things, I'm willing to try to help you achieve them."

3 Nothing is conceded or lost by agreeing to terms that will, over time, allow you and your loved one to safely determine if his or her participation *might be possible*. Agreeing to support your son or daughter trying to become an astronaut does not mean he or she will be lifting off from a launching pad at Cape Kennedy next week. Time will tell what the outcome will be. In the same way, agreeing to terms that permit your loved one to pursue an interest of concern is not detrimental either, even when that outcome could be either unrealistic or unsafe. Defining the necessary requisites for the process frees you to reinforce your loved one's pursuit, and your doing so allows your loved one "to pump" his or her own swing. Most importantly, it promotes equality in the relationship, a crucial component to getting to your final destination.

PERSON WITH APHASIA

3 You may not know the exact criteria that would allow you to feel comfortable in letting your loved one drive a car. That is OK, too; that step can be postponed. The decision cannot be that your loved one is simply told he or she cannot proceed on a chosen course. There needs to be more than simply a proclamation that such an endeavor is not possible. He or she needs to be told what stands in the way of moving ahead, and what must be achieved to permit his or her active participation in that pursuit. If the necessary criteria for defining that option is not present, then you need to set out on a course that would permit its specification. Ask your loved one's physician for the rules in permitting someone with a brain injury to drive a car; call the Department of Motor Vehicles and inquire about their procedures; speak to someone at a driving school who has experience instructing people like your loved one; and talk with physical or occupational therapists about their recommendations. **You simply do not want to say: "You cannot do that!" Work to assist, not hinder, your loved one's chosen paths in daily life.**

**PERSON
WITH
APHASIA**

WHAT YOU MIGHT DO

1–3 MOVING TOWARD EMPOWERMENT

The targets over the next year need to be toward "empowering" your loved one, that is, finding ways of turning over more of the living of daily life to him or her, stepping back and letting your loved one set his or her own agenda, and urging its slow expansion and development. By now, you have likely established some base from which to work. Quite likely, some parts of this process are working better than others. Your loved one is apt to have begun accepting ownership of minor roles and functions in daily life, but the pace is often awkward and the task too much. Many parts of a chosen activity no more than get launched than they succumb to some interfering obstacle. As a result, he or she must stop, regroup, rethink how and what to do, and then try again or select a different course. The fluidity of life seems constantly "ajar." Don't dismay over these symptoms, they are normal. In the months ahead, skills and participation in life will become increasingly smooth and familiar.

1–3 WHAT TO DO NEXT

We begin with suggestions for persons with aphasia whose outlook lies somewhere in the middle of the above continuum, simply because this is where most individuals are at this point. However, smaller numbers do fall toward either end of this continuum, that is, either mired in depression and inactive (**1**), or endowed with self-confidence and an undaunting eagerness to move forward (**3**). If your loved one's profile better fits one of these two extremes, you will want to read the specific suggestions that follow later in this section. However, do not skip over the fundamental principles laid out in this first section.

2 CREATING A SENSE OF "FLOW" IN DAILY LIFE

The earlier example of the gentleman playing golf serves as a metaphor, not as a prescription for every person with aphasia who has not chosen to participate in life. Certainly, there are more factors to regaining an enriched lifestyle than simply redefining skills and expectations in terms of current skills and challenges. How people with aphasia viewed and conducted their lives prior to injury, as well as their personal preferences at the moment, influence life now. However, coming to empower your loved one to act often involves some form of blending *what once was* with *what is* and striving to eliminate as much myth from the equation as possible.

2 WHAT TO DO

- Try to determine how empowered your loved one may feel at this moment.
  Ask your loved one, "How much of your day and week is spent the way *you* would like?"
    Have him or her rate this on a 10-point vertical scale, that is, a 1 meaning that none of his or her day is spent as he or she would like, and a 10 meaning that life could not be improved on.
- Write down this number; you will want to recheck its value months later.
    It is not uncommon that people with aphasia at 1-year postinjury spend very little of their day in activities of their choosing. Ratings between 1–3 are common. However, over time, and with some willingness to act, there is no reason that such ratings cannot reach the 6–9 range in the years ahead.
- Start seeking activities that strongly appeal to your loved one, regardless of their apparent feasibility.
- You might wish to probe:
    Things that your loved one derived pleasure from prior to injury.
    Things that your loved one always wanted to do, but couldn't prior to injury.
    Things that might link your loved one with other people and events while assisting *them*.
- Try not to let the current perception of *inability* eliminate a choice from consideration.
    It may be that gardening, sewing, traveling, cooking, fishing, exercising, dancing, etc., may fall within your loved one's list of preferred options. As the above example illustrates, the issue is not whether your loved one can do these activities, as he or she

**PERSON
WITH
APHASIA**

likely *can* in a modified form. It doesn't matter what the entry level may be as long as your loved one enjoys the activity and can forego evaluating his or her current performance in relation to what it once was.

- The first step is pairing current skills with an effort that is viewed as possible, safe, and potentially rewarding over time.

  You needn't figure this out alone. In fact, you most likely will need help from others—specialists in rehab or people knowledgeable about the particular areas of interest. However, in soliciting this help, it is important to focus first on identifying starting points within your loved one's existing skills, and second, on where such participation might lead over time. Usually, it is impossible to know an answer to the second question until you have clearly identified the answer to the first question.

- When meeting with rehab specialists (see earlier Recovery section), specify your loved one's areas of interest and ask *where* and *how* participation might be possible now. Second, ask where such participation might lead over time.

  Maybe gardening was a selected activity. Ask the PT, OT, and speech-language pathologist to specify the types of activities he or she might attempt in this realm. Ask that their suggestions be as specific as possible. For instance, can your loved one get up and down from ground level when planting flowers or weeding? If so, how? If not, what might be done to permit this? Maybe a special chair or bench could be fashioned. Gardening catalogs are full of adaptive devices to make this process easier and more enjoyable for many individuals with physical limitations.

- Plan to leavie this meeting with a plan of action.

  Possibly these specialists think your loved one could look through seed catalogs now and begin selecting several varieties of flowers. In early March, these seeds could be placed in small germination pots in a south-facing kitchen window and tended until early summer. Then, your loved one could transplant them in flower beds along the front walk.

- Focus on the act of doing and de-emphasize how much is accomplished or its value at this time.

- If any comparing is done, compare the value of acting versus *not* acting at all.

  A person who is empowered has a willingness to try. There need be no commitment beyond that . . . exploring something

PERSON WITH APHASIA

of interest! The truly important step is not whether the chosen activity ultimately remains a part of daily life or not. The value of trying is that it provides your loved one with an experiential reference from which to begin to better select and refine what he or she does want to pursue. Remember that, short of trying, nothing will change!

- From the outset, look for ways of involving other people and resources besides yourself.

  Maybe you have access to a local stroke or aphasia group, and one or two of its members likes to garden and would like to work with your loved one. Maybe there is a local garden group at a senior center. Maybe a member of that group, once introduced to your loved one, might elect to spend some time individually assisting him or her. Perhaps there are nonprofit agencies in your community that strive to advocate for individuals with disabilities and to address the needs of people with the goal of promoting their independence and self-sufficiency in daily life.

- Remember that when a good idea gets stalled in the "real world" . . . and it likely will, correction often involves a small adjustment, not a complete overhaul of the entire system. Often getting life moving again requires attention to a number of smaller issues:

  "How can I make whatever is *not* working even simpler?"

  "How can I do that without accentuating my loved one's disability?"

  "How can I keep the task fun and engaging?"

  "How can I start things in motion without doing the task entirely myself?"

- Step back, simplify, look for inviting parts of a preferred activity, and begin doing these *together*.

  The sole aim at first is to see if a chosen activity naturally leads to any desire on the part of your loved one to try to pump that swing. If not, it may be important to probe why the desire is lacking, as in the example of the gentleman rejecting golf yet inwardly still drawn to it. It is *necessary*, though, that your loved one agree to act rather than having this action imposed on him or her.

- Keep the process fun and continue probing until you or others find the right swing(s) that your loved one can and will pump.

- Every 3 to 6 months, re-examine your loved one's rating on that 10-point scale.

Check for gradual improvement. Don't expect anything more. Moving from 1 or 2 to 4 or 5 on this 10-point scale is a *huge accomplishment*. It may take many months or years depending on circumstances, personal needs, and style. The prediction of such gradual progress may appear disheartening at first glance; however, it is not so much the amount of gain that matters as it is coming to feel that life is pointed in the right direction. The constancy and momentum of this forward movement over time will ensure that your loved one will advance on this 10-point scale. If you reach your second anniversay with aphasia feeling as if you are assisting *from behind* rather than directing from in front, you will be where you need to be—regardless of the number on the scale.

2 WHAT TO SAY

- "Getting better means trying. If you could do anything you'd like, what would it be?"
- "Come on, help me, help you!"
- "Let's pretend we're about to go do something you'd like—in spite of this injury—what would it be?"
- "Come on, play along with me, let's give this a try. You really don't have a lot to lose."
- "I'll be right here to see that nothing goes astray."
- "If you don't like it, we'll either change it so you do, or we'll look somewhere else!"
- "By continuing to try, we are apt to figure out eventually what you really do like."
- "Short of doing something, nothing is going to change."
- "That is not good for you, but it also is not good for me."
- "Let's make things better *together!*"

1 WHEN DEPRESSION AND SELF-DEPRECATION DOMINATE

It is possible that your loved one may reach the first year's anniversary of coping feeling severely depressed. When this is the case, individuals often view themselves and their abilities as marginal. Such a debilitating state of mind frequently comes as a reaction to either perceived or real functional losses or from neurochemical changes in the brain that directly affect one's ability to monitor moods or emotions. In either case, people confronting severe depression are apt to withdraw from life and to refuse to act.

1 WHAT TO DO

- Search out a physician who is comfortable with treating *depression* as a lingering part of the aphasia.
  By a year postinjury, it often takes a trained specialist with knowledge, experience, and insight into the chronic nature and consequences of aphasia. **Too often, once a person with aphasia is physically stable, a mood or emotional problem is viewed as *a secondary problem*, or simply something the sufferer *needs to learn to live with*. When depression remains for months at a time, this is *not* the case! Professional help is needed!** Through a combined treatment approach of using an antidepressant medication, like Prozac, and behaviorial modifications at home, noticeable improvements are possible. The trick is in finding the medical specialist who perceives and manages this problem with the seriousness it deserves.
- For referral sources, ask:
  the physician who treated your loved one during rehab.
  > You need *not* feel obligated to ask this doctor to treat this problem, although he or she may be the best referral source. You may wish to begin by simply asking his or her opinion on the matter, what action it deserves, and who would be the recommended professional for referral. If depression has lingered on, do not back away or compromise on finding a professional who considers this a serious matter to treat and resolve such as:
  the rehab social worker or psychologist.
  community agencies dealing with mental health, aging, or personal rights for disabled adults.
  other people with aphasia in a peer support group who have had to cope with depression.
- Do know that the best qualified professional may fall within one of many medical specialties:
  physiatrist (rehab), neurologist (brain function), gerontologist (aging), psychiatry (mental health), internist (interal body dysfunction), or family practitioner (general medicine specialist).
- Look for the professional with the most knowledge and experience in treating *depression* in people with aphasia.

PERSON WITH APHASIA

- Getting life moving forward often requires more than medical intervention, it requires changes in one's living environment as well. Once again, the key here is gently urging the person with aphasia to become involved at some elementary, yet engaging, level of participation, even if it is only peripheral and somewhat sporadic to begin with. Getting a foot in the door is the aim. If you are stymied as to where and how to do this, turn once more to core rehab staff to point you in the right direction. No matter how severe your loved one's aphasia, there are always areas within his or her existing skills that can be called on. Your loved one's recovery is partially tied to putting these to use, even if minimally at first.
- **If you cannot find any satisfaction or any enduring answers and if your loved one remains despondent and nonparticipatory in life, call or write to me at Living with Aphasia, Inc. and let's discuss your particulars. You do not want to let this stay untreated!**

1 WHAT TO SAY

- "*Your* getting better involves *you*."
- "I know you may *not* feel up to doing anything at this time."
- "But, for *you* to improve, *you* need to try."
- "And if you won't do it for yourself, then please, at least *try* for me."
- "If you'll try two times at any one thing, and if you still want to stop, then, that's OK! "At least you tried!"
- "Short of trying, nothing is going to change."

3 WHEN EMPOWERMENT AND SELF-CONFIDENCE REIGN

If a person's attitude tends toward the postive end of the continuum, this is obviously advantageous. Feeling relatively in charge of one's destiny and current direction in life while trying to gain more function is the ideal position for making the most of the road ahead.

3 WHAT TO DO

- Review the earlier suggestions for fostering optimal participation in life.
- Being confident and motivated does not preclude the need for them.

- Acknowledge these strengths and try to help your loved one keep his or her confidence and ambition strong, active, and working in his or her own behalf.
- The key to doing this is:

  encourage activities at your loved one's level of ability and desire:

  > not *too* taxing.

  > not *too* easy.

  > of his or her own choice, and if at all possible, fun.
- Jointly settle on the terms or conditions you both need to feel comfortable pursuing a given course:

  Present the list of conditions that would influence your support and allow your loved one to react:

  > If he or she agrees with your list, move ahead.

  > If he or she disagrees, revisit that list to find out where the problem rests, returning to the earlier scenario about driving a car:

  >> Maybe your loved one doesn't feel that going to a driving school is necessary. Perhaps retaking the written and actual driving test is all that he or she wishes to do. You do *not* want to reject his or her position any more than you would have before the injury. As you likely would have done then, offer another compromise, for instance, maybe the entire driving school program would not be needed but at least several outings with a trained instructor would be. Should the instructor feel he or she was doing well enough then, you would be willing to forego the complete school program.

- Once these conditions are settled on, *support* your loved one's efforts as completely as possible.

  Again, you cannot be responsible for satisfying all parts of your loved one's needs, but to the extent that you can cooperatively reinforce a chosen direction, you have done your job. It is likely that your loved one will have to assume greater ownership of the task over time and that others will need to assist as well.
- Point out a probable progression that might follow if your loved one's skills improve over time.

  Sometimes entry levels for beginning a pursuit seem so menial and removed from the target that your loved one's motivation may wane. With the assistance of the rehab staff, lay out a possible path that skill levels may follow over time if he or she continues to improve. Such an overview gives your loved one a longer perspective of what may eventually come of this effort.

PERSON WITH APHASIA

**PERSON
WITH
APHASIA**

- Keep encouraging your loved one to do as much in his or her behalf as possible.

3 WHAT TO SAY

- "I understand where you want to go and what you want to do!"
- "And within reason, I'll do everything I can to help you get there!"
- "To do this, though, here is what I need in order to feel comfortable and to be able to help you in this pursuit:"
  (list the conditions that stand in the way of your support or participation)
- "Do these seem reasonable and agreeable to you?"
  (If your loved one endorses them, move ahead; if he or she doesn't, back up and find out where the point of contention rests; look for an agreeable compromise and proceed from there.)
- "Here's how we might start."
  (establish a beginning point from which to start this pursuit)
- "Here's where it might lead over time."
  (specify a possible course)
- "We'll just take a step at a time and see where it leads."
- "If it works out, fine; if it doesn't, we'll find something else that will."

RELATIONSHIP

1–I know you love the person I was, but do you respect the person I currently am?

*2–For me, I need to be **more** my own person.
Please allow me and help me to do more on my own.
That's what I need the most!*

WHAT TO KNOW

1 Your loved one is likely viewing him or herself as being *more deficited* than well. Given the longevity of your relationship, this person probably is not questioning your love or commitment, but rather worrying that his or her diminished skills may tarnish your respect of him or her. Since many people with aphasia struggle constantly throughout the first year after injury to regain some sense of self-worth and self-respect, it is not strange that this injured person may wonder whether you respect him or her under current conditions.

1–2 It may seem contradictory in a period of personal uncertainty that your loved one may be requesting more freedom to act in his or her own behalf. The simple truth is that most people with aphasia contend with opposing desires at about this time in recovery. On the one hand, present skill levels are not good, so acquiescing to someone "more capable" seems not only logical, but the only way to ensure the job gets done properly. There is often considerable embarrassment over not being able to do even simple tasks. On the other hand, your loved one is likely growing aware that his or her nonparticipation or quickly acquiescing to you or others, is not helping him or her either. The dilemma has led to inactivity, feelings of isolation, boredom, and personal despair. **Although present function may not be as complete or prompt as before, acting in some capacity feels more desirable than *not* acting at all! This second realization is a healthy, positive sign of recovery. It is one involving internal conflict and challenge, but ultimately an easier choice than having to deal with total inactivity.**

PERSON WITH APHASIA

2 Your loved one may remain "stuck" in a lesser inactive role, however. He or she may be concerned that performing "poorly" will *only diminish his or her value* in your eyes, or he or she may feel that you have *assumed responsibility* for parts of life that he or she couldn't. Although your loved one may have actively sought your assistance at first, it may well be that he or she is coming to want and need to do more in life on his or her own. There is often a clear plea to, "Please value *me* as I am (even though I may not totally value myself as I am), and please allow me to try to do more in my own behalf."

WHAT YOU MIGHT DO

1–2 ALLOWING YOUR LOVED ONE MORE RESPONSIBILITY

Transferring responsibilities to your loved one is nothing new, and, hopefully, you have been encouraging his or her developing levels of independence at home. At this juncture, however, it is even more crucial to reassess what you are doing

RELATIONSHIP

1–I know you love the person I was, but do you respect the person I currently am?

*2–For me, I need to be **more** my own person.*
Please allow me and help me to do more on my own.
That's what I need the most!

PERSON WITH APHASIA

unconsciously for your loved one and to determine which of these tasks might be turned over to him or her. Keeping in mind his or her concerns about self-respect, it is important to reassure your loved one that his or her level of skill is unimportant, but it is the willingness *to try* and to *extend effort* that is.

1–2 WHAT TO DO

- Write out a list of daily functions that you now provide or oversee for your loved one on a regular basis.
    Include only those functions that you did not provide prior to the injury.
- In each case, sit for a few minutes and rethink how you might shift a portion of what you are currently doing back to your loved one.
- Don't make any decisions alone, involve your loved one from the beginning.
    You did not unilaterally decide your loved one's fate before the injury, so try not to do so now. If aphasia is all that he or she has, it is likely that reasoning is relatively intact. Strive to keep your exchange about such matters much as it was pre-aphasia, that is, one adult addressing another adult. Avoid any exchange that diminishes his or her power or status by addressing or treating him or her as an "underling" or "child." By conversing as an equal, there is a much greater chance that your loved one will feel a sense of ownership from the beginning.
- Overview your list, ask if he or she can think of additions or changes.
- Ask which of these activities or responsibilities he or she might like to resume if supported.
- Ask whether he or she has any ideas about how such a transfer of responsibility might occur at this time.
- Don't concentrate solely on the mechanics, but convey your *confidence* in him or her as a person.
- Remember to avoid teaching per se. Try instead to facilitate function through demonstration.
- If you are unsure of any of the steps in a plan, get input from a trained specialist.
- As always, try to keep the endeavor positive and fun, not business-like.

WHAT TO KNOW

COMMUNICATION
1–I still want to talk!
2–How can I increase my progress?

PERSON WITH APHASIA

1 Of all the areas of remaining dysfunction, it is often within this realm—talking—that your loved one wishes to do more! If you've followed the earlier suggestions, it is likely that you've met regularly with a speech-language pathologist to plot ways of facilitating interactions at home, with others, or in the community. By now, a truer picture is emerging, to suggest whether or not your loved one may be one of those communicators who can make his or her basic needs known through speech. If talking is not functional to that degree, it still doesn't mean that it won't ever be. It may simply take longer. After a year, though, if talking is severely impaired, it lessens the likelihood that everyday usage will return to a functional level.

1–2 Regardless of the level of current function, it is likely that your loved one is still desirous of stimulation that might further his or her speech and communication. In Chapter 6, Person with Aphasia—Communication, we offered suggestions for promoting speaking or other desired communication skills since formal treatment was ending. Possibly, you have found a long-term therapeutic aid, such as attending a local peer group or individualized services through a university training program for speech-language pathologists. **For many people with aphasia, though, any treatment now is apt to involve exercises with you at home and natural, real-life contacts and situations with others outside the home. It is reasonable to expect that both of these environments hold potential for fostering change in the years ahead.**

2 It may seem to you that improvement in talking or communicating at home is slowing. This observation is likely true. However, this is not a reason to despair or to avoid attempting to add more. Even when functional gains from speech practice seem negligible, practicing may still be important to your loved one's self-esteem and self-image. For example, his or her repeating words in a conversation or reading them aloud may not seem to transfer to spontaneous everyday use. You may then question whether continuing with these "nudges" to the speaking "swing" makes sense. The answer is likely in whether your loved one still encourages your assistance! He or she may remain *starved* for any kind of verbal interplay that activates his or her speech machinery! Remember that talk-

PERSON WITH APHASIA

ing was a mainstay in daily life before, and being without it has only heightened his or her desire to do *anything* possible to promote it.

2 There is another reason for including some regular stimulation of speech at home. Specifically, if talking isn't improving adequately, your loved one needs some sense of its limitations to feel free to entertain other options for communicating. These methods were first introduced in Chapter 5, Caregiver—Communication, and then expanded on in Chapter 6, Caregiver—Communication. They are placed in a personal context for you in Caregiver—Communication later in this chapter. **If talking is not functional at this time, it is important that these augmentative means of interacting are in use, and that they continue to improve in the months ahead.**

2 If some talking is possible, it is best to find natural, meaningful ways of making use of it rather than just in contrived speaking tasks or drills. For example, if your loved one is able to repeat short phrases, then you might wish to provide choices in spoken pairs, and ask that he or she indicate his or her choice through that form of repetition. You can say, "Do you want to take a ride or stay home?" or "Would you prefer to go to a movie or eat out?" This format allows your loved one to respond by modeling your words. On the other hand, if you ask an open-ended question such as, "What would you like to do?" he or she may not be able to respond.

2 It is equally important to give your loved one opportunities to converse and communicate with others outside the home. In Chapter 8, we detail how to find or set up protective communities outside the home in which the collective membership in a small group knows and accepts your loved one's speaking limitations because he or she is *one of them*. That is, he or she provides an ongoing service, shared interest, or commitment that bonds him or her to everyone else in this forum because they, too, hold this service and interest in high regard. Starting to sample where in the outside world your loved one might feel most comfortable and willing to interact begins now.

2 Make sure he or she accompanies you whenever possible to outside settings such as the grocery store, bank, church, theater, restaurants, convenience stores, or shopping malls. From these encounters, you may learn where your loved one might wish to spend more of his or her time interactively. In the third case presentation in Chapter 14, you will meet a gentleman with aphasia who came to spend much of his communicative time outside the home as a volunteer at a daycare center. The idea for pursuing this target came from observing him interact freely and out of personal choice with youngsters when on shopping outings with a friend.

PERSON WITH APHASIA

WHAT YOU MIGHT DO

1–2 STRIVING FOR MORE TALKING AND BETTER COMMUNICATION

COMMUNICATION
1–I still want to talk!
2–How can I increase my progress?

Gains in this realm may come more slowly from here on out. This is *not*, however, a reason to back away from trying to keep this swing in motion. In fact, of the "swings" your loved one would like to try to pump, this is apt to be high on his or her list.

1–2 WHAT TO DO

- Revisit the speech-language pathologist who has been overseeing your care.
- Specifically request talking and communicating tasks that might be done at home to:
  increase your loved one's ability to talk.
  increase your "connectedness" as a couple.
  increase your loved one's ability to work independently on areas of his or her interest.
- Continue to look for resources outside the home that might provide some communicative stimulation.

WHAT TO KNOW

FAMILY/FRIENDS
1–What happened to our "supposed" friends?
2–How will we ever gain new ones when I cannot talk?

1 Over the past 6 months or so, you and your loved one have likely increased your contact with family members and friends. For reasons introduced in Chapter 6, Caregiver—Family/Friends, some close friendships from the past have likely changed in their form and constancy. Often this change involves less contact and less personal closeness. Most conspicuously absent, though,

PERSON WITH APHASIA are those individuals who your loved one might have felt were most vested in his or her well-being. This trend and realization often brings with it feelings of embitterment, pain, anger, and personal betrayal.

1 Some of the suggestions from prior chapters may have helped maintain or reinforce social ties that otherwise would have gone astray. If by chance, you and your loved one have not familiarized yourself with this information (Chapters 5 and 6, Family/Friends), it is not too late to do so, nor is it too late to approach certain important others with whom you might wish to try to reestablish contact and bonds. The main theme to remember is that this breakdown is *often not of either party's choosing*. It is due to an incomplete or inaccurate understanding of what has happened, a lack of understanding of what residual abilities remain, and a lack of confidence in how best to cope with them. With your very good friends from the past, it may make sense to invest *further effort* to reduce or eliminate some of the myths and fallacies that keep people apart. If an apparent breakdown or rift still remains, at least you can rest assured that knowing you did your part to try to hold the friendship together.

2 Not being able to readily communicate may indeed obstruct the ease with which your loved one may acquire new friends. However, not being able to communicate is actually less of a hindrance than he or she or you might think. **There are many people with aphasia who cannot talk or express their basic needs and yet can readily interact with others and form new friendships. What is more important than talking is how the person with aphasia views and presents him- or herself to others in an interactive situation.** If your loved one approaches others and life with a confident and "in charge" manner and attitude, it is quite likely that much of the outside world will reciprocate in a positive way too. Not every new acquaintence may be so kind, but many are! What astounds many normal interactants is seeing someone with aphasia make a concerted effort to share with others, even if his or her talking is not perfect.

2 Having the outside world be more receptive to interacting with your loved one, and making new friends are not the same thing. Finding people who truly choose to spend quality time with your loved one is usually a slow and somewhat agonizing process. As far as finding mutual friends, it often takes finding people who either share your predicament, that is, another couple confronting the dilemmas of aphasia, or finding others who *choose to look beyond* your loved one's communication problem and enjoy the person as he or she is. As your loved one becomes more mentally and attentionally astute, he or she is apt to do more communicating and interacting with others irrespective of whether talking comes readily or not. It is from these interactions that new friendships are likely to evolve. Much more is devoted to this process in Chapter 8.

PERSON WITH APHASIA

WHAT YOU MIGHT DO

1–2 REESTABLISHING FRIENDSHIPS

> **FAMILY/FRIENDS**
> *1–What happened to our supposed friends?*
> *2–How will we ever gain new ones when I cannot talk?*

It makes sense to put forth a concerted effort to stay connected with people who mattered the most to you before this injury occurred. To do this, you need to systematically give your collective swing a push by addressing their worries or concerns as well as your own. You may not want to abandon this effort until they have had ample time to adjust and to decide on an informed course of their own. If they decide to move farther away, it is important to understand that this action may not be *because of you*, but because of their own fears and feelings of inadequacy. They simply may not be able to change their frames of reference and comfort level. More importantly, with time you *will* find others who do relate to and value who you are, not who you once were!

1–2 WHAT TO DO

- Consciously revisit your connections with past close friends: mutually decide if any of these still warrant some time and effort on your part.
  If so, how might you wish to proceed?
  Recall how difficult this process is for everyone.
  Strive to eliminate feelings of personal rejection, and simply act on your desires to strengthen these ties whether they may be reciprocated or not.
- Begin exploring other situations where *new friendships* might evolve:
  Enroll in local aphasia/stroke support groups.
    The National Aphasia Association can aid you with the most current information about groups in your region of the country: 1–800–922–4622.

**PERSON
WITH
APHASIA**

The National Stroke Association may be another outlet to contact: 1–303–762–9922

Taking day or weekend excursions from local senior centers.

Enrolling in community adult education courses of interest.

Going on weekend outings to small, intimate settings, such as bed and breakfasts.

Attending elder hostel classes and events.

- Realize that establishing new friendships will take some time.
- Look for creative ways that might foster bonds with others.

For instance, your loved one may have liked to go fishing. However, since his or her injury you wonder how successful such an outing might be. You explore some adaptations to his or her fishing pole and reel that permit him or her to participate with the use of only one hand and arm. You begin visiting a local lake on summer weekends and renting a fishing boat. You typically ride along and read while he or she fishes. In the course of these trips, you meet another couple with similar interests. With time, the two people who like to fish go off on their own, while you lounge around with the other person reading and chatting. After a day's outing, you sit together and share that day's stories over dinner.

EMPLOYMENT

1–I couldn't go back to my old job but I sure would like to have something meaningful to fill that void!

2–What might that be?

WHAT TO KNOW

1 For most people with aphasia, returning to work has not proven possible. A smaller number has either returned to their old jobs, usually with more restricted duties and less responsibilities, or moved to new jobs where the duties better match their existing skills and interests. Whether paid or not, roles within the world of business are rewarded for efficiency, productivity, and quality of performance, standards that place people with aphasia at a clear disadvantage. It is not that individuals with low productivity cannot contribute meaningfully or significantly, it is that monetary compensation is society's reward system, and it is often interpreted as a measure of "worth." For most persons with aphasia, tasks take longer and require more concentration and effort, and certain outcomes may not be as refined or complete as they once were. Yet, none of these restrictions need stand in the way of your loved one's perceived ability to work or his or her perceived value in the workplace.

1–2 It is likely that some form of work was and still is important to your loved one's self-worth. Because of this, it is important to recapture the personally rewarding elements of working even if its form is much different now. I once knew a gentleman who had made his living prior to his aphasia converting a never-ending list of ideas into practical realities. Since he had far more ideas than actual plans or money to implement his notions, he typically "sold" them to others who had the means and desire to develop them. His joy in working was problem-solving. After his aphasia, he could no longer easily communicate his thoughts to others. In fact, in the beginning months, he could not readily understand what was said to him. And yet, he longed to return to some form of his old occupation of problem-solving.

PERSON WITH APHASIA

1–2 Through the aid of a volunteer who was an executive for a large service-related company, it was possible to provide this gentleman with some real-life dilemmas to resolve. At first, this executive volunteered to be trained in how to understand and interact with this gentleman having aphasia. After a couple of months of learning and practicing their interactive skills, this gentleman began attending some lower level managerial meetings at this executive's company. At first, he tape-recorded conversations for later review so he could be sure he understood the nature of the problem. Then after mulling them over for several days, he sat with the executive and shared his notions of how the company might improve its operations. It was not so critical to him that every idea be perfect or accepted; what was important to this person was resuming a process he dearly loved.

2 Putting people with aphasia back to work in ways of their own choice is actually a part of creating "flow" in their lives (See Person with Aphasia: Emotions—Feelings About Self—Daily Life in this chapter). As with this gentleman, this process means trying to recreate the daily challenges that so inspired your loved one to act in life before his or her injury. Whether these activities are of the same form or manner as before is less important. Whether they lead to any financial remuneration is also secondary, although getting paid may be a requisite in your loved one's mind.

2 What is needed now are environments where your loved one's contribution is sufficiently valuable to warrant the time and support that others must provide to keep it going. In other words, you need to look to *partnerships* in real life that work to everyone's benefit. Chapter 8 expands on the practical and logistical considerations for achieving these ends.

EMPLOYMENT

1–I couldn't go back to my old job, but I sure would like to have something meaningful to fill that void!

2–What might that be?

PERSON WITH APHASIA

WHAT YOU MIGHT DO

1–2 FINDING WORK AGAIN

Often, it is not so much returning to your loved one's former job that is important to him or her. Rather, it is restoring the underlying process that yielded personal satisfaction from working. **Finding work now requires identifying the satisfying parts of a task and matching them with current skill levels. Over the next year, you and your loved one will only begin to "explore" outside settings where his or her participation might be possible. Your loved one is likely only beginning to sense what may or may not be possible in his or her newly acquired sense of being.** Chapter 8 is dedicated to helping you get reconnected with the outside world. For now, though, you need only concentrate on fun, exploratory excursions that might evolve later into something more meaningful. We offer a broad overview of this process through another example.

1–2 AN EXAMPLE

Maybe your loved one was a trial attorney before his aphasia. These demands and duties are now totally beyond his current scope of function, and he is left idle much of his waking hours, longing for a similar experience. It was the process of ordering the unmanageable and unexplainable and presenting it in a more understandable and workable form that your loved one thrived on. Now, through some joint exploring of alternatives, he elects to begin volunteering at a food bank one morning a week. He begins by learning and observing the operative parts of this puzzle, much as he would if taking on a new case. As he understands more, he naturally begins "ordering" and "presenting" new options for collecting and distributing food supplies. A year and a half later, he is working three mornings a week as a volunteer supervisor, checking incoming and outgoing food supplies to see that they are ordered, arranged, and disbursed in a timely and proper manner. Besides being rewarding to him, this position allows the food bank a quality service it previously lacked. Both parties benefit!

1–2 WHAT TO DO

- If a work-related activity is desired, look first at the broader picture to see what most appealed to your loved one's personal interests and motivations prior to injury.

- Seek out your loved one's input.
- Begin sorting out together what factors were most rewarding and important in his or her prior work.
- Start looking at possible environments and activities where current skills might support limited participation in a manner desired.
- Consult with rehab specialists about how current skills might be matched to preferred outside activities.
- Keep initial outings exploratory and fun.
  At first, you want to explore possibilities but not get overwhelmed with how they might work.
- Look for a way that planned activities might be built into a *partnership*.
  That is, the activity needs to benefit all parties. Chapter 8 details this process more fully.
- The goal now is simply to identify some areas of life where flow from working might evolve over time.

WHAT TO KNOW

> **RECOVERY**
> *1–How can we make things better, they seem stuck to me!*
> *2–I cannot accept that our lives may not get any better than this!*
> *3–There has got to be **more** possible . . . but **what** and **how**?*

1–2 Near the end of the first year, caregivers often experience the first alarm that recovery may be over. Most had hoped for *much more* by now. In truth, they had hoped to see a close semblance of the person they once knew. During rehab or even the first 3 or 4 months at home, there was simply too much to do or think about to worry over recovery's eventual outcome. Instead, every ounce of energy was channeled into getting back as much function as possible. Quite likely, these initial efforts yielded consistent and visible signs of improvement all along the way. Now, though, physical and communicative gains are becoming limited both in their frequency and magnitude. It is this "plateauing" of returned function and the amount of remaining dysfunction that frightens, even discourages, many caregivers at this point.

CAREGIVER

2 What is happening, though, is a healthy and necessary stage in the course of recovery. It is a new phase of "awareness" that you *are only beginning* to see and internalize. Yes, you were told repeatedly that your

CAREGIVER loved one's disabilities would come and stay! Yet these words carried little meaning: They were devoid of a personal context in which to place
them. It is not dissimilar to hearing stories of people victimized by crime
and then coming home one evening to find the door of your *own* house
wide open and its contents strewn about and violated. Coming to understand the reality of your loved one's permanently disabled self requires
the same thing; you needed to see and experience its consequences *in
your own terms and manner*. You have needed to see the debris throughout the house and your prized stamp collection gone before your loved
one's injury would compute. And, yes, although these stamps are gone,
likely forever, it doesn't mean that putting the house back together, or
restoring a different collection, is gone. It is *not!*

2–3 It is not strange that caregivers arrive at this juncture embittered and
angry: "I cannot envision a life *like this*. What can we do to make it different!" Not relinquishing your hopes until now was important. It provided you and your loved one with the strength to put your house back
in order. It is likely that this obsession provided the impetus to keep moving and trying over the past year. **Now, however, it is unavoidable that
you take stock before you try to shape this configuration to your
advantage. Yes, subsequent gains *will* likely be smaller and less frequent, but they are *not* over!**

3 The most important thing to know is that recovery's course and outcome is not dependent on what does or does not return. Recall the words
posted on your refrigerator that you have been looking at daily for the
past 6 to 9 months: They still are as true today as they were the day you
wrote them! Remember that recovery is more about making use of what
does work, than fretting over what doesn't, especially from this point
forward. Recovery depends more on reassembling and reordering the
contents of the disheveled house, than fixating on how perfect the house
once was. The truth is, your loved one has likely only begun to turn the
corner on his or her changed self. In this climate, it is not surprising or
wrong that you may need to recalibrate, too. The "whys" are covered in
more detail in the next section entitled: Emotions—Feelings About Your
Loved One—Daily Life.

WHAT YOU MIGHT DO

1–3 SEEING RECOVERY IN A DIFFERENT LIGHT

RECOVERY
1–*How can we make things better, they seem stuck to me!*
2–*I cannot accept that our lives may not get any better than this!*
3–*There has got to be **more** possible . . . but **what** and **how**?*

Your loved one's recovery is not stuck even if gains in daily function are beginning to slow. Recovery's course depends more on discovering and actively pursuing what is or might be, than ruminating over what is not present or not working (see Person with Aphasia—Emotions-Feelings About Self-Daily Life)! No matter how severe your loved one's aphasia, there *is* potential for keeping the recovery process moving forward.

1–3 WHAT TO DO

- **Realize that the current stagnation is not about recovery's path or longevity . . . but about coming to terms, *your own terms*, with your loved one's *permanent injury*.**
- **Accepting its permanence takes nothing away from the recovery equation.**

  Giving up returning to one's old self is not synonymous with giving up on recovery. Just the opposite, it frees the two of you to work with what is possible and to build from there. There is *no longer an expectation* that he or she will or should be more. Recovery is not bound to your loved one's resumption of past or normal functions, although these are welcomed and likely to continue to occur on a much reduced scale, but solely on making the most of what is and what might be.

- Begin looking for smaller gains in daily performance.

  It is *not* that functional return has stopped. It is that the extent and frequency of change has diminished. **Gains now are apt to come in spurts. Nothing will happen for months at a time, and then another series of improvements will emerge. These gains, although undetectable on a larger scale of function, will likely continue for years.**

- Acknowledge and reward these gains whenever they occur.

CAREGIVER

Nothing prompts your loved one to try harder than realizing the swing is moving in the right direction. As well, nothing keeps you more oriented to recovery's presence and progress than looking for and noting such outcomes.

- Keep noting change in a written log.

  Slower change does not eliminate the importance of keeping your past records. Nothing provides a better overview of where you have been or where you likely need to go next than this.

EMOTIONS—FEELINGS ABOUT YOUR LOVED ONE—DAILY LIFE

One of several scenarios is likely evolving:

1–**DISCOURAGED**—*He or she has given up: What kind of existence is this? The good life is **over**!*

2–**STYMIED**—*He or she is still trying but little is changing: There's got to be more, but **where** and **how**?*

3–**DETERMINED**—*He or she isn't giving up and neither am I: We've always managed before, we'll manage this too!*

WHAT TO KNOW

1–3 Caregivers differ, as well, in their reactions and adjustments to their loved ones' injuries. *Their emotions* may range from severe discouragement to a strong determination. A majority, though, remain perplexed over how to proceed from here. *Views of their loved ones* range from "He or she isn't even trying anymore!" to "He or she is staying with this, and so will I!" Again, though, most fall in a middle ground: "He or she is still wanting to change, but little seems to be happening!" *Their view of daily life* may range from resignation to a lesser existence to a strong will to push forward. The more likely scenario is not wanting to give up, but being uncertain where to move next.

1–3 In a similar way to the earlier profiles of people with aphasia in this chapter, caregivers likely vary from moment to moment in terms of their characteristics. But like people with aphasia, a predominance of one characteristic may enhance the likelihood of another. Above you find three descriptive profiles of caregivers. Quite likely, most travelers reside in a middle range at this point in time.

1–3 Note, too, that your profile may not mirror your loved one's (see Person with Aphasia—Emotions—Feelings About Self—Daily Life). That is, just because his or her dominant view of life at the moment may be restricted, does not mean that yours is. Also, just because he or she may be feeling empowered and eager to move on, does not preclude that you may feel highly discouraged at the moment. However, a majority of people with aphasia and their caregivers are apt to fall within middle ranges. As a result, many *do share* some similar characteristics.

CAREGIVER

1 *Discouraged and seeing life as over.* Should you be here and have been here for any duration, you need to address this situation immediately! Nothing threatens the journey's completion more than prolonged bouts of mental or emotional despair. You, as a caregiver or friend, are only as good to your loved one and yourself as your mental and physical health allow. For this reason, it is imperative to get to the source(s) of conflict contributing to your decline.

1 Caregivers' discouragement typically originates from one of several sources: (a) realizing that your loved one's *gains are slowing*, (b) *feeling overwhelmed* with existing demands and responsibilities, and (c) *feeling entrapped.* Regardless of whether your despair is tied to these or other sources, the journey cannot continue without your support and well-being. To start with, moving forward likely requires ridding yourself of any feelings associated with your loved one's injury that engender guilt, shame, obligation, anger, or false hope. Fundamentally, to get back on track, you need to let yourself *lay claim to who and what you are*, even if, by doing so, it seems oppositional to your loved one's basic needs and requirements. Quite likely, the past months of coping have cast you into roles and responsibilities that neither fit nor totally work. Your getting better begins with you confronting your "true" feelings and needs alone and then mutually with your loved one.

1 If you can expunge yourself of wrongdoing, then you are in a better position to attend to what is needed, identifying the true sources of your despair and setting about to ameliorate them. We offer a number of suggestions in the next section for helping you with this. If your discouragement is severe, prolonged, or predates your loved one's injury, however, you need to immediately enlist professional guidance, from individuals such as your physician, or the former rehab social worker or psychologist. **Do not wait on this!** The journey cannot proceed without your emotional well-being intact.

CAREGIVER   **2** *Stymied and uncertain where to go from here.* It is in this realm of existence that many caregivers find themselves at 12 months postonset. Usually there is a somewhat predictable pattern to daily life, but much remains askew, rough, and uncomfortable. Much has been offered about moving your loved one ahead (see Person with Aphasia—Recovery and Emotions—Feelings About Self—Daily Life), but little has been said about making *you* better. Quite likely, as much of the current immobility in life rests with needing to "treat" you as it does in finding solutions for your loved one's problems or needs.

2 Getting yourselves to your ultimate destination involves more than empowering your loved one to do more; it requires that you grow and select routes along the way, as well. No one ever intended your loved one's aphasia to be a *life sentence*, nor should it be! Getting home requires that you get "equal billing," that is, that you acknowledge your needs as no less important than your loved one's. Sacrificing continuously in your loved one's behalf, when it fails to satisfy your wants and desires, is a sure formula for mental and emotional fatigue and breakdown. This is a mutual process the two of you are dealing with: addressing *your needs* is not a nicety, *but a necessity.*

3 *Determined and eager to do more.* If you are here after 365 days, you are on a preferred path. Should your loved one feel equally empowered and desirous to move forward, you are ideally equipped to travel the roads ahead. Keep doing whatever you have been to make yourselves feel strong and confident. Don't ignore your own needs.

WHAT YOU MIGHT DO

1–3 ALLOWING YOURSELF TO ACHIEVE YOUR VERY BEST

Let's repeat the last section's theme once more: *your* feelings, perceptions, and outlooks on daily life are no less important in the recovery process than your loved one's. If you are not psychologically and physically well prepared and fortified, you are apt to fall short in your attempts to aid him or her or to fulfill your own needs. Truly getting to your destination requires that you *consciously nurture and take care of yourself*. We begin here with suggestions for caregivers in the middle of the above continuum: the more likely position of many travelers, and then follow with advice for those discouraged or determined individuals.

> **EMOTIONS—FEELINGS ABOUT YOUR LOVED ONE—DAILY LIFE**
> *One of several scenarios is likely evolving:*
> 1–*DISCOURAGED*—He or she has given up: What kind of existence is this? The good life is *over*!
> 2–*STYMIED*—He or she is still trying but little is changing: There's got to be more, but *where* and *how*?
> 3–*DETERMINED*—He or she isn't giving up and neither am I: We've always managed before, we'll manage this too!

CAREGIVER

2 GETTING PAST FEELING STYMIED

Moving out of feeling entrapped in something that was not of your choice requires creating something that *is* of your choice!

2 WHAT TO DO TO GET "UNSTUCK"

- Take out a writing tablet and tear off 5 or 6 sheets.
- Draw a vertical line down the center of each sheet.
- Label the columns:
  Obligated time—when assigned duties or responsibilities dictate your presence and participation.
  Free time—when you are free to pursue activities of *your* own personal choice.
- Beginning with Sunday, enter the activities that describe a typical week in your life at the moment.
- For each entry, specify the prime benefactor(s) of your action (you, your loved one, both of you, or someone else).
- When finished, repeat the same task characterizing a week in your loved one's life now.
- Finally, redo this task for typical weeks *prior to injury* for both of you.

CAREGIVER

- Lay these four acountings out on the kitchen table:

  YOUR LIFE NOW   YOUR LOVED ONE'S LIFE NOW

  YOUR LIFE BEFORE YOUR LOVED ONE'S LIFE BEFORE

- Compare obligated versus free time *for you* now versus before the injury.

  This is a crucial comparison! Quite likely, considerably more of your time now falls on the commited side of the ledger than before. As well, more time is likely being directed toward benefitting your loved one's well-being. And most telling, less of your obligated or free time is directed toward addressing *your own needs or desires*. Although you have been told in a number of different recovery contexts that recapturing the past is not a reasonable expectation, this is *not* the case here. That is, it is not unrealistic to think that over time the two of you could closely approximate *the relative percentages* of obligated and free time you had before injury. Certainly, the activities that led to your previous percentages of obligated and free time will *not* be the same. Quite likely, your loved one's obligated time was tied to work, something that is not possible now. However, finding activities that obligate time and are of choice, regardless of whether they qualify as paid employment, is still possible.

  Quite likely, your obligated time is different, too. Now your daily routine is filled with more time dedicated to your loved one's care. During the summer, you may not feel the comfort to play golf every weekend as you once did. But it is not unrealistic to look for activities that your loved one would choose and that would free you up to play during the week, or maybe every other weekend. With a concerted effort toward redistributing how time is spent now, it *is* realistic, and likely beneficial to both parties, to bring these relative percentages closer to what they once were, knowing that the actual activities are apt to be different. Also, since more of your obligated and free time is apt to be directed toward assisting your loved one, it is crucial that *something of your own* constantly sit on your side of the ledger. It is important that an event or occasion be selected solely because it promotes *your* well-being.

- Next, compare your loved one's present and past profiles.

  The difference here is that percentages now are apt to be the opposite of yours. That is, your loved one has lots of free time (80% or more of daily life) compared to little prior to injury (20% or less). Also, current obligated and free time activities are apt to benefit his or her needs more than yours. Usually, this does not mean that your loved one has not begun helping around the house; he or she likely has. It is just that time spent in those efforts, compared with a time before his or her injury, is much less. While it is unlikely that your loved one's preinjury levels of efficiency are attainable, establishing a *more equitable split* between his or her obligated and free time is reasonable. Obligated time *is not* simply adding "household chores," but daily activities of choice in and outside the home (see Chapter 8). With these, a 50–50 ratio or better is possible between obligated and free time.

CAREGIVER

2 WHAT TO DO NEXT

- Now take a couple more sheets of paper.
- Write out some reasonable *short-term goals* for categories of behaviors that differed in the above pre- and postinjury comparisons. For example:

     OBLIGATING MORE OF YOUR LOVED ONE'S TIME TO ACTIVITIES OF CHOICE:

     Reintroduce him or her to some meaningful role on a church committee once a week.

     Increase his or her participation in helping you weed flower/vegetable gardens.

     FREEING MORE OF YOUR TIME FOR ACTIVITIES OF YOUR OWN CHOICE:

     return weekly to your yoga class.

     return to an hour of pleasure-reading two nights a week.

     FREEING MORE OF YOUR TIME FOR
     ACTIVITIES THAT YOU MIGHT DO TOGETHER:

     every other Saturday morning or afternoon select a new activity to explore outside the house, e.g., taking in a movie, visiting the zoo, or going to a craft fair.

- Strive to make modifications in each of the above categories simultaneously.

     It is important *not to simply do one part and ignore the others*. You need to modify each category over time. In this regard, it is better to make smaller changes in all categories than a huge change in just one. For an enduring solution to evolve, finding and maintaining a BALANCE between all of these is required.

CAREGIVER

- Don't expect *big changes* all at once.

  It is not the size or speed of change that is important, but the recognition and attention to these realms of daily life on a consistent basis. Once attending to all of them becomes habitual, the rest of the journey will take care of itself.

- Finally, skip ahead and examine the profiles for people with aphasia and their caregivers at 2-years' postonset (in the first portion of Chapter 8).

  Start planning your trip so that it keeps you within the center or upper end of the ranges described in these profiles. The severity of your loved one's injury may affect the amount of change that is possible over the next year. Even with severe aphasia, though, routines made up of daily choices are possible after a much longer period of time, perhaps years. To a large degree, the final outcome relies more on your perceptions of injury and chosen ways of confronting daily life than on what remains "broken."

- Recalculate your obligated and free time percentages every 3 or 4 months over the next year.

  Use these percentages as a gauge of your progress and a guide for planning your next targets. After a year's duration, the percentages need to be moving closer to preinjury levels.

1 WHEN DISCOURAGED

Giving up what once was, especially when it was endearing and special, is not without anguish and despair. Furthermore, these feelings usually do not occur once or twice, and then nicely fade away. Instead, they return repeatedly over a period of months and years. Thus, recurring bouts of discouragement are to be expected. However, when these moments in life persist, you need to address them directly.

1 WHAT TO DO

- Rest assured that, if you were not a discouraged person before this injury, you need *not* be now.
- Recall that common sources of discouragement come from:

  Feeling permanently *stuck* in something too large or difficult to manage.

Feeling permanently *stuck* in something that fails to address or satisfy your basic needs.

CAREGIVER

A combination of these.

- *You* will need to make changes in whatever part is not working.

   No source of discouragement is unchangeable, even though it may seem that way! You needn't condemn yourself for needing to make changes in daily life, even if they appear to directly impact your loved one or his or her care. As a simple rule of thumb, if your participation and support of your loved one continue to detract from certain critical realms of daily life, it is far better for everyone concerned to *find a different solution*, regardless of whether it satisfies your loved one completely or not. You need to look for solutions which meet your joint needs! Thus, if enrolling your loved one in an adult daycare or senior center one or more mornings a week allows you to cope better with the rest of life, it is likely not an "unkind" act, but an absolute necessity! Besides giving you what you may need, it may, as well, provide him or her with a greater sense of independence and personal freedom away from you. It is not encumbent on you to give up living life to attend to your loved one or his or her needs.

- Actively seek out, join, and participate in realms of life being at your loved one's side.

   They will add to your sense of self, and free up and reward the togetherness of you as a couple.

- If your discouragement is so pervasive as to disallow any action, it makes sense to seek out a knowledgeable professional of choice: rehab social worker, psychologist, physician, or clergy.

   Do not let this arena go unaddressed, this will jeopardize the journey's outcome.

3 WHEN DETERMINATION AND PUSHING FORWARD REIGN

The earlier suggestions about mapping your course ahead still apply here. You are in favored position to move ahead. Just keep to the course you're currently on!

RELATIONSHIP

1–I **still** sense I'm not allowing my
loved one to do all he or she
might. How can I "let go" further?
2–How can we make **us** better?

CAREGIVER

WHAT TO KNOW

1 This topic was presented from your loved one's perspective earlier. How it differs from yours is that you likely were encouraged, and even prompted, to support your loved one's functions in the early going. Two unwanted consequences may have evolved from this: (a) your loved one saw your efforts not only as superior, *but necessary* to permit his or her attempts to work at all and (b) you saw your loved one's efforts *as insufficient to stand alone*. Even if your loved one has assumed greater responsibility now, it is likely that these early supportive efforts have distorted your loved one's sense of what is possible. Whereas he or she quickly recruited your support or help at first, now there is enough autonomy and use of basic skills that he or she is saying, "Let me try more on my own!" However, given your past support, it may seem unsafe or uncaring not to remain close at hand.

1 Letting go involves more than allowing your loved one to participate. It involves assuming a different perspective about his or her ability to take part in life. Whenever possible, it involves taking a proactive rather than a reactive or questioning stance. For any activity of your loved one's choice, there is cause to approach the situation as an enabler, rather than as a discourager or disenabler. Even when participation seems to require skills beyond his or her current abilities, it is better to start from a position of not just *allowing*, but actively *encouraging* participation. **When someone usurps another's choice in life, even if it is with that person's well-being in mind, it undermines that person's ability to try, or to gain access to what he or she might be able to do. For this reason, you want to extend *every opportunity* to your loved one to act in his or her own behalf, even when you wonder if that choice is totally sound.**

1 With this notion in mind, recall our earlier discussions of your loved one's ability to drive a car and how you might support his or her efforts even though they conflict with your own desires. In the current context, however, we need something more illustrative of "letting go" of your loved one's personal choices in life! Suppose, for instance, that he or she came home one evening prior to this injury and announced that he or she was going to start sky diving! You likely would have panicked! Yet, even though your inner desires might have screamed out, "I'm sorry, but I forbid it, you simply cannot," you would have looked for an explanation for his or her considering this unsafe, choice! You might have gone further and expressed your own reservations, but it is unlikely that you would have forbidden his or her participation. Your relationship, then, permitted each of you the freedom to decide what you would pursue in life.

CAREGIVER

1 Your loved one is probably not going to jump out of a plane in the near future. But whether the chosen activity is sky diving, driving an automobile, or walking unaccompanied to a nearby convenience store to buy the morning newspaper, there is probably some risk involved. To help you "release yourself" from monitoring every aspect of your loved one's participation in life, you need to consider each request, not as an action about to happen, but as a request to try. Just as people do not jump from a plane without intensive on-the-ground instruction and being strapped, piggyback style, to a licensed instructor, so too, your loved one's requests are statements of intent and desire rather than imminent action. They need to be honored as such!

1 Your goal, then, needs to be to examine every way possible *not to deny* your loved one's request to take part in life. To feel comfortable with this, you may need to consult regularly with "sky-diving experts" or other instructors. What you want from these experts are *reasonable and well-defined steps* for allowing your loved one the right to try! You want a safe and specified course that permits your full support of his or her efforts to do more. It does not matter whether all parts of the chosen pursuit actually come to pass. What does matter, though, is that you permit him or her every opportunity to learn and experience *what is possible*. With time and some accumulated experience in trying, he or she will elect whether to continue, switch, or discontinue any pursuit. Quite likely, these are the same options that he or she exercised in life before injury. Licensing your loved one's participation was not something you did before and it is not something you wish to do now!

2 Making your relationship stronger depends on *mutuality*. Chapter 8 lays out how mutuality begins with communication and extends to treating each other as equal partners in daily life. **Sometimes it may seem that with all your loved one's communicative, physical, emotional, or social barriers, that equality is not possible. You can counter these notions best by viewing and thinking about him or her as being no less as a person, but simply outwardly changed or different!** Most

CAREGIVER certainly, some functions or processes *are less* in terms of their ease, availability, or accuracy, but the person inside is not. You may need to supplement these impaired processes, but always give full respect to the individual. This will ensure that you grow as a couple, or as friends.

2 Finally, you need to have as much faith in yourself as a couple or pair as you do in your loved one as an individual. You, as a twosome, have been provided with lots of suggestions on how to augment the parts of life that still seem the most impaired (see Caregiver—Recovery in Chapters 5, 6, and 7). Don't feel discouraged if certain barriers remain substantial. Some of these breakdowns are apt to never *fully disappear*, but your understanding, willingness, and ease *in confronting them together* will help make them less prominent or obstructive over time.

RELATIONSHIP
1–I **still** sense I'm not allowing my loved one to do all he or she might. How can I "let go" further?
2–How can we make **us** better?

WHAT YOU MIGHT DO

1–2 LETTING GO AND MATURING AS A COUPLE

The time is right to give your loved one every opportunity to assume greater responsibility and choice in daily life. It will take many months or years to uncover your loved one's full potential to act in her or his own behalf. Look for, ask for, urge, and support your loved one's effort to move in this direction. As well, search out ways of improving the quality of your time together.

1 WHAT TO DO

- From your earlier lists of current and past activities in daily life, review current entries for your loved one to see whether more function or greater responsibility might be added.
- Look hard at those activities where your loved one might be most interested and willing to do more.
- Look for ways of increasing his or her participation or facilitating greater involvement.

  Maybe he or she has begun helping with the laundry but cannot get the dirty clothes down the basement stairs unaided. By pro-

CAREGIVER

viding a laundry bag with a pull-string, he or she can hook the bag around his or her involved arm and still get up and down the stairs safely. Because of his or her compromised stability, it requires two or three trips to fill the washer. Free time, though, is a commodity that your loved one has plenty of, and if he or she is willing to make multiple trips, it greatly enhances his or her contribution at home.

- Look at your weekly or monthly logs to identify areas where your loved one's activity has increased over the past 6 months and in what way.
- Make sure that you are making the most of your loved one's increased participation in daily life.

  Try to use more of his or her free time in something you do together! This is a tangible way of letting your loved one know that his or her contribution *does make a difference.*

- Review your findings and discuss how you, together, might further improve his or her participation in life.

  Sometimes changes occur in daily life, like beginning to physically manage stairs or carry objects, and yet these accomplishments have not transferred from one setting to another. Using the earlier example, perhaps your loved one is beginning to go up and down stairs to do the laundry at home. Yet, on review of your logs, you notice that he or she is still avoiding stairs in public places because he or she cannot negotiate them quickly or because other people are around. Knowing this, you may decide to visit some public places where the stairs are few in number and traffic minimal. Offer to negotiate them with him or her, and go slowly at first.

- Look for areas within existing, working, preferred areas of daily life where small, additional changes might enhance matters further.

  Maybe over time your loved one begins adopting the laundry as his or her responsiblity. It is obvious that he or she would elect to do more in this realm! From what you can tell, he or she possesses the necessary skills to fold and return the clean laundry to its proper place upstairs. You ask if this addition might be something of his or her choosing. It is! You set about establishing a plan for incorporating it into his or her existing routine.

- Acknowledge gains, regardless of how small they may be.
- Point out how increased use in one area has supplemented use in other areas of daily life.
- Stay positive, share with one another, and try to maintain a constant sense of forward momentum.

COMMUNICATION

1–We figure out almost everything now at home . . . however, occasionally we still get stuck!

2–Is there anything more we might do that we haven't already?

CAREGIVER

WHAT TO KNOW

1 You and your loved one have had a year to fashion your own communication style. We urged you to begin this process early on (see Caregiver—Communication, Chapter 5). By now, the two of you have likely developed a communication style that addresses most basic functions in daily life. If your loved one's talking is restricted, hopefully an experienced speech-language pathologist has aided you in selecting and using methods to circumvent this problem. For example, you may provide printed or pictured options from which your loved one can make an expressive choice. You may encourage his or her writing or drawing of parts of the message. Whatever the process, you are likely settling into a mode of interaction that works for you. Within this constellation, though, there are still moments when parts of messages get lost or misinterpreted.

1 You have likely already heard from experts (physicians and speech-language pathologists) that most of your loved one's language and communication improvement is over. Although this statement may apply to some, and maybe even in the larger percentage of people with aphasia, it does not apply to all! There are individuals with aphasia who only begin to show changes in their speech or other forms of expression at about this point in time. In addition, it is encouraging to find that most people with aphasia continue to show small gains in their language and communication for months and even years to come. As a result, it may be better and more accurate to cast the above pronouncement in a slightly different light, that is, the likelihood for *sudden* or *dramatic resumption of function* in language or communication diminishes after a year postinjury, but further change in communication is still possible—and likely!

1–2 Bridging your own communication breakdowns depends considerably on how important they remain in your daily lives. Quite likely, speech and language improvement in your loved one is slowing. **However, you need to know that whatever your loved one's language ability, even if it is severely impaired, his or her level of communication is not at its full potential! That is, *communication* can still be enhanced within whatever ability level your loved one has.** Moving forward from here, though, often requires a slightly different focus. Instead of "repairing" your loved one's broken parts, it requires consid-

ering existing abilities and singling out the parts of your shared commu-   **CAREGIVER**
nication that might be improved further. For example, you may feel that
your loved one usually understands your messages and that you typically understand his or her general topics. However, most of your communication breakdowns occur in missing or misunderstanding details of his
or her message. Thus, it is this area that, cooperatively, you may need to
target in the months ahead.

**2 The integrity of your communication as a couple is not dependent
solely on your loved one's ability to communicate. It is a joint
process of knowing how to circumvent the limitations in your interactions together.** During the first year after injury, the primary focus of
treatment is usually on restoring as much verbal communication as possible. It is not until the permanency of loss becomes clear that either the
person with aphasia or the caregiver can truly become dedicated to augmenting communication with other techniques. When taken seriously,
these strategies can often make communication a truly shared, interactive process rather than one where speaking is not enough. These augmentative strategies include: (a) pointing (selecting options from a list of
pictured objects and/or printed words), (b) pantomiming (acting out
basic needs according to their associated function and bodily movements), (c) writing (identifying words by printing their initial letters in a
known or familiar context), and (d) drawing (conveying ideas or
thoughts through simple cartoons using stick-figure depictions).

2 When blended in their proper proportions, these other expressive
means often aid adults with aphasia who cannot fully achieve communication through speech. However, it is more than just access to other ways
of expression that matters. It is how these forms are used cooperatively
that makes their added influence so valuable. In Chapter 6, we mentioned the importance of "staying connected" while communicating with
one another. When nonspeaking ways of communicating are attempted,
it becomes imperative that their use allows for a mutual connecting of
interactants. Sometimes such techniques only serve to single out the person with aphasia as being less of a participant and more of a reactant in
the communicating process. For these techniques to be truly effective,
their use requires that both people interact as mutual players. Chapter 8
highlights the type of "back and forth" communicative process that you
need to pursue if speaking is no longer readily available to your loved
one.

CAREGIVER

COMMUNICATION

1–We figure out almost everything now at home . . . however, occasionally we still get stuck!
2–Is there anything more we might do that we haven't already?

WHAT YOU MIGHT DO

1–2 IMPROVING YOUR COMMUNICATION AS A COUPLE

Although the repair of your loved one's speech and language may be slowing down, the potential for continued improvement of *your own communication as a couple* still remains strong. Efforts to further your interactive style and success were suggested in earlier chapters (Chapters 5 and 6, Caregiver—Communication). In addition, we urged you to seek out a speech-language pathologist regularly over the past year to refine your communication skills. If you have done so, the two of you should have a functional communication system of your own by now. If you have not had this support and your communication remains problematic, you need to retrace these steps. They are likely very important, as will be highlighted in Chapter 8.

1–2 WHAT TO DO

- Revisit your current communicative strengths and weaknesses with an experienced speech-language pathologist.
  By now, you should know what does and does not work for you as a couple. In addition, you should have some sense of how you have tried to make your communication better and which efforts have and have not worked. The emphasis now needs to be on perfecting ways of augmenting speech with other nonspeaking methods that might allow for a more active and successful "give and take" between you.
- Keep asking the speech-language pathologist *to demonstrate* any recommendations.
- If they involve significant modifications to what you have been doing, you may want this professional to observe your attempts and to take several treatment sessions just to practice incorporating these changes.
- Ensure that any changes in your communication system still allow you to relate first as people and, within that process, to gradually promote a better or more complete exchange of information.

WHAT TO KNOW

FAMILY/FRIENDS
1–What, if anything, might make past friendships better? *2–How might we **add** new ones?*

1 In Chapters 5 and 6, Caregiver—Family/ Friends, we offered suggestions for fostering ties with past friends. If you are like a majority of others confronting aphasia and its associated disabilities, a limited number of these ties still remain. Too frequently, the very people who knew you best cannot separate the past from the present in spite of an inner desire to do so. All too often, they can neither confront nor accept the changes that now exist. These changes are simply too painful and uncomfortable for them to see or too complicated for them to react to. And as a result, these individuals tend to drift away rather than move toward a mutual renewing of past ties.

CAREGIVER

1 There are exceptions to the above generalization. Sometimes *friends of yours*, who were not particularly familiar or tied to contact with your loved one, may remain active and close. Even with these friends, though, there is often a difference or an adjustment in the frequency or depth of your interactions. To the degree desired, though, it is terribly important to keep these ties active and strong. You likely need outlets where you can talk freely and openly with others, especially if you find conversing in certain realms of life impossible with your loved one. Without the same depth or ease of exchange with your loved one, it may be important to know of other people with whom you can talk and explore thoughts and ideas.

2 As alluded to earlier, *new friendships* are apt to develop from others who know you and your loved one only as you are now, and thus, can accept you quite readily (see Person with Aphasia—Family/Friends in this chapter).

WHAT YOU MIGHT DO

FAMILY/FRIENDS
1–What, if anything, might make past friendships better? *2–How might we **add** new ones?*

1–2 MAKING YOUR TIES BETTER WITH OTHERS

Improving your relationships with others likely involves a combination of blending the old with the new. Because much of the old may not feel or work as it once did, it is particularly important to search out new areas of interaction and sharing with others.

CAREGIVER   **1-2** WHAT TO DO

- Revisit the suggestions in Chapters 5 and 6, Caregiver—Family/Friends for fostering past tics with others.
- Take time to meet with some of your former friends.
  In terms of adding free time activities of your choice, this may be one pursuit you need to foster.
- Review suggestions earlier in this chapter, Person with Aphasia—Family/Friends.
- Scan Chapter 8; it describes ways of getting the two of you more engaged in life with others outside the home.

EMPLOYMENT (YOURS)
1–Thank goodness, I still have my work!

WHAT TO KNOW

1 Keeping your employment, if you elected to do so, is probably paying dividends by now. It has likely taken 6 to 9 months to assess and arrange daily life at home so you could feel some ease in being away through much of the day. By now, though, some pattern is developing and you are realizing the importance of having your work. Contrasted to life at home, it may represent one arena in life where you still can continue to grow and enhance your self-image without ongoing concerns about your loved one's well-being.

1 Also, being away from your loved one is apt to have fostered his or her greater independence. Like it or not, when you are there and he or she knows *you will attend* to things that others might not, there often develops a kind of dependency that works against both of you. Being away regularly, when your loved one is properly supported, likely *benefits everyone*, whether or not this arrangement was fully endorsed at the time of discharge from formal care.

1 Finally, if you have elected to retire from work to be with your loved one, that does not mean that *you have made a poor choice*. Perhaps your work was not personally rewarding, nor particularly promoting of your energies or potential, and spending time with your loved one is! If absence from work is financially possible and of benefit to both of you, then maintaining your employment contact is less concerning. However, it is important, even under these circumstances, to keep a watchful eye on how you spend your mutual time. As discussed in the earlier section, there likely needs to be well-defined joint and separate activities that permit a healthy balance between free and obligated time.

CAREGIVER

WHAT YOU MIGHT DO

EMPLOYMENT (YOURS)
1–Thank goodness, I still have my work!

1 KEEPING YOUR WORK IMPORTANT

A healthy balance is needed between attending to your loved one and deriving from life what you most need for your own well-being. When working is a prime part of your identity and purpose in life, you need to find ways to continue it. If there is still guilt over your devoting time and effort to such an endeavor, you likely need to look for ways of changing your loved one's daily routines so they, too, are of your own choice.

1 WHAT TO DO

- Review earlier suggestions for creating states of "flow" in your loved one (see Person with Aphasia: Emotions—Feelings About Self—Daily Life).
- Look to other people who might help support your loved one and other settings where this support might be available.
- Review suggestions in the next chapter for establishing activities outside the home.

WHAT TO KNOW

HEALTH
1–This all happened a year ago. Are we doing everything we can to ensure it doesn't recur?

1 Your loved one's physical health has likely stabilized since his or her injury. What likely remains most worrisome is whether or not his or her chances for further injury have been minimized. Depending on what caused the initial brain damage, there are various precautions one might wish to consider. What these are and how to attend to them are reviewed in Chapter 13.

> **HEALTH**
> *1–This all happened a year ago.
> Are we doing everything we can to
> ensure it doesn't recur?*

CAREGIVER

WHAT YOU MIGHT DO

1 MINIMIZING YOUR LOVED ONE'S RISK FOR FURTHER INJURY

Besides medical precautions that might help lessen your loved one's risk of further injury, the standard considerations include regulating diet, exercise, and daily stress. Within what your loved one's medical condition permits, careful attention to these concerns will minimize his or her risk of further injury.

1 WHAT TO DO

- Review Chapter 13 for details that are applicable to your loved one's condition.
- Be sure to talk to your loved one's physician about plans to address these concerns.
- Carefully regulate and monitor his or her prime risk factors.
- Usually, over time, even severely *threatening factors* can be modified, often to acceptable levels.
- Do not ignore or neglect prime threats. Recurring injury is more likely in the first 3 years after initial injury, and more so in individuals who don't attend to these concerns.

Getting more familiar with traveling these roads

You should be getting a better sense of traveling these roads by now, even though they may not feel totally comfortable or be your personal choice. The truth is, they may not feel comfortable for some time to come. That prospect may not feel encouraging, but it has nothing to do with anything you have done wrong; it simply takes time to derive the right formula for you. What is more important is that, at every juncture along the way, there is a growing sense that you have matters moving in the right direction. You may not feel wonderful, but you feel far better than you did, and you feel as if tomorrow may be better. **Keep building on what you have; keep revamping what isn't working; keep participating instead of**

withdrawing; and keep moving ever so slowly ahead. You *are gaining* **the upper hand on aphasia and its associated disabilities. You are beginning to sense that these additions need not rob you of** *your* **lives, separately or together.**

      CAREGIVER

The next 12 months are critical! As urged in this chapter, you need to systematically start reordering some of the working parts of your daily lives. You need to be sure that more free time evolves on your ledger to pursue activities of your own choosing, and that on your loved one's ledger more obligated time evolves for pursuing finding desirable activities that may add "flow" to daily life. Hopefully, a year from now, your combined profiles of time spent will be more in line with your preinjury percentages (see Caregiver—Recovery). You want to keep checking these gauges on your vehicle in the months ahead. In fact, you may wish to scan ahead through Chapter 8 right now and see if you might arrive at next year's crossroads on, or ahead of, schedule. The road ahead contains some of the most fertile and promising countryside so far.

Remember, though, it is not the distance you travel, it is whether you are moving ahead. If your journey takes several years to get to the next juncture in the road, don't fret as long as you are progessing along a desired path. **There is something inherently better about being the "tortoise" in this venture rather than the "hare."**

❖   **CHAPTER 8**

Two years later . . . keeping life meaningful and rich!

By 2 years into this journey, there should be increased ease and comfort in living daily life, especially in those environments where the two of you spend the bulk of your time and share freely. Quite likely, if you will reflect back to a year ago, life today is not as daunting as you might have envisioned it would be. If the two of you have continued your pursuit of a better lifestyle, you probably have broadened your scope, manner, and depth of sharing. Because of this, not only are you more connected as a couple, but there is actually some discernible pleasure, comfort, and fun in life. And whereas no more than 20% of your shared time was likely judged as *enjoyable* or *of choice* a year ago, you are likely beyond this level of mutual satisfaction by now.

Even so, life's pleasures are not as complete or as diversified as they might be, not by a long shot! In fact, if current daily pleasures are even half of what they were prior to injury, you are doing exceedingly well. Quite likely, today's rewards are coming in environments and situations where you have generated them alone or with each other, and contact with others is minimal. It is likely in this latter realm of life, finding your own place and style outside the home, that the greatest change still awaits you. Although everyone must foster new ties to the outside world as he or she sees fit, seldom do travelers get to their ideal destination without confronting this part of daily life. Put slightly differently, you may have come to feel some ease with life at home, but if you are not moving freely and comfortably in and out of everyday society, an essential part of life is still missing. Even if both of you preferred minimal contact with the outside world before, this restriction was of your own choosing, and participating in outside activities did occur at times. **The same freedom and opportunity needs to exist in your lives now; you need to discover and select ways that permit you and your loved one, separately and together, to move in and out of society with ease. This choice should not be constricted or changed *because of aphasia or its related impairments*, but only if *you elect* to have it that way.** If you desire to do more with others, but simply *don't* because of your loved one's injury, then the journey is not over. In that regard, you should know that your traveling may extend over many years to come, if not a lifetime. Seeing, learning, and adding onto what currently exists often is a chosen way of life!

By now, the two of you have probably ventured outside known and friendly environments on a number of occasions. For many, going out into the world for the first time calls on the strategies you have developed at home. For instance, you probably began with a commonly held interest or desire that you thought might yield a mutually favorable outcome, like eating in a favorite restaurant from the past. Most likely, some parts of this adventure went well, other parts proved challenging, and some were simply impossible. From this experience, you decided to try again, try something different, or not return at all. If you decided to revisit this experience, you slowly began accruing a new road map for eating out. And although this pattern is probably much different from before, it has become more comfortable and acceptable over time, especially if the experience *added* to life's pleasures. The accrued knowledge from repeated visits molded new ways of making these outings more mutual and shared, and by the time of the fourth or fifth visit, your initial feelings of apprehension and awkwardness had slowly faded.

Eating out is just one small piece in a much bigger puzzle of putting together life outside the home. More than likely, there are many other settings and occasions in real life still awaiting your exploration, but many of these may appear beyond your current reach or means. In some ways, your view may be absolutely right. People in everyday society naturally tend to value, seek out, and reward others who look, think, and act as they do. As a result, people with aphasia and their caregivers often find themselves feeling and seeing themselves *as oddities* or *uninvited participants*. Whereas you and your loved one attended social forums with ease before, your entry now appears to be a different matter. In truth, though, there are other routes awaiting you, and you still can take part in life outside the home! It simply means that there is a different set of rules, and for many, a different route, to make them feel desirable and worthy of pursuit.

Gaining access to the outside world is what this chapter is about. Even if routes outside the home still feel awkward, scary, and even hostile at times, know that they are within your means and skills. In many ways, they are no more difficult to learn or manage than the routes you've already traversed in the hospital, in rehabilitation, and at home. They likely require adopting a few common sense changes, like making sure you know how to use four-wheel drive in certain difficult and slippery terrain, confining your initial excursions to routes where others know of your needs and can assist you, and learning to travel these routes for your own reasons rather than worrying what others might think. By risking to venture out on these roads, you not only elevate your own skills and confidence, you provide access to opportunities that many travelers unfortunately forego. Once again, it is unlikely that alone, restricted to the safe havens you already know well, you can ever push life's pleasures beyond half of what they once were. You must determine your ties with others and the outside world in order to free yourselves to be fully who you are independent of those influences. In the end, you and your loved one may not choose to participate any more in these settings than you currently do, although most travelers typically do! However, what is important is coming to this determination on your own, and *not* having it imposed upon you.

You have done a remarkable job getting to this juncture in the road. It has been no small feat! So don't lose heart now, keep plugging along! If moving outside the home seems simply too much, then skip ahead to Chapter 14 and read some of the stories of people who have already done so. Their accounts may help nudge you into trying. Redefining your new selves requires traversing some rough road ahead, but don't stop now! You are about to gain access to country that may elevate life's pleasures to a completely different level and define a far more desirable way of living life. Stay with it!

Profiles

PERSON WITH APHASIA

- realizing aphasia and its consequences are a part of daily life . . . whether fully accepted or not
- still experiencing slow, but consistent gains in most impaired realms, especially if dedicated to their pursuit and resolution
- beginning to notice that many gains are now too small for casual observers to even notice
- realizing that some small changes, though, *add* significantly to daily life; for example, the addition of a simple greeting might permit contact with people that wasn't possible a month ago
- gauging change over time in reference to performance *since,* rather than *before*, injury
- coming to see well-being, recovery, and relationships with others as bound to assuming greater responsibility for self and actions in life
- watching daily life evolve in one of several directions:

MEANINGLESS AND EMPTY
relying on others to determine life's course; acting as a passive observer unless called on; experiencing bouts of depression and anger; not having others besides the caregiver to turn to.

CAREGIVER

- feeling settled into a new and different daily routine
- still adjusting and negotiating with self and loved one over long-term changes
- not seeing as many major changes in loved one as earlier although still aware of minor improvements
- not attaching as much function significance to loved one's possibilities as before or as he or she is still apt to
- growing more resigned to the fact that one's prior lifestyle is a thing of the past; noticing your loved one's change since injury, although unable to stop comparing current functions to those prior to injury.
- accepting the permanence of injury, but perhaps unaware of the amount of independence still possible with current levels of function
- seeing daily life evolve in one of several directions:

STARK AND EMPTY
thinking that life will be *less* and deciding to "make do" with what remains; perceiving that little is modifiable *now*; feeling angry, resentful, or entrapped; occasionally displaying such feelings to aphasic partner; pessimistic about future; withdrawing from life and past activities and friends

RESTRICTED BUT STILL IMPROVING

sharing responsibility for determining what constitutes daily life with caregiver and others; participating in a limited number of activities where personal comfort is assured; most new activities are within a familiar setting and with family or friends; viewing life as *less* and seeing this as "reality" rather than something of choice; increasing self-confidence and motivation to do more independently if permitted and properly supported; finding new friendships but still highly isolated from the outside world

MANAGEABLE WITH LOTS MORE TO DO

assuming the bulk of responsibility for daily life; engaging in a broad range of activities, most of these in familiar settings but venturing out more into the real-world; less preoccupied with aphasia as a hindrance or an excuse not to take part in life; actively looking for options; self-confident in established realms of activities and trying to do more alone; evolving new friendships

RESTRICTED BUT STILL IMPROVING

adapting to a lifestyle that is *less* but also with more harmony than at first; accepting that this is the way life is going to be; coming to embrace loved one's condition as disabled or restricted; striving to find ways around current limitations; still feeling victimized; hoping for more but unsure whether it is possible; finding few old or new friends available to interact with

MANAGEABLE WITH LOTS MORE TO DO

redefining life as simply different and *not* necessarily more or less; focusing on improving participation in life regardless of form, accuracy, or completeness; emphasizing equality by empowering both parties to fully participate in life according to personal choice; looking for how to expand current options; not allowing life to be less because of current limitations; slowly gaining new set of friends

Primary concerns

PERSON WITH APHASIA AND CAREGIVER

DAILY LIFE

1–Life at home or in other familiar and shared environments is beginning to take form, but how do we expand further on these realms?

2–How do we reenter society when all the things that were so automatic and natural before now feel uncomfortable and unwelcoming?

DAILY LIFE

1–Life at home or in other familiar and shared environments is beginning to take form, but how do we expand on these realms?

2–How do we reenter society when all the things that were so automatic and natural before now feel uncomfortable and unwelcoming?

PERSON WITH APHASIA AND CAREGIVER

WHAT TO KNOW

1–2 The categories of concerns laid out in previous chapters have gradually blended. This merging of areas of concern was evident in the last chapter where emotions, feelings about self or loved one, and daily life were more easily addressed together than separately for the person with aphasia and the caregiver. This merging has continued as all areas of concerns from before are now encapsulated under a single entity: quality of daily life. This blending of concerns, though, does not mean that prior categories no longer exist or are unimportant, but rather that the distinctions among them have become less striking and more integrated into ways of living daily life (see earlier profiles of person with aphasia and caregiver). Thus, while coping suggestions needed to be more specifically tailored in the past, most have always related to some aspect of either making life better and more productive.

1–2 Certainly by now, the two of you have some plan of action, whether formal or informal, for coping with daily life. The success of this plan depends considerably on your willingness and skill to address certain concerns along the way, especially those detailed in Chapters 5, 6, and 7. Of these, probably the most influential is your comfort and ease *in sharing* with each other. Certainly the proficiency with which the two of you *can exchange facts* is a vital part of this process. Even more than that, however, the success of the process depends on whether or not you can freely approach and engage one another in an interaction, enjoy the exchange, and make daily decisions regardless of whether all aspects of your messages were understood or not.

1–2 To help you visualize this process, examine Figure 8–1. Here you will find three ovals layered on one another. The base, or first oval, represents your skill in staying communicatively connected as a couple while engaging in and enjoying interactions in daily life. The oval resting on this first one, and thus likely somewhat dependent on it, is your skill as a couple in honoring, relating, and respecting one another as independent and competent people in daily life. The final oval, resting now on top of the second one, and likely dependent on both, is your skill as a couple in approaching and promoting your ties with others outside yourselves and with matters pertaining to the outside world and society.

1–2 Now look at Figure 8–2, which contains an enlargement of the prime contents of these three ovals, but now displayed separately so you

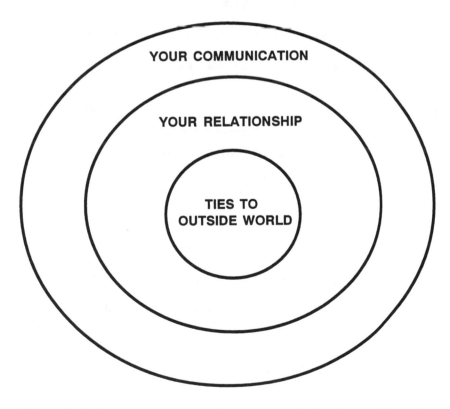

Figure 8–1. Viewing your communication, your relationship, and ties to the outside world

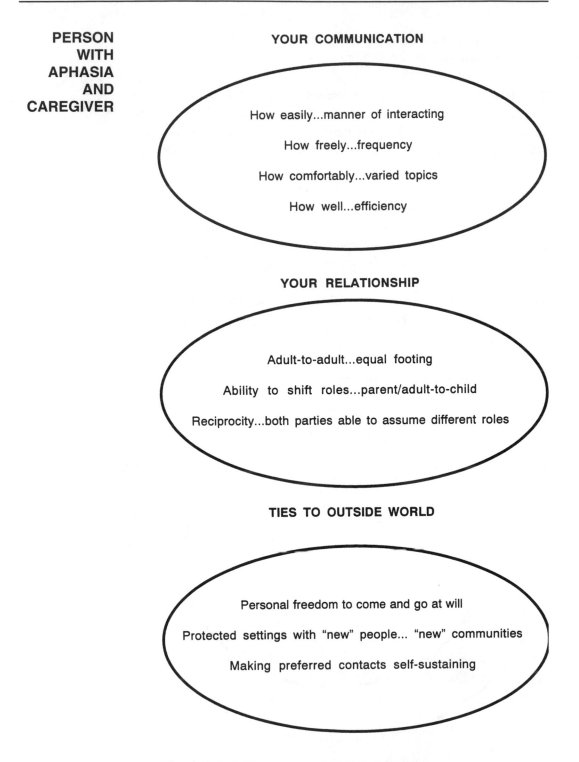

PERSON WITH APHASIA AND CAREGIVER

YOUR COMMUNICATION

How easily...manner of interacting

How freely...frequency

How comfortably...varied topics

How well...efficiency

YOUR RELATIONSHIP

Adult-to-adult...equal footing

Ability to shift roles...parent/adult-to-child

Reciprocity...both parties able to assume different roles

TIES TO OUTSIDE WORLD

Personal freedom to come and go at will

Protected settings with "new" people... "new" communities

Making preferred contacts self-sustaining

Figure 8–2. Main component parts to daily life.

can see their main parts. In the first oval—your communication—it is your joint skill in knowing how to communicate and share with one another that is apt to influence how frequently, which topics, and how well you exchange thoughts and feelings. In the second oval—your relationship—it is your skill in perceiving and treating each other as one adult to another that is apt to influence whether both participants can assume other important relational roles, such as nurturing and advising. In the third oval—your ties to the outside world—it is your joint skill in feeling the freedom and right to act as you would choose in life that is apt to influence whether you can establish "new," and protected "communities" in daily life, and whether these supports can become permanent and self-sustaining.

PERSON WITH APHASIA AND CAREGIVER

1–2 *The form and quality of your communication.* Communicating with other people often seems driven by *a need to share information.* Whereas this motive is the more visible component, it is not always the most crucial one! People communicate with one another for many reasons, not the least of which is to stay socially connected and bonded with each another. This role and its importance in life was detailed earlier in Chapters 5 and 6 (Person with Aphasia/Caregiver—Communication). **It is this component of being able to share mutually with one another, more than any other, that is now apt to set the tone and tenor of how your communication as a couple is working in the real world. Basically, the more you and your loved one are able to converse in a manner where there is *equal recognition and importance* afforded each person's contribution and participation, the more likely communication will occur over a diverse range of subjects. With more opportunity and reason to converse, it is likely that your skill and success at exchanging information will increase too.**

1–2 Think of this process as two people wanting to hit a tennis ball back and forth when one of them is no longer able to use his or her preferred hand, run, or change directions. The most important game strategy then, especially in the beginning attempts, would not be to worry about keeping score (noting how much information was exchanged)! Instead, it would be to find ways of just keeping the ball in play (keeping participants interacting and sharing). To do so, you might confine play at first to just one side of the court, remove the net, and hit the ball only to your partner's forehand (slowing your rate of speech, writing out key words, and drawing portions of messages). If such adaptations permit you and your partner to hit the ball back and forth, you might slowly progress toward putting up a net and keeping some type of score. However, it is unlikely that you would ever care to play an "official" game of tennis together again. The rules have changed, and you have your own set now that permits a connectedness to remain under mutually agreed upon rules of your own. Keeping that connection is more important to you than playing conventional tennis. If the two of you have found ways of keeping that ball moving back and forth, you are exactly where you need to be. If you haven't established ways of interacting with ease, then you need to back up, take down the net, and review past suggestions (see Chapters 6 and 7, Person with Aphasia/Caregiver—Communication). Remember that, to continue on your journey from here, you need a well established way of staying bonded with one another regardless of the level of information exchanged.

1–2 It is important to realize that, although your communicative connection is imperative to future progress, the level of communicative skill of your loved one is *not!* You do not need to play a full-fledged tennis match in order to keep the tennis ball in play. If your loved one's speech or language remains severely impaired, you may not be on opposite sides of the net. Interactively, you may be limited to hitting balls back and forth to one another from several feet away: The reciprocal volley is far more relevant than playing by the rules, or even playing "well."

1–2 *The quality of your relationship*. The quality of your communication significantly influences the quality of your relationship. Assuming you freely and comfortably shared life with one another prior to injury, *you can* achieve a comparable level of sharing again, in spite of aphasia. **Strong relationships depend foremost on treating one another with** *mutual respect*. **In more practical terms, this means viewing and conducting personal interactions** *in an equal manner:* **adult-to-adult rather than adult-to-child or parent-to-child.**

1–2 Aphasia and its related consequences can threaten previously equal interactions. When language level becomes overly influential in the partnership, the person with aphasia may become cast in a much lesser role in both communicative interactions as well as in power or status. For this reason, acknowledging your loved one as a viable and equal participant in the relationship, in spite of current communicative barriers, is fundamental. As shown in Figure 8–1, restoring equality typically begins with how you communicate with one another. If the two of you can communicatively hit that tennis ball back and forth freely and equally, you set a precedent for doing the same thing personally within your relationship. Certainly, the easier it is to discern each other's messages, the easier personal relating may be. But even if your informational exchanges are limited, this does not preclude treating one another with mutual respect.

PERSON WITH APHASIA AND CAREGIVER

1–2 Realize, too, that the health of your relationship involves more than interacting in *a single set of roles*. There are occasions in life when one or the other person in a partnership must assume roles of parenting, nurturing, or advising the other. For the nonaphasic partner, though, relinquishing such roles can prove challenging. The person with aphasia too often is viewed as not possessing the necessary requisites (competencies), either communicatively or interpersonally, to take on the role of a nurturing adult or advising "parent." As a result, the caregiver may not relinquish these roles once assumed, thus keeping his or her aphasic partner entrenched perpetually in the role of a "child." Receiving advice or support from a loved one is not necessarily "childlike," or beneath the dignity of an adult. In an equal relationship, a balance of various roles prohibits type-casting. However, if one partner is *always* in a receiving role, there is the danger that he or she will feel unequal and more like a child. It is vital to relationships that neither party becomes cast *in a single role*, and that both participants are able and willing to assume different roles at different times.

1–2 People with aphasia must not only be kept out of the role of a "child," but they must be encouraged and permitted to nurture or advise their nonaphasic loved one in times of need. Often, though, restricted communication, perceived inability, and a seemingly self-absorbed view of life interfere with aphasic adults easily assuming a nurturing or advising role. Even if it takes more time and effort on both of your parts, placing your loved one in these roles is essential to constructing a better relationship. You, as the caregiver, not only need to bring your interactions with your loved one to an adult-to-adult level, but solutions in life need to be derived from his or her support and advice as well. As part of this input, you may need to nurture your loved one's nurturing along. For instance, because communication is apt to hinder his or her participation, you want to suggest ways that he or she may have helped you before this injury. You may, for instance, help him or her by saying: "Oh, yes, you used to tell me: Back up." "Take a moment and relax!" "Guess that's what you would be saying now, right?"

PERSON WITH APHASIA AND CAREGIVER

1–2 Finally, the form of your relationship now is likely bound to what it was prior to injury. If the two of you *did not share equally*, adult-to-adult, before your loved one's aphasia, it is unlikely that you will now! If you tended to parent or oversee your loved one previously, that tendency is apt to remain. Even though your loved one's communication may interfere, if he or she governed your choices, he or she is apt to attempt to do so now. Occasionally, though, individuals who dominated before but who cannot communicate now acquiesce to their "subordinate" partner. The long-term well-being of your relationship is something you define. As much mutuality and respect that you can restore—*in your terms*—the more equal your relationship is apt to be.

1–2 *Your ties to the outside world*. It is in this realm of life that the greatest potential change still awaits you. Even if the two of you have found ways of sharing and maintaining an adult-to-adult relationship, the ability to move freely in and out of spheres outside the home is often limited. There are few settings or people outside of the home where you can turn with any ease or comfort in the beginning years after injury. Although, it may feel as if access to these resources in life is permanently beyond your reach, it is not!

1–2 What is apt to interfere most with moving outside the home *is your own perception* of that process. Quite often, it is a perception of either inability, disability, increased visibility, or limited viability that restricts movement outside the home. It is how you see your changed selves and how this perceived change fits or doesn't fit with *your view* of the outside world. Experiences up until now may not have encouraged "lots" of participation outside the home. Self-sustaining routines that exist at home have required significant modification, and few of these modifications *automatically work* in the outside world. Additionally, most successful ventures require that others have *some knowledge* of aphasia and *a willingness to accommodate* specific communicative differences. Not surprisingly, faced with this view of life, you and your loved one may hesitate to venture out the front door!

1–2 Hopefully over the past year, you and your loved one have sought out activities that might add "flow" to daily life (see Chapter 7, Person with Aphasia: Emotions—Feelings About Self—Daily Life). You may have had some success as well in establishing a better balance between obligated and free time (see Chapter 7, Caregiver: Emotions—Feelings About Loved One—Daily Life). From these efforts, you likely know the types of activities that might add further value to life. However, it is likely that most of these arenas probably occur in or near home and under your direct supervision. If so, it is extremely important that this base be broadened *to other settings* and *with people.*

1–2 The target in the years ahead is to keep adding chosen activities to daily life, your loved one's, yours, and yours as a couple or pair. Regardless of where you find them, it is important to look for ways of getting these chosen activities up and running. Although the focus here is on exploration outside the home, the rules for doing so work equally well within the home. Basically, the aim is to make chosen activities pleasurable, beneficial to everyone involved, and over time, self-sustaining. Accomplishing this typically requires identifying an interest, finding an activity that supports that interest, exploring where and how it might be introduced, deciding who will take part and in what manner, searching out ways to keep it in motion, and promoting it to a self-sustaining level. Although this list may seem substantial, it is actually less complicated than it first appears.

1–2 In the beginning, you need to keep expectations minimal and choose pursuits that everyone finds agreeable or better. Once you find a protective setting where the activity might take root and grow, try to foster ways of making it more self-sustaining. Being more self-sustaining means either building something over time that will naturally maintain itself or building a supportive environment, that is, a protected "community," where participants have sufficient knowledge and skill and derive sufficient benefit to elect to keep it up and running.

1–2 One example involves a gentleman I know with moderate to severe aphasia, who wanted to do more in everyday society. This gentleman lived alone at home, could not talk easily or fluently, but understood others well. Through some initial probing, it became apparent that a prime interest of his was animals. Relying initially on a friend who was familiar with him and his restricted communication style, a plan was devised for the two of them to begin visiting a local Humane Society animal shelter to see whether some mutually satisfying activities might be found. After examining a number of options, this man chose to spend a half-day weekly unfolding newspapers for the bottom of cat cages and socializing with animals brought to his work room.

1–2 After several weeks of having a friend accompany him to the shelter, a self-sustaining routine emerged that no longer required an aide.

PERSON WITH APHASIA AND CAREGIVER

PERSON WITH APHASIA AND CAREGIVER

This gentleman and the staff had devised *mutually beneficial ways* of keeping existing activities in motion, ones that served everyone's interests. The gentleman with aphasia devised a way to transport newspapers from a storage room through several spring-loaded doors by using a canvas bag strapped to his paralyzed right arm. In addition, staff members at the shelter assisted him in selecting and bringing cats and dogs to his work area. The shelter benefitted from week's worth of unfolded newspapers, a job the staff found tedious and unrewarding. The other benefit was someone who attended "personally" to lonely pets, a prime theme of the shelter. The gentleman with aphasia experienced the satisfaction of devoting more "obligated time" to a task that was highly personally rewarding and helpful to others. Besides the personal satisfaction it added to his daily life, his efforts were recognized in a quarterly newsletter that honored volunteers in that setting.

1–2 This example underscores the ease and simplicity of moving a person with aphasia from the home to outside settings where mutually beneficial activities might be explored, modified, agreed upon, and implemented. This gentleman *did not have a caregiver*, nor could he do the chosen task alone at first. However, with a friend who was willing to devote several hours a week over a month's duration, a common plan was devised that benefited everyone. Within this *protected setting*, this gentleman has not only become an active participant, but after some longevity, *an accepted member* of that "community." Whether or not he can manage all parts of a particular task on a given occasion is no longer an issue! Other staff members there now know him, his manner, and his communication! They see him as one of them, rather than someone with a strange communication problem. As a result, the regular staff at this animal shelter know *how* to help and would come to his aid immediately in a time of need . . . he is not "aphasic" so much as he is someone who shares their love for animals!

1–2 Having such communities outside the home, even if they are small and insulated from the rest of society, is important. We all need to find purpose in what we do; knowledge of how our efforts contribute not only to our own lives, but to the lives of others as well. Most of us are wedded to society through a number of "assumed" communities, that is, small collections of people we like, with whom we relate, and in whose presence we feel better. These communities may be related to our work, church, recreation, education, children, community, government, or hobbies. **Because aphasia commonly interferes with a person's viability within groups, it is not strange that making daily life better now**

requires finding and establishing communities where people with aphasia feel accepted as full-fledged members.

PERSON WITH APHASIA AND CAREGIVER

1–2 As the caregiver, though, you may say, "I'm not comfortable serving as a coordinator who might find or implement activities outside the home. I don't even know *how* to go about doing such a thing!" Whether your reluctance is due to constraints of time or expertise, it is perfectly understandable! There are many reasons why serving in such a role might be hard, if *not impossible*. However, in the above example, there was *no caregiver*, but that did not prevent its implementation. If you cannot act yourself, there are others who often can and will. Some suggestions follow in the next section on how to find and recruit such people.

1–2 Finally, it is important to emphasize that reinvolvement in the outside world is not an issue confined to your loved one; it is yours, both individually and as a couple. Too often, meaningful parts of life are lost or abandoned because of a perception that they may no longer be possible. If the two of you spent 2 months each winter in Florida, quite likely there is nothing standing in the way of you doing so now, even if your loved one's injury *is severe*. Winter in Florida before may have meant 18 holes of golf every day and the thought of *not* playing now may seem like a waste of time. Well, strolling along a paved, beachfront path (whether in a wheelchair or walking slowly), putting together your own collection of seashells, feeling the freedom of being in 70° weather versus the four stark walls of your northern winter-bound home, taking in an occasional preseason, major league baseball game, arranging to hit golf balls at a driving range, visiting parts of the Everglades you never saw—and the list goes on—*are all possible!*

1–2 The same principles you applied to modify daily life at home now work in "other" settings. It may seem like the effort and expense is too great for the amount of return, and sometimes, this is true! However, "the doing," the participating in life at whatever level may be possible, typically outshines *not participating* at all. If your daily life remains significantly *less* than it once was, recognize that this is not a edict you were handed; it is partially, if not fully, self-imposed. There are alternatives, better ways of spending and living your hours and days, than "vegetating." They require a willingness *to change* something that either doesn't work or is largely unsatisfying. As long as you *insist* on making those changes, changes that refuse to let daily life be retarded by the presence of aphasia, you *will* find options that promote rather than "demote" your sense of self and life.

PERSON WITH APHASIA AND CAREGIVER

WHAT YOU MIGHT DO

1–2 MAKING DAILY WORK BETTER

Making daily life better depends on you and your loved one having access to cooperative and effective ways of relating and working together. At the beginning of this chapter, we profiled several patterns that may be evolving for the person with aphasia and caregiver at this point in time. Should you or your loved one see life as predominantly stark, meaningless, or empty, then these symptoms need addressing before proceeding. In Chapter 7, we offered ways for coping with life when it appeared particularly gloomy (Person with Aphasia: Emotions—Feelings About Self—Daily Life and Caregiver: Emotions—Feelings About Loved One—Daily Life). You need to return to these suggestions if either of you still feels highly immobilized by aphasia's presence. Should this be the case, it is quite likely that you need professional guidance. On the other hand, if you and your loved one have established patterns that permit your loved one to act somewhat in his or her own behalf, and free you to do more on your own, then you are ready to proceed.

1–2 HOW TO EXPAND ACTIVITIES OF DAILY LIFE

- Reexamine the obligated and free time percentages in your daily lives at this time.

  By now, this procedure should be familiar. In the previous chapter, you were encouraged to repeat this process several times yearly (Caregiver: Emotions—Feelings About Self—Daily Life). The purpose of this exercise was to direct you and your loved one in identifying places in life where further change might be advantageous. Over the past year, these percentages should have inched closer to preinjury levels, that is, obligated/free time ratios should now more closely approximate obligated/free time ratios from before. Additionally, it is important that this trend has added to life's pleasure. If so, it suggests a positive direction for future modifications.

- Single out which parts of daily life require modification.

  It may be that your loved one's free time has steadily diminished *in favor of obligated time* to take part in activities of choice. Even so, free time remains excessive, and most activities at the moment are in the home or *under your supervision*. Thus, the next step entails finding other settings or activities where you are less present. It may be that your obligated time has decreased as your loved one has assumed more responsibility around the house, but your free time is still not adequate, either to fulfill your needs or to allow quality time with your loved one. Look carefully at these time ratios and how you and your loved one might add balance to daily life. Quite likely, you need to increase your time interactively outside the home.

PERSON WITH APHASIA AND CAREGIVER

1–2 VENTURING OUTSIDE THE HOME

Venturing outside the home is not something to dread or avoid. You do, though, want to carefully consider and gauge your initial steps; they are often the most important. If you can orchestrate them well and successfully, the rest often follows naturally and with minimal effort.

1–2 HOW TO VIEW THIS PROCESS

Think of undertaking outside activities as similar to riding a bike for the first time.
- The first outings are the most unsteady and scary.
- Even when carefully planned, the bike may tip over and you might get scraped up.
- However, there comes a magical point along the way when you can say:
  "Aha! I've got it!"
- Once the concept and the feel are there, subsequent trips are *not nearly as threatening*.
- Remember that the beginning moments that are the toughest!

1–2 SETTING AN OUTSIDE ACTIVITY INTO MOTION

Table 8–1 lays out areas of concern for setting up new activities of choice outside the home. It is divided in focus between: (a) activities intended to benefit just your loved one and (b) activities intended to benefit you as a couple. Both forms of expanded involvement are likely important in the years ahead. Key issues in getting such activities up and running involve the type of activity, where to begin, who should be responsible, and how to ensure success and longevity.

Table 8–1. Prime considerations in establishing activities in daily life outside the home.

INTENDED BENEFACTOR	SELECTING AN ACTIVITY	WHERE AND HOW TO BEGIN	WHO IS RESPONSIBLE	MAKING THE ACTIVITY SELF-SUSTAINING
You as a Couple	Look for activities that might yield "flow" states: former interests untapped interests helping others Look at what you would have done in retirement without loved one's injury	Look for setting(s) that permit maximal use of what does work Identify worries or concerns Slowly add on to successes Reassess each additional step Decide together where to move next	Distinguish between taking part and being responsible Be fair and caring, but most important, be honest	Fight lethargy not to act Don't expect immediate pleasure Don't abandon an activity too quickly Focus on the doing Extend and support one another
Your Loved One	(same as above)	Start in a "protected setting" to see if existing skill levels permit participation outside home Build a viable base inside this setting before venturing outside Check into outside setting: receptivity other options Visit chosen outside setting Keep "your role" in mind Don't expect perfection at first Interpret loved one's actions . . . not defend them Withdraw slowly Make sure the working parts fit	Don't obligate beyond what is everyone's choice Look for support beyond yourself: in that setting other social agencies advertise Value to you may not be in less time spent, but *how* that time is spent Don't hurry the process Arrange to see outside setting Break task into component parts and examine each ahead of time Work in small increments over time	Have a sustainable target in mind from the beginning Include *lots* of repetition Look for other ways to make chosen activities more self-sustaining

1–2 HOW TO SELECT AN ACTIVITY

- **Look for activities that excite the participant(s), and may yield states of "flow."**
  In Chapter 7, we introduced the concept of "flow," the personal absorption in a chosen action to the extent that one totally "forgets" about one's self. In that discussion, we detailed likely areas to probe with your loved one when searching for areas that might yield flow states. They included: prior interests or hobbies, areas of interest unexplored before now, and opportunities to help others through some form of volunteering. Whether the activity involves just your loved one, or you as a couple, these areas may be natural places to search for actions that might sustain "flow" outside the home.

- If none of these areas elicits your loved one's clear or strong endorsement, ask, "What kind of activity would you have chosen if this injury hadn't occurred?"
  Such a question may seem insensitive at first glance, because many people no longer see such pursuits *as even plausible*. Maybe your loved one would have chosen to take trips abroad, spend more time outdoors hiking, fishing, hunting, working in a backyard garden, or reading and writing for pleasure, things that now seem *too involved* to pursue. However, *portions* of these pursuits, if carefully crafted and reconstructed around existing skills, are not only still desirable, but possible as well.

1–2 WHERE AND HOW TO BEGIN AS A COUPLE

- **Start activities in settings that provide the greatest opportunity for their continuation and expansion.**
  For example, if traveling abroad was a common interest and desire previously, embarking on a trip to Egypt by yourselves may not be the best first step. You may want to begin with day trips by car to nearby locations of interest. From these outings, you may want to identify and begin working on ways to solve common problems you encounter along the way.

- Discuss and jointly decide what might be done about problems that arise.

- **Make problems your joint responsibility, not yours or his or hers alone.**

**PERSON
WITH
APHASIA
AND
CAREGIVER**

For instance, maybe your loved one is generally confined to a wheelchair, but he or she can stand and walk short distances assisted. From your outings, you realize that by learning to walk unassisted 20 to 50 feet, or up and down 5 to 10 steps, you might greatly enhance your travel options: boarding of planes and buses, and staying in lodges where ramps and elevators are not standard. Knowing this, your loved one may elect to work harder at home and welcome your assistance.

- **Even if some problems are not fixable, do not forego preferred experiences.**
- Look instead for alternative options that permit their occurrence. If changes in your loved one's walking are not possible, this may restrict the type and extent of travel you elect to undertake. However, much of the outside world is increasingly more oriented toward people who have physical limitations. In larger metropolitan areas, it is common to find city and destination buses that accommodate people in wheelchairs. A variety of cruise ships offer complete packages of accommodations for people using wheelchairs. The boarding of planes and buses may be more involved and time consuming, but, if they are of your choice, they are usually still possible if arranged ahead of time!
- **Keep adding onto a known, established base.**
  Staying with the earlier example of traveling abroad, you may elect next to expand your day trips to weekend excursions and to stay at bed and breakfasts that can accommodate your specific needs. Such settings are not only removed from the congestion of larger hotels or motels, but give you a chance to interact in a home-like atmosphere with unfamiliar people. Seeking out a somewhat familiar setting may prove helpful in diminishing your concerns about interacting with total strangers.
- **Reassess and revise your joint desires and priorities after each outing.**
- Decide from these shared discussions where to go next.
  In this example, you might choose next to attend an elderhostel outing which focuses on a topic of joint interest. Such an event would allow you to share time with a small, likely unfamiliar, group of people in a setting where you might get to know some of them. Depending on what comes from that, you might elect, then, to take a small group trip, possibly with family or friends, or members of a stroke/aphasia group. The aim here might be to

see how well you travel with a group of people you know. Down the road and depending on your experiences, you may decide to take a chartered trip, again with a small unfamiliar group of people, yet with your travel requisites well-provided for. In this latter category, maybe you would decide to board a small cruise liner in Seattle and travel up the inside passage to Alaska and back.

PERSON WITH APHASIA AND CAREGIVER

1–2 WHERE AND HOW TO BEGIN OUTSIDE ACTIVITIES FOR YOUR LOVED ONE

- **As with joint activities, begin the activity of choice in a setting where success is most likely to follow.**
  Activities outside the home often require probing their key parts before undertaking them in real life. For instance, maybe your loved one is interested in joining a group of Euchre card players on a regular basis. He or she played Euchre prior to his or her injury, but that was years ago. His or her participation now depends on his or her current skills, and thus, laying out some dummy hands at home seems like a reasonable place to begin . If difficulties arise, you can figure out their nature and severity before proceeding. If problems occur, your loved one probably does *not* need to be retaught the game of Euchre, only refamiliarized with its rules and given ways of compensating for his or her communication problems.

- **Keep adding to what you know works.**
  Now that Euchre's rules are familiar, you may wish to invite a foursome of family members or friends over for an actual game. You may find that your loved one can play reasonably well as long as he or she is given a little more time to make decisions and a way of indicating trump. For the latter, you devise a picture card with symbols for the different suits and verify that he or she can easily indicate a choice.

- Look for settings outside the home where his or her participation might be possible.
  You may know that Euchre is played weekly at the local senior center and yet not know much about the group or requisites for playing in it.

- Find out whether your loved one's current skill levels permit his or her participation.

- Be honest, but cast his or her current skills in a positive light, not in an apologetic one.

Next, you might call the Euchre coordinator at the senior center and review your loved one's skills and needs. It is important to *not* emphasize only what doesn't work, but instead to emphasize *what does*, how you have dealt with what doesn't work, and, most important, your loved one's desire to participate and improve his or her game. In general, people are far more receptive and extending in life when they know that their efforts matter!

• **Listen carefully for receptivity to your loved one's presence and participation.**

You never want to select a setting, for whatever reason, that is uninviting or hostile. Even if you may disagree with others' reactions toward your loved one or his or her abilities, it is important to listen to whether his or her participation will be welcomed.

• **If a setting is not welcoming, do not forego the activity; look instead for a setting that is welcoming**.

In this example, maybe the Euchre coordinator at the local senior center is sympathetic to your loved one's desires but worries whether his or her skills are adequate in their highly competitive atmosphere. This person suggests that there may be a subset of players from the center, people who simply love to play Euchre at almost at any time or place, who might elect to play occasionally with your loved one simply to assist him or her. As another alternative, maybe there are residential or adult daycare facilities nearby where Euchre is played, but their membership is less competitive. Thus, it is not your loved one's skill level that should determine whether participation occurs, but rather finding a setting where his or her skill more evenly matches the needs of the others involved.

• **Visit and observe the outside setting before your loved one tries it out.**

Once a setting is identified, it's advisable to visit it prior to your loved one's participation. Nothing helps defuse potential problems more than seeing the whole situation firsthand. You may not be able to foretell all of its dangers, but going and observing helps predict what might happen. In addition, your attendance helps set a foundation for your joint return later. You both won't be strangers on that first visit and you can concentrate more on orienting him or her to this new setting.

• **Keep your role and level of participation well in mind.**

The next section, "Who is going to take responsibility?" addresses how to determine your role and involvement in outside activities. In this example, though, you likely want to let others know your intentions and level of involvement *from the beginning*. As such, it may be appropriate to indicate your desires: (a) to accompany your loved one to this setting until it is apparent whether or not he or she can participate successfully and (b) to help others adjust to and, hopefully to accept, his or her manner of play. If you are able to accomplish these objectives, your hope is that this activity will become self-sustaining over time.

- **Don't expect everything to work immediately!**
- Anticipate that others may not be as sensitive to your loved one's needs as you are.

  It is not to be expected that others will be as understanding of your loved one's difficulties as you are. When this occurs, you can help out the most, not by defending your loved one or attacking his or her detractor, but by translating the part in the exchange that was misunderstood or misinterpreted. Try to think of ways that others in the group might better understand your loved one's situation and communication. Sometimes you may not even know why he or she misunderstands certain rules or conventions. You do know, though, that such errors do not interfere with his or her overall ability to participate if the activity is approached in certain ways. These interpretations of his or her behaviors may help others the most to "catch on" and to interact more easily.

- **Try to promote your loved one's participation, diminish your own, and still not impose on others.**

  You want to work toward a sustainable mix that does not rely on you *or* impose on others. It is likely to involve a combination of your loved one identifying a role that is possible and successful in this setting and others learning and adjusting to your loved one's skills and needs. After a while, you need to slowly relinquish your position of support and let your loved one begin playing the game with others while you support *their* efforts. You do not want to entrap anybody in anything that isn't of their choice, but you do want to encourage participation from others when it is willingly extended. A protected environment outside the home *must* have others to sustain it. Nurture these environments and people when you find them.

- A square peg won't fit in a round hole, but over time, you can slowly whittle its corners down until it does.

  The aim here is *not* to do the impossible or to impose your loved one on someone else or interject him or her into another environ-

PERSON WITH APHASIA AND CAREGIVER

**PERSON
WITH
APHASIA
AND
CAREGIVER**

ment. The aim is to find a setting and an event where your loved one's contribution is viewed, not just as sufficient, but as valued, and where others view him or her as a full-fledged member. Protectively looking and carefully encouraging such an evolution is not as hard as envisioned. Remember, it's like riding that bike for the first time. Once you've got the knack, the next trip around the block is not nearly as difficult.

1–2 WHO IS GOING TO TAKE RESPONSIBILITY FOR YOURSELVES AS A COUPLE

- **Participating and being always responsible are two different things.**
  Adding meaningful activities to your daily life as a couple requires that the responsibility be shared. Although your loved one may be limited in his or her communicative and physical abilities, that does not preclude his or her sharing the burden of making them happen or making them eventful.

- **Be honest, fair, and caring.**
  Sometimes the hardest part of adding to daily life means being honest. If it is done in a fair and compassionate manner, however, it is the best option available to you. If adding a new activity of joint interest only adds to *your* burden in life, then it is critical to readjust the formula so that both the burden and the pleasure are equally shared. If traveling abroad is of your choice as a couple, it may mean that your loved one needs to agree to certain conditions that might lessen your burden or increase your pleasure. Maybe it means giving you every other day "off" so you might sightsee, fish, shop, play golf, or just relax and read. The joint activity must be joint in all respects—pleasure and burden!

1–2 WHO IS TAKING RESPONSIBILITY WHEN THE ACTIVITY INVOLVES YOUR LOVED ONE

- **Find solutions that do not *obligate* anyone more than he or she chooses.**
  Many of the suggestions so far have focused on *your* participation or supervision as well as involving others in protected settings or "communities." To the extent that these recommendations coincide with the choices of those involved, they deserve considera-

tion. However, when they exceed such limits, for whatever reason, it is best to *look for other solutions*.

- **Do not hesitate to look beyond yourself for assistance.**
  If your loved one has an interest outside the home, but you do not have the time, ability, or desire to pursue it, look for others who might. Depending on what that activity is and where it might occur, begin by looking for support in the very settings where the activity might occur. Remember the earlier example of the gentleman wanting to volunteer at an animal shelter but not having a caregiver to assist him. The people at the animal shelter did need someone at first to help them decipher his basic needs and wants. But within several visits, a couple of staff members had "caught on" to his communication system and simply adopted this gentleman's situation as their own. The friend continued to accompany this gentleman to the shelter over the next month, but it was the staff who willingly assumed and carried the burden of work in getting him involved and comfortable in that setting.

- Look to multiple sources if necessary.
  If support is needed beyond your abilities and time and if others in particular settings cannot provide such assistance, then consider recruiting a temporary liaison. Perhaps a friend or family member might assist you. If these resources are not readily available, look to supportive social organizations in the community that provide voluntary assistance, like church organizations, senior citizen agencies, aging coalitions, stroke/aphasia clubs, and senior centers, or consider placing an ad in the local newspapers. When the latter course is chosen, look for someone who is willing to volunteer 3–4 hours weekly over 5–6 months to help your loved one become situated in an specific outside activity of choice.

- **Finding someone else still requires time and effort on your part, but in a different way.**
  Getting an activity up and running outside the home takes time. You might wonder why you would want to invest so much time in someone else when you *could* accomplish the task alone in the same time period. However, it may be that weekly meetings with a volunteer to discuss establishing an activity fit comfortably into your evenings, yet you cannot be available during the day when the desired activity actually occurs. Also, it may be that you cannot help overseeing the desired process if you are present, which only inhibits your loved one's participation. For whatever reason,

**PERSON
WITH
APHASIA
AND
CAREGIVER**

this type of effort, although just as consuming of your time, may be better for both of you.

- **Don't hurry the process along too quickly.**
  Remember how scary and difficult the beginning stages of adapting to your loved one's communicative and physical disabilities were for you. Anyone who is not familiar with your loved one, even if he or she is willing to help and be present, is going to need considerable time and a lot of encouragement to learn and adjust, too.
- As mentioned before, arrange to visit and observe the outside setting and activity with this person.
- Use whatever you envision might be needed outside the home to help give you a common focus to talk about and work on at home. Maybe your loved one wants to learn to ride the city bus to the YMCA so he or she can participate in an exercise class. You begin with the friend or volunteer by breaking down that process into its likely parts: walking two blocks to the bus stop, climbing three steps onto the bus, paying the driver, getting a transfer ticket, knowing when to get off, alerting the driver when to stop, getting off, knowing which bus to catch next, and repeating the above process once more to arrive at the exercise class.
- **Review every one of these steps, one by one, until all parties feel comfortable with them.**
  Maybe from riding the bus route earlier with the friend or volunteer you noted that the entry steps on the city bus were higher than your loved one was used to. Although there is a railing for support, you want to be sure that he or she can negotiate these. Thus, at home, you arrange for your loved one to try to step up onto a 10-inch step rather than a 6-inch step.
- **Begin outside the home in small increments and with parts that you know are possible and safe.**
- Meet regularly to discuss every outing:
  what happened.
  what did or did not work.
  how enjoyable it was.
  whether it can work now by itself.
  if it can't, what more can be done:
    to make your loved one's performance better.
    to recruit someone else in that environment to assist.
- Slowly, add on to what is working and fun.

1–2 HOW CAN WE MAKE OUTSIDE ACTIVITIES
SELF-SUSTAINING AS A COUPLE

**PERSON
WITH
APHASIA
AND
CAREGIVER**

- **Fight any lethargy that might lead to not participating at all.**
  In the beginning, it may seem easier to say, "What's the use?
  With things like this, why even try? With all the demands on
  everyone to make this work, why not just get up each day, get the
  essentials done, and vegetate in front of the television?" Well,
  being alive and *living* are not the same thing. Your shared daily
  routines need to have periods of flow if life is to improve. If they
  don't include "flow" at present, retracting from participating is
  the quickest way to ensure that matters will remain the same . . .
  indefinitely!
- **Don't expect immediate pleasure and reward to come from
  your initial efforts; these are the hardest to undertake.**
  Often, because it takes time for the two of you to adapt and to
  build a new experiential base from which to operate, the beginning stages may seem unrewarding and maybe even a bit dull and
  arduous. Remember, though, that it takes a lot of repetition and
  revision to truly set joint activities into motion.
- **Try not to abandon a chosen activity too quickly.**
  Even when an "adventure" didn't work, if there is a sense of pleasure and an inclination to return to it, do so. Keep probing and
  revising its parts until you have it in a form that works for you. It
  still may not be something you ultimately *choose* to keep and do
  every day. However, if you don't invest sufficiently to know this,
  you are apt to skip from process to process without ever finding
  sustainable states of "flow." Even if only 1 or 2 ventures out of 10
  are "keepers," over time, you stand to accumulate a preferred and
  sustainable list of activities.
- **Focus on the "doing" and *not* so much on yourselves or the
  outcome.**
  Putting matters into states of flow requires just this—acting for
  the sake of the pleasure derived from simply *doing* an activity, not
  focusing on its reward or your performance within it. Finding sustainable activities in life demands that the pleasure of doing them
  be sufficient to keep them going.
- Extend toward, and support, one another.
  Your supporting of your loved one is likely not in question.
  However, you need to support yourself as much as you do him or

PERSON WITH APHASIA AND CAREGIVER

her, and probably most important, you may need to assist your loved one in relearning how he or she might support you. The latter means finding ways in which he or she can offer you the consideration and support he or she used to, but now with an altered communication system.

1–2 HOW TO MAKE OUTSIDE ACTIVITIES SELF-SUSTAINING FOR YOUR LOVED ONE

- **Have a self-sustainable target in mind from the beginning.**
  It helps if everyone understands and agrees on a mutual goal for your loved one's participation from the beginning. By doing so, it does not mean that all parties are "locked in" to doing just this or that the chosen objective is even attainable. It simply helps the people involved to stay focused on a process of working together toward a common end. Maybe your loved one would like to try to have a small vegetable garden this summer, join an adult non-credit automobile repair class, volunteer to help others at church, enroll in a low-impact exercise class, attend afternoon matinees at a nearby theater, assist with a local "Meals on Wheels" program, or grocery shop independently. What the outside activity may be is not as important as having *something* to do that is interesting to your loved one and engages his or her participation.
- **Go slowly, build in a lot of repetition, and try to make it successful and fun for everyone!**
  These criteria have been emphasized before—they are the keys to finding and keeping something self-sustaining. Continuation of an activity depends not so much on level of performance or ability as on matching skills to settings, and to activities, and making the results *fun* and *rewarding* to all parties.
- **If an activity is fun and of choice but not self-sustaining, look for ways to make it stand alone.**
  Maybe your loved one loves to weed gardens but his or her standing balance is not sufficient to leave him or her unattended. An effective system has been devised at home with help from a friend. However, this system still requires someone to assist your loved one in getting up or down and traversing uneven ground. The friend was happy to assist in the beginning to see if gardening might be possible, but is not available indefinitely. You need to find a solution that permits the activity to continue and the friend to conclude his or her participation. It so happens that there

is a neighbor four doors down the street who has a lovely garden and is constantly working outside. As one possible option, you approach this person about having your loved one assist her. You indicate that your loved one loves to weed but needs a little assistance to do so. You wonder whether your loved one might assist your neighbor, and if that works, whether your neighbor might be willing to assist your loved one. You indicate that you or a friend would detail the precise nature of assistance your loved one would need. Also, you assure this neighbor that there are *no obligations* to do more than just see if something mutually beneficial might evolve.

PERSON WITH APHASIA AND CAREGIVER

Getting out into society permits exposure to countryside needed to reach your ultimate destination. Again, it doesn't mean, or even suggest, that you need to become socialites; it simply means that you need to become free to be fully who you are! Just as we've repeatedly acclaimed about your loved one, who you are, as a pair or couple, is no less than who you once were! New environments outside the home should come to feel as free and inviting in your select ways as old ones did. Stay with it. It will take some time for you to feel such comfort.

The roads ahead

We have come to the end of our suggestions for guiding you to your destination on this journey. As emphasized earlier, where you are now isn't likely to be the end of your road or your final destination. There are still many roads and routes before you that promise to offer you *more in life*. In fact, it may be most productive to think of what lies ahead of you not in terms of when you'll get home, but in terms of establishing a routine or way of life that offers a comfortable and harmonious blend of endeavors of your choosing. For many, this combination doesn't come at some magical point along the way; it slowly accrues over years of living with aphasia and its co-occurring impairments. Also, getting home doesn't mean that you won't be doing some remodeling or changing of house sites down the road. Rather, it means that the two of you have worked out effective ways in life that do not let aphasia and its consequences stand in the way of continuing to do and be more. **Instead of having something less than you did years ago, you simply have something** *different* from before. Among the many parts of what you now have, some are apt to be viewed as *positive,* and some perhaps even better than before.

Many changes still await you, and many of them *are* for the better! Seeking them out requires ongoing diligence and courage, but even more challenging at times, it requires that you continue to believe they are still there to be found. In the beginning, the drive to find solutions was often strong and relentless. As time living with aphasia accrues, making changes in life may seem less likely or possible. However, the *greatest* changes so far probably occurred only after you and your loved one realized that many of his or her basic functions were not apt to change a lot. What it meant was a "giving in," not fighting the status quo, but rather, setting about to build a better life within the existing boundaries. There will still be times when it appears as if no more changes can be made, but this statement is no different from similar statements you made before the injury. Just as with anyone in life, aphasic or nonaphasic, further improvements *can* always be made as long as you elect to search them out!

The chapters immediately ahead provide specific information about the nature of aphasia, its consequences, and related impairments. If you haven't already, scan these chapters in the months ahead for the parts that pertain to you.

The final chapter, Chapter 14, contains several case examples of people who are in the process of making this journey or have completed it. Their stories are each unique to them, as yours will be to you. Each is included to illustrate how different people under different conditions have chosen to cope with aphasia and to provide you with further incentive to continue your journey. **We began this journey with a sense of direction and hope. We leave you with the same themes, but also, with the knowledge that you now have the means to travel these roads independently in your own unique way.** Our best wishes on reaching your final destination safely and successfully!

CHAPTER 9

How the brain handles speech, language, and communication

Aphasia involves selective injury to the brain. When aphasia occurs, it typically results from an impairment in the flow of blood to the portion of the brain that regulates language. Generally speaking, such an injury does not mean enduring dysfunction to other prime brain functions such as thinking, reasoning, or memory. Instead, this injury selectively affects the areas of the brain where one retrieves words from a mental dictionary and arranges them for the purpose of communicating. Because of breakdowns in these functions, aphasia impairs one's ability to speak and communicate. This chapter explains how the uninjured or normal brain deals with speech, language, and communication. Later, in Chapters 10 and 11, we address the specific impairments incurred with your loved one's injury, and their causes. First, though, you may be uncertain how the related, and sometimes interchanged, terms of speech, language, and communication differ. We begin this chapter by defining them and their specific functions.

Speech

Speech is *a form* of language, that is, its *spoken version*. Quite likely, your loved one relied heavily on this form of expression to convey every-day messages to others. We all do, because of the ease and efficiency with which speech works. Shortly after birth, we began making speech-like sounds. Over the next 12 to 18 months, these sounds gradually became more refined until they became recognizable words in our own language. By age 2, 3, and certainly by 5, most of us likely were proficient talkers, users of speech.

Language

Language refers to more than talking. In a formal sense, language is an agreed on system of symbols and rules that permits us to share thoughts, ideas, desires, and feelings. As mentioned in Chapter 2, the ways of using language are many: listening, reading, writing, gesturing, and of course, speaking.

Acquiring language

As you acquired speech in early life, you simultaneously acquired language. With repeated exposure to language spoken by your parents and siblings, you learned and incorporated its use. You learned, for example, that only certain word orders in a sentence were acceptable. If you deviated from those, the sentence made no sense. For example, the words in the phrase, "House over come to my on" only made sense when you reshuffled their order to say, "Come on over to my house!"

In school, you were taught other uses of language. These involved *printed forms*, such as reading and writing. By the time you graduated from high school, you had gained sufficient skill in the use of these modes of communicating to comprehend thoughts recorded by people hundreds of years before and to write down your own thoughts to share with others hundreds of years later. Your uses of language were no longer limited to just listening and talking, you were also well versed in written forms; *you were literate.*

Gesturing

The use of gestures is related to language, but may not actually **be** language. For instance, when normal communicators talk to others, they are apt to use hand and head movements and a variety of facial expressions while conveying the spoken content of their message. These gestures alone probably would not be enough to convey the full meaning of a message. Yet, these nonspoken and highly visible "signals" would convey some of the meaning even if the more obvious agent, their spoken words, was totally absent. These additional signals often tell listeners which parts of messages are the most important and how to interpret what is said. For instance, one hand or facial gesture might indicate that your words are quite true; another gesture might suggest that others should doubt your spoken words.

At times, you may chose to pantomime or act out certain happenings in detail, for example, pretending to swing a golf club or to smell a bouquet of newly cut flowers. These facial and limb movements are not made up of words either, but many experts in language maintain that they are mediated or modified by your language system. In this regard, know that some parts of gesturing may be more dependent on language than others.

Gesturing as a part of language

For some communicators, gestures represent the "heart" of their language. This is true for children and adults who are deaf and unable to hear spoken words. Instead of speech, they rely on sophisticated hand and finger gestures, or "signs," to convey complex ideas quickly and accurately. These signs are coded in a language system like American Sign Language. When adults who are deaf acquire aphasia in later life, they, too, abruptly stop communicating their thoughts to others because their signed gestures are no longer accessible—much like your loved one's reduced access to spoken symbols.

As this example demonstrates, language is a far more inclusive system than just listening and speaking. It is made up of symbols and rules that govern how people might share their innermost thoughts regardless of form. As has been discussed in this chapter, the forms and uses of these symbols involve more than spoken communication. They also involve reading, writing, and gesturing. Although aphasia typically involves all these forms of language use to some degree, it does not necessarily impair all to the same degree. This means that there are many avenues or communication forms to explore to help your loved one reestablish a workable communication system.

Communication

When you share information or feelings with another person, you communicate. This interaction may or may not depend on language. Besides talking, writing, or gesturing, you may interact through forms that may be free of words entirely, such as drawing, painting, sculpting, dancing, pantomiming, playing, or sharing music. When it is shared, enjoying an art exhibit or an evening at the symphony can capture as much feeling or emotion as talking for hours about ideas. And none of these alternative activities *depends on language!* Thus, although language represents the spoken and written forms of communication, pictures, photographs, dance, music, and touch are equally feasible ways of communicating. How this relates to aphasia, a disorder of language, is that other "non-language" ways of communicating are less impaired. **It may well be that your loved one's overall communication might be enhanced through the use of such modes as drawing, pantomiming, or singing, because they are more intact and accessible!**

Having explored how speech, language, and communication both relate and differ, we move next to our primary aim, providing an explanation of how the brain normally handles these functions. However, if even thinking *about the complexities of the brain* is enough to make you break out in a "cold sweat," sit back, relax, and take a long, deep breath! Understanding the next sections is not a complicated or demanding affair; all of their content is well within your grasp. They contain only what *you* need to know! If some parts still seem too involved or unrelated to you, skip over them to something that does make sense. They will be easier to understand after the next chapter, which explains the nature of your loved one's injury.

Mapping out normal brain function

Sitting in the top of your head within a protective bony covering is your brain. Until recently, we had no easy way to look inside this covering to find out which part performs which function. As a result, most of what is known about brain function today comes from studying people who have survived injuries to their brain. In the past two decades, though, new, innovative equipment has permitted scientists and researchers to begin viewing "the workings" of the normal brain. The more sophisticated tools, such as *positron emission tomography* (PET) provide color pictures of brain activity while the patient performs mental activities like speaking, listening, singing, or looking at pictures. From monitoring which areas of the brain seem more active during a particular activity, scientists have begun mapping out normal brain functions.

What is apparent so far is that *many parts* of the brain participate at any one time when a complex activity is going on. For example, if you were asked to talk or to do simple math problems, multiple areas throughout your brain would show immediate activity. A broad area, consisting of the overlapping of many smaller areas of activation in the brain would be evident for both of these tasks. When a person is talking, there usually is one area that is more intensified than others in its involvement. As well, doing math problems yields a specific, and different, region of increased activity. What this suggests is that multiple parts of your brain work jointly and harmoniously on many functions, especially those that tax the mind, body, or emotions. Additionally, with certain functions like language or math there are discrete areas in your brain that contribute more to that whole than others. This added involvement does not mean that *all* of language ability or *all* of math ability resides in just these specialized areas. It means, instead, that these specialized areas are likely *more* crucial in carrying out those functions. This issue of localized function becomes more important in Chapters 10 and 11.

Structures and functions of the normal brain

The normal adult's brain has far too many parts and functions to consider here. We've limited the following discussion to those that relate directly to speech, language, and communication. It is important for you to gain this understanding in order to better understand the nature, and potential outcome, of your loved one's injury. As you begin, keep that relaxed attitude we spoke of earlier as we delve into the normal workings of your own brain.

Envisioning your cerebral hemispheres

To begin with, simply put your two fists together so your thumbs touch. Now, keeping your fisted-hands pressed together, move them around so you can observe them from all viewpoints: left, right, top, and below (see Figure 9–1 **(A)**). Now look at Figure 9–1**(B)**, and notice the general resemblance of your fisted-hands to the ***hemispheres of the brain***. Like your bonded fists, there are left and right halves of the brain that are tied together with nerve fibers. It is within these cerebral hemispheres that most of the complex planning and executing in daily life actually occurs.

Working together

Some higher level functions, like your thinking and memory, require a sophisticated interplay between these cerebral hemispheres to work at peak efficiency. An isolated injury to one hemisphere of the brain, either

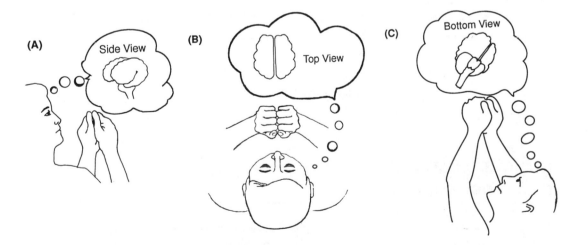

Figure 9–1. Comparison of joined fists to hemispheres of the brain.

right or left, *is often not enough* to permanently incapacitate reasoning and memory. Typically, there must be injury to *both hemispheres* before higher thinking and recall functions begin to erode. Such is the case when someone suffers from ***dementing diseases***, like Alzheimer's disease or Pick's disease, or has multiple head injuries to both sides of the brain. The word "dementing" actually means lowered mental activity, which is associated with injury to both hemispheres of the brain.

Working separately

As highlighted earlier, certain higher level functions of thought, like language, speech, drawing, painting, mathematics, music, or singing, depend more heavily on the participation of one region of the brain than others. Because each of these functions is more dependent on one cerebral hemisphere than the other, each such function is said to have a ***cerebral dominance***. We begin by examining which of the above functions is associated more with the left side of the brain than with the right.

Envisioning the left side

Imagine slipping on a pair of boxing gloves. With the gloves on, look at your right hand from above. Rotate the glove until it looks like Figure 9–2. This configuration, oddly enough, closely resembles the outer surface of your *left cerebral hemisphere*.

Looking for language in the brain

Chances are 90% or better that your own use of language depends more on functions carried out in the left hemisphere of your brain than in the right. This does not mean that the right side plays no role, however, it just means it is a less significant one! If you are left-handed, the likelihood increases that a more evenly distributed or right-sided dominance might exist. In fact, greater than 95% of the people having a right-sided dominance for language are left-handed! However, the opposite does not hold true: More than 80% of left-handers are still left-side dominant for language use. Right-handers have a higher probability of a left-sided language preference, 97% or greater. **Thus, in general, most people depend on greater participation of the left side of their brain than their right when listening, speaking, reading, or writing.**

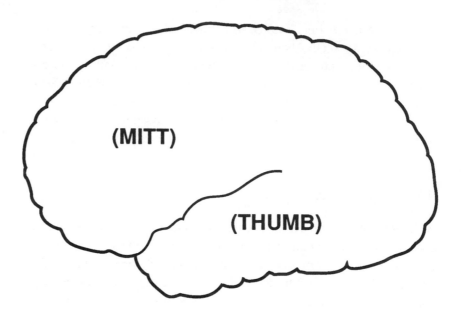

Figure 9–2. Comparison of the left hemisphere of the brain to a boxing glove.

Looking for language on the left side

Not all parts of the left hemisphere *are equally involved* with language. It turns out that the outer surface of the left side of your brain contributes more to language than do areas deep inside. In addition, not all surface areas of the left hemisphere are equally participatory. Language is most active in the *surface* areas toward the center of Figure 9–2 where the thumb and the remainder of the glove meet (see Figure 9–3). The outer perimeter of the left hemisphere serves a variety of other functions, for example, the back region involves "seeing," some upper areas toward the back deal with one's sense of movement or position in space, and some areas in the front aid problem solving, and starting and maintaining functions. But it is the central surface areas of the left side of the brain that directly oversee language.

Looking for speech and other uses of language

Within this central surface or *language area* of the left hemisphere, it is possible to speculate about certain uses of language more specifically (see Figure 9–4). For example, notice that the dominant region for talk-

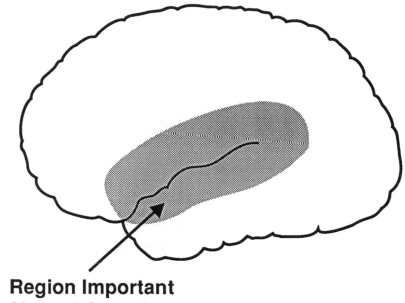

LEFT SIDE (HEMISPHERE) OF THE BRAIN

Region Important to Normal Speech and Language Functions

Figure 9–3. Region of the brain that is of prime importance to normal speech and language functions.

ing is a position where the thumb and the mitt of the glove meet. The prime listening region is further back and underneath the crease where thumb and mitt meet. Specialized areas for reading and writing, although much harder to pinpoint because they are so closely tied developmentally to speaking and listening, are governed by regions all along the central crease of the glove. But when reading and writing are severely impaired while listening and speaking remain more intact, the injury often involves an area beyond the tail end of the glove's crease.

Another quick note about speaking is in order at this point. Although using one's spoken language seems tied to the area discussed above and shown in Figure 9–4, the act of talking requires a rapid interplay between the brain and mouth, lips, tongue, and larynx or "voice box." Both sides of your brain must work together to coordinate the movements needed

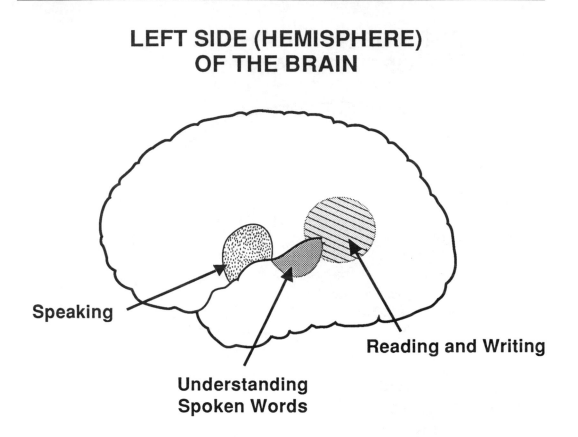

LEFT SIDE (HEMISPHERE) OF THE BRAIN

Speaking

Understanding Spoken Words

Reading and Writing

Figure 9–4. Differentiated areas within the normal speech and language area and their associated functions.

for talking. As will be discussed in the next chapter, disruption can occur to speech signals after they leave their language origin on the left side. When this occurs, a person's language system for talking is still working but his or her speech is not.

Envisioning the right side

The outer surface of the right hemisphere of the brain roughly mirrors the left one. Envisioning your boxing gloves again, the glove on your left hand now serves as the model of the outer surface of the right side of your brain. What is strikingly different about this side, compared with the left, is how cerebral dominance *is less bound to specific locations*. Thus, functions that prevail on the right side such as drawing, painting, or sculpting; music, particularly the melodies of songs; dancing; and parts of mathematics are less bound to specific regions of function.

Instead, the right side of the brain participates in greater unison during these functions than does the left side when performing language tasks.

Looking for communication in the brain

From our definitions at the beginning of this chapter, it should be obvious that communication is widely spread throughout the brain, that is, on both left and right sides. Nevertheless, much has been written over the past two decades about "left-brain" and "right-brain" personalities. Those who are considered more left-brain oriented tend to be more verbal people who depend on language to organize their world and their perceptions of it. Right-brain people may talk less and rely more heavily on visual, pictorial, or intuitive impressions about their world and environment. Often, right-brained people are more interested in the "Gestalt," or the whole, while left-brained folk are more analytical and sequential in their thinking. These notions, although oversimplified, reinforce the notion that the brain deals with communication in self-determined and specific ways. It would seem that for most of us communication involving language tends to be left-side dominant, while art, music, and parts of pantomime and math predominate on the right side.

In this chapter, we have introduced you to ways that the normal brain acquires and deals with speech, language, and communication. Whereas these terms and functions *are related*, there are *distinct differences* in where and how they operate in the brain. Knowing these fundamentals allows us to move on to changes that likely have accompanied your loved one's aphasia. Quite likely at this point, you can almost predict some of what we will discuss. You may need a little time to just let this information settle before moving onto the impaired states. Quite likely, though, these normal distinctions will become more evident as you grasp the nature of your loved one's injury, and how speech, language, and communication might be best approached. The next chapter, Chapter 10, overviews these issues.

How speech, language, and communication change with aphasia

You may have been told that there is "a picture" of the injury to your loved one's brain. Most likely, this reference is to a CT (computerized tomography) or MRI (magnetic resonance imagery) scan of his or her brain that was taken days or weeks after the onset of aphasia. Depending on your personal preferences, you may wish to see this picture. With the assistance of your loved one's physician, you may be able to better grasp the nature of the injury, especially its size and location in the brain. Sometimes, though, this picture may not reveal the full extent of damage, especially if it was obtained in the early hours or days after injury. In fact, a CT scan performed then may not look abnormal at all. You may wonder about the purpose of such a test. The reason for scanning the brain in the beginning hours after injury was not to determine the site of injury, but rather, to ensure that open bleeding was not occurring. Your loved one's doctor should be able to tell you how accurate and complete the existing picture is.

As you sit looking at this image, you may wonder about other aspects of your loved one's injury: Just how severe is this? To what extent will his or her speech and language be impaired? What caused this injury? What can be done? This chapter deals with the first of these questions: where the injury occurred and what it means in terms of speech and language disruptions. Chapter 11 addresses the causes of aphasia, and Chapter 13 provides an overview of what can be done to prevent further damage or recurrence. For now, we focus on how this brain injury has altered your loved one's speech, language, and communication.

Identifying the site of impairments

From Chapter 9, you know that it is the left side of your loved one's brain that most likely oversees his or her speech and language skills. Not surprisingly, then, it is here, on this side of the brain that the injury has probably occurred. You know, too, that normal language relies more on the outer surfaces of the left side of the brain than its inner or deep structures. As a result, more severe, persistent forms of aphasia typically follow injury to outer surface areas near or on the crease of the "boxer's glove" displayed in Figures 9–2 and 9–3. However, it is important to know that aphasia can, and does, accompany injury to areas inside the left side of the brain. Because this type of injury often results in rather unique speech and language features, we overview them before turning to the more common forms of surface-related aphasias.

Dealing with injury deep inside the brain

If you have elected to look at the brain pictures of your loved one's injury, they should help pinpoint the location and extent of damage. Figure 10–1 is a depiction of a horizontal "cut" through a person's brain in which the injury lies completely inside the left hemisphere (the dark or blackened area). Again, there is a greater likelihood that your loved one's injury is nearer the surface of the brain, or if somewhat deep, that the injury extends to the surface. But if it resembles Figure 10–1, and if your loved one's speech and language totally ceased in the beginning days and weeks, and he or she slept constantly except when aroused

Horizontal Slice Through Brain at the
Level of Speech and Listening Regions

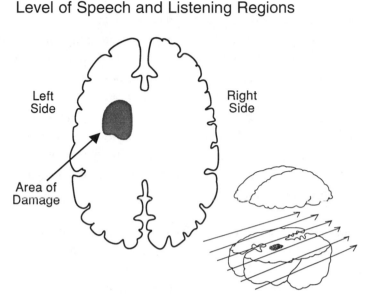

Figure 10–1. Deep lesion inside the left hemisphere of the brain.

through pain or discomfort, then you may wish to scan this section more carefully.

Coma-like symptoms are typical of people with deep lesions to the brain in the early going. People in this state appear totally "out of it." At first, they do not communicate, or recognize their surroundings or important others. If their injury is confined to just this impairment, and if they continue to improve, many of these individuals suddenly "awaken" days or weeks later. When this occurs, you may arrive one morning at bedside to find your loved one awake and talking. Although not all of his or her spoken words may make sense, their flow and usage suggest more of a problem in coordinating thought and speech, rather than an underlying language breakdown. Out may come complete sentences, although their meaning may be confused or unclear, for example: "Can't you undo my wallet hanger!" when, in truth, the intended message might be, "Can't you come visit me tomorrow." Over time, though, self-monitoring skills will likely improve to a point where most thoughts can be readily exchanged. In the months and years ahead, certain word selections may remain slightly ajar.

Dealing with injury to the outer surface of the brain

The more likely site of injury with aphasia is to an outer segment of the brain near the crease created by the "thumb" and "mitt" of the boxer's glove (see Figure 9–3). Look at Figure 10–2, and notice that the outer quarter inch is darker than much of the inner portion of the brain. This outer section is known as the ***cortex,*** and it, more than any other single structure, differentiates mankind from other species. It is the extensiveness of this portion of the brain that makes our brains so structurally different from those of other species. Functionally, then, it is not strange that higher human functions of thought and language rely heavily on cortical regions of the brain.

This outer lining is actually grayish in color because it contains a high concentration of cell bodies, central mediators of incoming or outgoing brain signals. The actual transmission of nerve impulses happens along what are called ***nerve tracts***. These fibrous extensions from cell bodies typically are white in color and rest more within the inner portion of the hemispheres of the brain (see Figure 10–2). You may have heard the saying, "He certainly has all his gray matter up there!" This means one views a person's mind or thinking as exceptional, and reflects our knowledge of the color and location of the brain cells in question.

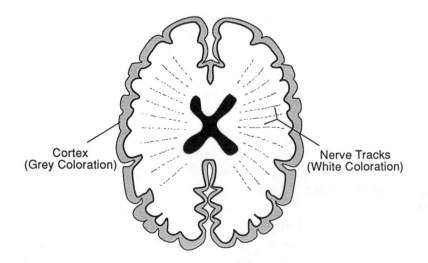

Figure 10–2. Cortex (gray matter) and nerve tracts of the brain.

Identifying the type of aphasia

In America today, a system of labeling types of aphasias prevails. Its origin is a group of noted neurologists/doctors, scientists, and specialists in aphasia who, in the late 1970s, worked together in Boston, Massachusetts to lay out these categories of aphasia: It is called the *Boston Classification System for Aphasia*. Like most other labeling systems in science, its true roots extend farther back to other documented clinical cases of aphasia in the literature more than a century prior.

Your interest with this classification system need only be to *better understand your loved one's aphasia*. To help you, we've suggested that an experienced speech-language pathologist point you in the proper direction here. Do not be surprised if your loved one's aphasia doesn't seem to fit neatly into just one or even two of the categories below. The aphasia of many people does not. This is not because you or the experienced speech-language pathologist are not practiced enough to make such distinctions; it is because many people with aphasia do not have pure forms of aphasia. Most have a combination of symptoms from one or more categories. Also, you need to know that types of aphasia change over time. That is, what appears today to be the proper labeling of your loved one's aphasia may, in several months or a year, no longer apply. Instead, his or her symptoms may better fit into a different category! In fact, many people with aphasia are classified as having one of the more severe types of aphasia in the beginning weeks or months, only to improve to a less-impaired form of aphasia down the road. Again, your loved one's speech-language pathologist should be able to assist you with these distinctions.

Keep in mind that placing a label on your loved one's aphasia only helps if it helps you, your loved one, or others. Knowing more about how other specialists refer to your loved one's aphasia may diminish your own confusion about their terminology. Above all, you needn't feel responsible for figuring out your loved one's type of aphasia; use this solely as an informational source to help the two of you through recovery.

Distinguishing between fluent or nonfluent aphasias

There are two broad categories within the Boston Classification System of Aphasia. They depend on the ease with which the injured person can talk. If speech flows from your loved one's mouth in an uninterrupted manner, similar to how it did before the aphasia, then his or her aphasia is likely ***fluent***. If speech, on the other hand, is nonexistent, minimal, not easily started, or filled with pauses or hesitations, then your loved one's aphasia is more likely ***nonfluent***. What may be confusing is that "fluent" and "normal" speech are not synonymous. In fact, in the initial days and weeks of injury, people with a fluent aphasia may use many totally *unrecognizable* sounds or words. Their speech sounds like gibberish or jargon, yet the flow of these vocal sounds and utterances comes without any apparent difficulty. It is this latter feature, *the ease with which speaking occurs*, even though the final result may not be recognizable, that determines whether your loved one has a fluent or a nonfluent aphasia.

A fluent aphasia exists if your loved one were asked "Did the doctor come today?" and immediately out came the spoken utterance: "Fibber moe is making my nist!" Not many of these sounds or words make sense! Yet the ease with which they occurred closely approximates a normal speaking rate, and your loved one is described as having a fluent aphasia. A contrasting example exists when asked the same question and he or she struggles for several minutes to utter a list of several descriptors like, "Can't. . .he. . .no!" In this case, the message is equally unclear, but the ease of talking is severely impaired; spoken words don't come out in a normal flow or pace, and your loved one is apt to have a nonfluent aphasia. In truth, though, you need to know that there are many people with aphasia who have some flow to their speech, but their spoken fluency is not the same as it was prior to injury. Also, there are some halting aphasic speakers who occasionally exhibit short bursts of three or more words. Thus, making a clear distinction between "fluent" and nonfluent categories is not always easy. What experienced judges do in these cases is to ask: "Which feature is more dominant, the person's ease or lack of ease of talking?" If confused at all, do not struggle over this distinction; ask your loved one's speech-language pathologist for assistance.

Types of fluent aphasias

If your loved one's speech flows with relative ease, two other features of his or her speech and language contribute to a decision about classifying his or her aphasia according to the Boston Classification System. The first is *the ability to listen or comprehend spoken language* and the second is *the ability to repeat spoken phrases and sentences.* As stated in Chapter 2, aphasia typically results in some impairment to both of these areas. Once again, trying to decide whether your loved one's remaining skills qualify as "good" or "poor" may prove challenging. If so, do not hesitate to consult with the speech-language pathologist.

Anomic aphasia: Good listening, good repetition

If your loved one's aphasia is ***anomic***, it literally means that his or her speech is without words. A better description, though, is that he or she cannot access and retrieve the precise symbols of choice from the dictionary in his or her head. For people with an anomic aphasia, the symbols for the *most meaningful parts* of their message are the hardest to retrieve. Thus, your loved one, when attempting to describe a recent family picnic, might say:

> "We were all out like . . . (gesturing a big area with her hands) . . . it was good for me . . . it was good for some I know . . . we did a lot of nice things. . .you know . . . there was . . . (gestures eating). Then, this thing started all at once . . . (gesturing something falling from the sky . . . to indicate that it was raining)."

Although precise terms are lacking, that is, the most meaningful elements like proper nouns and verbs are absent, much of the content of the message is still interpretable through its context and accompanying gestures. Because of this, most people with anomic aphasia are able to make most of their basic needs and wants well known. Even so, communication often takes more time and some listeners are not always willing to attend sufficiently to the aphasic speaker to discern the tone or complete message. Occasionally, even when communication is not significantly impaired, your loved one may *agonize* over his or her restricted command and usage of words and be less willing to interact with others.

Conduction aphasia: Good listening, poor repetition

It is possible that your loved one's speech may be fluent and somewhat interactive, that he or she understands most of what you say, yet *repeating* your spoken words is extremely difficult. When this is the case, your loved one may have a ***conduction aphasia***. For example, your loved one might say something quite freely, like: "Didn't see you come nearst my room." Although the meaning of this utterance may not be fully discernible unless you knew that it was said as you entered your loved one's room, much of the spontaneous speech of people with conduction aphasia is understandable. What isn't possible, though, is repeating the words of others. If you were to respond to the above statement by asking, "Try to say: Come into my room," a person with conduction aphasia might only be able to repeat this in a diminished form, if at all! In fact, instead of saying the same words he or she uttered moments before, your loved one might struggle to even say: "comst . . . im . . . man . . . rome." The injury to your loved one's language system directly interferes with the transfer of your spoken words to his or her own speech. In the early weeks and months after injury, though, most people with conduction aphasia are able to converse in everyday conversations with spoken words. Over time, their speech may come to resemble that of an anomic aphasic speaker.

Transcortical sensory aphasia: Poor listening, good repetition

This combination of abilities is sometimes confusing to understand. How can someone repeat complete sentences and yet not understand what is being said? Obviously, people with this type of aphasia retain a familiarity with how words sound, but they lose the ability to extract meaning or interpret the relationships between words. Not surprisingly, transcortical sensory aphasia often accompanies injuries that temporarily or permanently interfere with thinking.

In Chapters 2 and 4 (Person with Aphasia: Thinking), we discussed how the initial injury to the brain may initially interfere with reasoning or mental alertness. If your loved one is repeating your words in the beginning days of injury, but seemingly not understanding their meaning, he or she has a component of transcortical sensory aphasia. Usually, such injuries to thinking and integration are temporary, and so too, may be his or her limited ability to comprehend language. On the other hand, some injuries can occur either deep or toward the surface of the left side of the brain, which result in a more permanent version of transcortical sensory aphasia. However, even when these occur, most individuals show gradual improvement in their "understanding" and use of spoken words. This tendency toward improvement contrasts with people who have progressive diseases of the brain, like Alzheimer's disease, that interfere with thinking while allowing word repetition to continue unimpaired.

Wernicke's Aphasia: Poor listening, poor repetition

This form of aphasia is named after a famous German neurologist who first described its symptoms and location in the brain in the late 1800s. It is one of the more severe types of the fluent aphasias and often terribly frustrating for everyone involved. Should your loved one struggle to understand the simplest of statements or questions, be unable to repeat your words, and yet speak in an unending stream of jargon (meaningless words and nonwords), he or she likely has a *Wernicke's aphasia*.

Under these trying circumstances, you are apt to realize quickly that communication is all but impossible. Remember your communicative attempts in Chapter 2 while traveling abroad in a country where nobody understood you and you didn't understand them? Now your loved one doesn't understand your words and you can't understand his or hers. But, unlike being in South America where you realized the problem *was one of language*, your loved one is apt to be totally *unaware* that there even is a communication problem. People with severe Wernicke's aphasia outwardly act and feel as if they understand your words and feel that you *should* understand theirs. For example, such a person might say: "It's neherst fer you to fly coy?" when wanting to ask, "Should you be away from work?" Because nothing in that spoken message helps you figure out its intent, you are apt to request that it be said again. Now the speaker looks at you oddly, seemingly wondering, "Why didn't you get that? What is your problem?" Rather than aggravate the situation, you shake your head agreeably and sit quietly hoping that by reducing further communication you will not prompt a similar episode. Although such a strategy may diminish the quantity of your loved one's communication, it is not apt to eliminate his or her expressive attempts. With each, you face the very same dilemma over again.

Knowing how to deal with severely impaired communication when your loved one is unaware of the problem or its severity is challenging not only for you, but for others as well! Even experienced speech-language pathologists may find interactions with people having severe Wernicke's aphasia difficult to manage. As overviewed in Chapters 4, 5, and 6 (Person with Aphasia—Communication), there are ways of reducing the frustrations of interacting even though the meaning of messages may remain unclear. Pretending to understand your loved one when you do not, is *not* one of them. Instead, you want to look to other interactive ways that might increase his or her comprehension of messages, like using gestures, writing, or drawing. Probably, though, you will want to minimize the amount of talking you do. It only prompts more speech from your loved one, thus adding to the confusion of the exchange. By all means, seek out assistance from the speech-language pathologist in learning how to bridge this challenging communication gap.

Types of nonfluent aphasias

When speech doesn't "flow" with ease from your loved one, it is likely that his or her aphasia may fit into one of three nonfluent types. With the fluent aphasias, classification depends on your loved one's skills of listening and repeating words. Also, as with fluent aphasias, nonfluent forms may change over time into other, usually less-involved, forms.

Transcortical motor aphasia: Good listening, good repetition

It is possible that your loved one may understand speech, repeat your words well, yet struggle to get his or her spontaneous words to come out in everyday exchanges. It is as if the motor that drives speech has a "short" in it. Sometimes the power is there and a few words spurt out, but as soon as they do, something interferes and the next several words won't come. You can see your loved one struggling to get this speaking machinery back in use. Often the "on-off" nature of successful talking and the frustration of trying to get the system working is enough to curtail communication. The good news, though, is that people with *transcortical motor aphasia* often improve to a point where they can control their use of speech. They learn to hear and monitor their own speech production sufficiently that its halting and broken qualities are less apparent, and more controllable through a reduced speaking rate.

Broca's aphasia: Good listening, poor repetition

This nonfluent form of aphasia derives its name from the French neurologist, Paul Broca, who first described its symptoms and the location of its associated injury in the brain in the mid-1860s. If your loved one understands much of what is said, cannot repeat common phrases or sentences, and has limited access and use of speech, he or she likely has a *Broca's aphasia*. You need to know that there are varying degrees of severity of this type of aphasia. Some people with a "severe" Broca's aphasia cannot utter a single, purposeful word. They may occasionally put forth an automatic word like "hi" or "bye," but true content words in a statement or question are not possible, now or, in the most severe cases, even later after months of therapy or recovery. Other people with a more moderate form of Broca's aphasia may be fairly proficient communicators although their speech is clearly abnormal, broken, and telegraphic. For example, such a person might describe visiting an Italian restaurant as: "good . . . noodles . . . sauce . . . red . . . meatballs . . . hummm!" Small parts of speech, such as prepositions (of, with, to, from), conjunctions (and, but, or), and pronouns (he, she, they) are apt to be omitted or used inappropriately. It is not strange to find a Broca's patient referring to ladies as "he" or "him" and gentlemen as "she" or "her." Also, writing skills are apt to be no better than talking. When writing is *considerably better* than speaking, the communication deficit likely contains another condition known as ***apraxia of speech***. This speech disorder is discussed in greater depth at the end of this chapter.

The lasting challenge for many people with moderate to severe Broca's aphasia is communicating as fully as they might when speaking is less than desired. Throughout the journey chapters, especially Chapters 5, 6, and 7 (Person with Aphasia/Caregiver—Communication), we repeatedly discuss how to cope with communication when talking is not readily possible.

Global aphasia: Poor listening, poor repetition

The severest type of all aphasias, whether fluent or nonfluent, is ***global aphasia***. In its most literal sense, this term may suggest that all of language is interrupted. However, as stated in Chapter 2, this is seldom the case. When global impairment does exist, it generally occurs in the beginning days, weeks, or possibly months of injury. With time, the initial total interruption of language changes to some use, even if it is minimal. Hopefully, your loved one's language and communication skills are *not* this impaired. Be aware, though, that the label global aphasia is used frequently to mean *any* severe interruption of language and communication in the early stages. It is not uncommon to have a physician or nurse use the term "global" to refer to any marked interruption of understanding and talking. It is important to withhold judgment about the severity of injury until weeks or months down the road. **Many patients begin with a global profile, and slowly evolve over time toward a much more favorable and functional category of aphasia. This term may be used to describe either fluent or nonfluent forms** of aphasia. **Even if your loved one's language impairment is severe, this does not mean that communication is no longer possible. The journey chapters include support and suggestions for building onto whatever language your loved one still has.**

Picturing the actual injury to the brain

In Chapter 9, we introduced some pictures of the brain which displayed areas of increased activity during normal speech, language, and communication. Now we turn to several simple views of the brain that may help detail the injuries that accompany fluent and nonfluent types of aphasia. Keep in mind that structure and function in the brain vary considerably from person to person. The pictures here illustrate current notions and trends in thinking about aphasia. Your loved one's injury and aphasia may or may not be represented here.

Looking at front and back halves

In Chapter 9, we used a boxing glove comparison to discuss major landmarks within the left side of brain. In Figure 10–3, we revisit that basic illustration, but notice that there is another indentation or crease in the "glove." This division extends upward from midway where the "thumb" and "mitt" meet to the top of the glove (Figure 10–3 [**a**]). In fact, if viewed from above, this crease extends all the way to the midline, thus effectively dividing the brain into front and back halves (Fig 10–3 [**b**]). This division proves significant anatomically in that it "roughly" divides the types of aphasia as well. It turns out that most *nonfluent aphasias* result from injuries to the front central part, and most fluent aphasias come from injuries to the back central half.

Looking within front and back halves

You may wonder whether front and back halves of the left hemisphere can be subdivided further. Can we specify places in the front where injury is apt to occur with nonfluent aphasias? Similarly, can we locate distinct regions in the back half for the fluent aphasias? To a rather limited degree, we can. Look back at Figure 9–4 in Chapter 9 and refresh your memory about locations on the left side of the brain for common language functions. Using this same figure realize that injury to the prime speech area

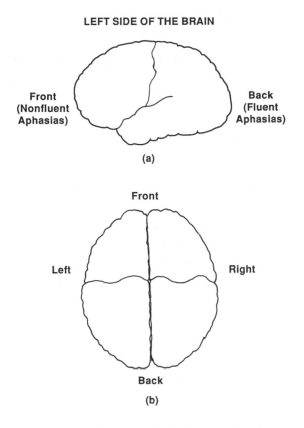

Figure 10–3. Front and back halves of the brain and their relationship to types of aphasia.

contributes to a Broca's aphasia, and injury to the prime listening area results in a Wernicke's aphasia. The fluent aphasias of anomic and conduction, *cannot* be pinpointed more specifically other than to smaller regions in the back half of the left side. Quite often, anomic aphasias evolve from improving conduction and Wernicke's forms. Transcortical forms (motor in the front and sensory in the back), likewise, can occur either deep or on the surface. As you might suspect, global aphasia typically involves a large area of injury, often encompassing much of the front and back language areas displayed in Figure 9–3 .

Speech impairments that are not aphasia

Injury to the brain can selectively *impair speech* while not impairing language. Two such speech disorders are ***apraxia of speech*** and ***dysarthria.***

Each of these conditions can occur apart from other impairments such as aphasia, but very often, one or the other, or both, are found *with* aphasia. When one occurs concurrently with aphasia, it is likely that the injury that caused your loved one's aphasia caused this speech impairment, too.

Apraxia of speech

If your loved one understands spoken words well but can't talk, he or she may suffer, in part, from a condition known as ***apraxia of speech***. The difficulty speaking is not due to an inability to access one's words; desired words are readily available "inside" one's head. What prevents the saying of these words, though, is that their speaking movements are no longer automatic. It is not that the muscles of the tongue, lips, mouth, or throat don't work; they do! It is as if someone erased or jimmied with how to talk!

People with apraxia of speech can readily move all of their speech structures rather quickly and freely. The problem exists further "upstream" where the planning and executing of movements of speech occur. To better envision this, pretend that you were once a well-accomplished ballroom dancer before acquiring an "apraxia" of dance (no such designation actually exists). As such, you would *know* what a fox-trot is and *how it should look and feel*, but your body simply will not move unthinkingly through the proper sequence as it had before, hundreds of times. You can readily walk, slide, skip, or make use of any other dance movement in isolation, but when strung together in a complex array, the template for these sequences no longer exists. Such is the case with *talking* for people having apraxia of speech; they simply no longer have a proper conversion formula in their heads for making words become realities at their mouths. Instead of a perfectly clear "What a beautiful day!" in one's head, out comes: "Putt . . . ta . . . poo . . . ta . . . able . . . kae!" at their mouths.

In its purest form, people with apraxia can *write out their messages* even though they cannot say them. More often, though, people with apraxia of speech also have an aphasia. It is their aphasia that prevents them from being able to write their impaired spoken messages. The good news is that, if it is an apraxia of speech that is most interfering with your loved one's ability to talk, it is a treatable condition. That can often be aided. Your loved one's speech-language pathologist should be able to advise you and help you with this matter.

Dysarthria

It is possible that your loved one's speech may be highly distorted and unclear, not due to aphasia or an apraxia of speech, but due to a speech disorder known as *dysarthria*. This speech impairment is not due to a breakdown in language (aphasia), nor is it due to planning or executing movements of speech (apraxia); instead it is due to the interruption of nerve impulses intended for the mouth, lips, tongue, larynx and chest (breathing muscles). When this occurs, the quality of one's speech is directly affected. It is as if this person's tongue and mouth won't move with the ease they once did. In truth, though, motor messages from the brain simply are not arriving in full at the level of the speaking machinery. If asked to say: "Billions of dollars won't guarantee happiness!" you may hear: "bi . . . on uh ah . . . uh on ga . . . un . . . dee ha . . . pi . . . us."

Notice that the speech of dysarthric speakers, compared to apraxic speakers, sounds somewhat familiar although by no means correct! It is as if all sounds are emanating from somewhere *in the middle* of the mouth. Also, whereas the mouth and tongue move reasonably well for people with apraxia, dysarthric speakers show clear signs of muscle weakness and incoordination. Saliva may run freely from one side of their mouth and wetting their lips may be a real struggle. For these people, their breakdown in talking is not due to recalling and executing the movements of speech (apraxia), their problem is in getting speech signals to their speech muscles. Some arrive; some don't. The good news for people who have dysarthria early on is that substantial improvement in talking may follow in the initial months after injury.

Sizing up your loved one's injury

Hopefully you have not arrived at this juncture terribly confused! You may find yourself asking questions such as: "Gee . . . what kind of aphasia does my loved one have? Does he or she have an apraxia of speech or dysarthria, too?" Do not struggle with these issues; turn them over immediately to your loved one's speech-language pathologist to answer. The explanations here are only intended to provide brief clarifications of what your loved one has, once it has been determined by an experienced expert. Don't struggle to comprehend parts of this chapter that do not relate to your loved one's condition. Study only those parts *that do*. It may help you understand where the communication problem resides. How specifically to cope with whatever type of aphasia your loved one has, is detailed in the journey chapters.

You likely will need some time to put this information into a workable framework for your purposes. Do not be surprised if you need to revisit the pertinent pages from Chapters 9 and 10 several times before they truly begin to make sense. At another time, you may want to know more about what caused this injury. When that time arrives, the next chapter details this information. For now, give yourself a little time to assimilate what you've learned so far.

❖ CHAPTER 11

What causes aphasia

By now, you understand something about the injury to the brain that caused your loved one's aphasia. Other impairments as well, like a weakened or immobilized arm, leg, or side of the face, all originated from this same fortunate injury. In this chapter, we overview the *cause(s)* of these impairments. Know that a *complete explanation* of injury may prove more elusive than you might first imagine. The most obvious part, that is, what caused the physical injury to the brain, is often known within hours or days of onset, and as a result, is typically the *easiest* and *most verifiable* portion of the causation equation. The origins of this physical injury, though, may not be as easy to track down or determine with absolute certainty.

Take, for example, one scenario: perhaps the physical injury occurred from blockage of a blood vessel in the head. Whether this blockage developed slowly over time from a "damming" in that particular vessel, or whether a piece of floating debris came from somewhere else in the blood system and lodged there, may not be known. Even when this second level of causation is definable, for example, when the injury was due to a piece of floating debris, the source of the floating debris may not be easily pinpointed. The debris may have came from a clot around a valve in the heart or it may have come from a chunk of fatty deposit breaking free from the lining of a vessel downstream from the injury. In the end, you may be left with a list of possibilities, but no one certainty. Even if you are able to make this determination, you may ask again: What caused the blood clot . . . or the fatty deposits?

Sooner or later, you will arrive at a list of *general health and aging factors* that were less than ideal. Possibly your loved one had a history of high blood pressure, cholesterol, or intake of salt, sugar, alcohol, or tobacco. These factors may seem vaguely tied to the true injury, and they may seem somewhat irrelevant now that the damage has occurred. Yet these third- or fourth-level causes are still of importance; it is through revisions in these aspects of daily life that your loved one might minimize the risk of further injury. Chapter 13 delves into these influences in greater depth. For now, though, we focus on the first two causal levels of injury: what caused your loved one's physical injury and where that problem most likely originated.

Identifying causes of aphasia

When injury to the brain results in aphasia, it commonly originates from one of several sources: (1) an interruption of blood flow to the brain, (2) a growth or tumor, and (3) a blow to the head. In this chapter, we address each of these causes separately. Before discussing injuries that involve blood flow, it is essential to glean a quick understanding of normal blood flow to the brain. Don't become overly consumed with the technical parts of what is about to follow. Simply scan this information to orient yourself to whatever pertains to your loved one's injury. The more technical aspects can be explained or elaborated on by your loved one's physician. This information is here to help you become comfortable and familiar with important constructs you may need to know.

Normal blood flow to the brain

Blood vessels that carry blood away from the heart are called *arteries*. Their counterparts, blood vessels that return blood to the heart, are called *veins*. Typically it is a blockage of vessels that carry blood to the brain, the arteries, that causes aphasia. To replenish oxygen to the brain, your body relies on two major passageways: a front route and a back route. The front or neck route involves a pair of arteries known as the *carotid arteries*. The back route consists of another set of arteries that ascend through the spinal cord to the base of the brain. This latter pair is called the *vertebral arteries* (See Figure 11–1 [**A**] and [**B**]).

Arterial blood flow via the front route

The two carotid arteries, one on each side of the body, originate in the front of the body near the breastbone and course upward on both sides of the neck. Although it is not shown in Figure 11–1, these major frontal passageways divide into two branches near the "voice box"; on both sides, they become the *external* and *internal carotid arteries*. The external carotid arteries supply blood to the face and outer skull. The internal carotid arteries follow an internal path through the lower face

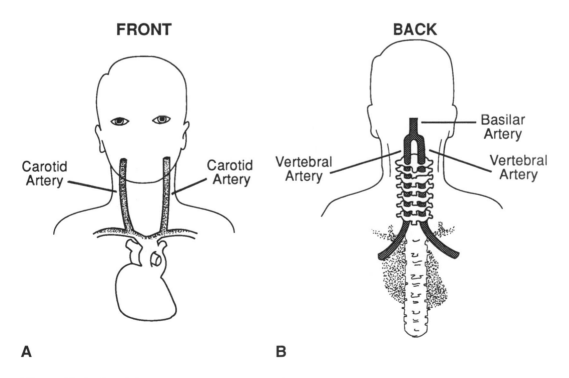

Figure 11–1. Arterial supply of blood to the brain.

until they eventually convene with the back passageway at the base of the brain. As detailed in the next section, this common shared "loop" at the base of the brain then provides blood to the entire brain by way of three *cerebral arteries*.

Arterial blood flow via the back route

At the rear of the body is the backbone or spinal cord. The vertebral arteries, both left and right, enter this bony structure near the chest level (see Figure 11–1 [**B**]). They follow the spinal cord upward to the base of the brain where these two arteries combine to form a single artery known as the *basilar artery*. The basilar artery supplies blood to lower brain structures that regulate basic life-support functions like breathing, balance, eating, and walking. From there, this artery ascends to connect the back portion of this shared "loop" with the front passageway. This circular communication of front (internal carotid arteries) and back (basilar artery) blood systems is called the *Circle of Willis*, resting at the base of the cerebral hemispheres (see Figure 11–2).

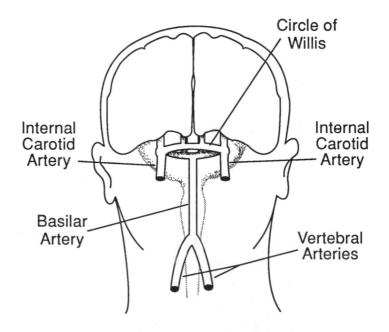

Figure 11–2. Ascending front and back arteries merge near the base of the brain at the Circle of Willis.

Blood flow through the Circle of Willis

The Circle of Willis is a fail-safe system for providing continuous, uninterrupted blood to the cerebral hemispheres; it provides an effective way of circumventing gradual blockages that might occur over time in any one ascending artery. Assume, for example, a person's left internal carotid artery became occluded by fatty deposits accumulated over many years (see Figure 11–3). Via the Circle of Willis, the resulting gradual reduction in blood flow most likely would not result in brain injury as blood from the right internal carotid and basilar arteries could compensate. In fact, this person's right internal carotid artery might become gradually occluded, as well, without signs of dysfunction as long as the vertebral/basilar networks remained fully able to compensate.

Blood flow to the brain

There are three major sets of arteries that supply blood to the brain from the Circle of Willis (see Figure 11–3 again). Each set contains

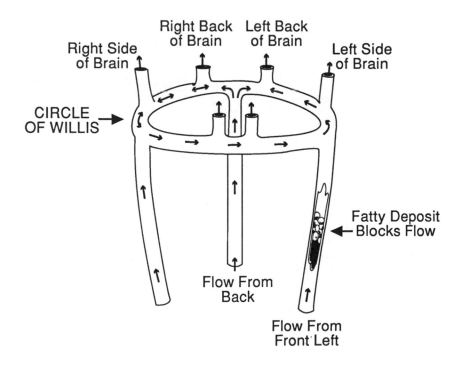

Figure 11–3. Gradual blockage in a lower arterial branch.

right and left sides and these sets are: (a) the *middle cerebral artery* (side vessels), (b) the *posterior cerebral artery* (back vessels), and (c) the *anterior cerebral artery* (front vessels). As you know, though, it is interruption in the *left-sided distribution of blood* to the brain that usually influences language and communication breakdowns. For that reason, we confine our discussion here to these pathways.

In Chapter 9, we compared the outer surface of the left side of the brain to a boxer's glove. Using the same referent, ***the middle cerebral artery*** emerges from between the thumb and mitt of the boxer's glove. This artery and its subsequent branches supply much of the blood to the surface areas where functions of language dominate (see Figure 11–4). As a result, it is not surprising that interruption of blood from this vessel, or a portion of it, often results in aphasia. The severity of the victim's aphasia is frequently related to the extent of the blood interruption. If the entire left middle cerebral artery is compromised, then the aphasia is likely quite severe. However, if only portions or smaller branches are involved, language functions are apt to be more selectively impaired or spared. Depending on where the interruption is, different profiles of listening, speaking, reading, and writing impairment are apt to occur (see Chapter 10).

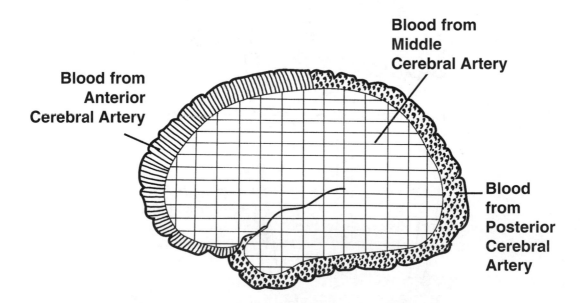

Figure 11–4. Distribution of blood to the outer surface of the left side of the brain from the anterior, middle, and posterior cerebral arteries.

You need to know, though, that the degree of loss of speech in the beginning days or weeks of injury is *not* predictive of the extent of injury! That is, complete cessation of talking at first does *not* mean that your loved one's *entire middle cerebral artery* has been blocked. Many **brain attacks**, in different and more limited locations of the brain, often result in a total loss of speech in the initial days after injury. It takes some time before a clearer picture of injury is known. Some of the images from brain scans may aid in this determination over the subsequent weeks, but it will likely be months, and a trial period of therapy, before you and your loved one truly know *the functional consequences* of this injury.

The **posterior cerebral artery** supplies blood to the back of the brain. It may seem from Figure 11–4 that the posterior cerebral artery has little influence on speech and language centers. This drawing, though, is a bit deceiving because there are actually many branches of the posterior cerebral artery that supply "deep" regions near primary speech and language areas in the back of the brain. Interruption of blood to any of these internal branches can produce aphasia. Often when this happens, the aphasia is more fluent than nonfluent in form. Besides disturbances to the clarity of spoken words, disproportionate losses commonly occur to listening, reading, writing, and visual perception. If large areas of the left side or both sides of the brain are compromised in these posterior or back arteries, the conceptual integrity of words, problem solving ability, and memory are likely to suffer as well.

The **anterior cerebral artery** supplies blood to the front of the brain. Because blood flowing through this artery supplies areas which are removed from primary language areas, its interruption seldom results in aphasia. Occasionally, though, smaller interruptions to specific vessels can cause an abrupt cessation of speech and voice. When this occurs, the injured person's language is usually intact; it is just the initiation of speech that is a problem. The result is a condition known as a **mutism**. When mutism occurs, it is often transitory and vocal tones spontaneously return in the weeks or months that follow.

Interrupting blood flow to the brain

Aphasia follows when blood flow is suddenly interrupted to language areas of the brain. Whenever sustained injury occurs from a blood flow problem in the brain, the person is said to have suffered a ***cerebral vascular accident*** or ***CVA***. When blood flow is stopped, the portion of the brain supplied by that vessel ultimately dies or becomes ***necrotic***. This dead tissue is slowly reabsorbed over time leaving a resultant "hole," or vacant space in the person's head. This destroyed portion of the brain is commonly referred to as an ***infarction.*** Not surprisingly, infarcted brain areas usually result in some diminished state of function. Impaired functions, then, must either be transferred to or supplemented by noninjured brain regions.

There are three types of blood flow injuries that may produce a CVA: (1) a constricted blood vessel that ultimately interrupts blood flow, (2) a plugged blood vessel, and (3) a ruptured blood vessel.

A ***constricted blood vessel*** may result from a gradual accumulation of debris (blood clots) and/or fatty deposits within the vessel's inner lining until blood flow is no longer possible. The accumulation of debris and deposits causing this blockage is called a ***thrombus***. When the reduction of blood flow is sufficient to interfere with normal functions, the injury or pathology is called a ***thrombosis*** (see Figure 11–5 [**A**]). The effects of a thrombus above the Circle of Willis are irreversible because there is no way to compensate for this blockage. But as mentioned before, a gradual occlusion of a blood vessel beneath the Circle of Willis may not adversely influence brain functions if other routes to the brain remain open.

A ***plugged blood vessel*** results from a piece of debris breaking off from a point downstream, either in a larger vessel or the heart, and floating freely upward until it wedges in a smaller vessel in the brain. The floating mass is called an ***embolus.*** The embolus then migrates outward toward the surface of the brain, where arteries become smaller and smaller. Eventually the size of the arteries is no wider than the embolus itself. When this occurs, the debris becomes lodged, much like a cork in a bottle, shutting off blood to brain regions beyond. The cessation of blood flow, or the injury itself, is called an ***embolism*** (See Figure 11–5 [**B**]).

Unlike the gradual evolution of a thrombus, the embolus enters the bloodstream abruptly and without warning. Because of this, its effects, even when trapped below the Circle of Willis, may produce a brain attack. Although blood flow to the brain may still be possible through the other major arteries, the *abrupt cessation* in a major vessel is often too much for the other arteries to offset all at once.

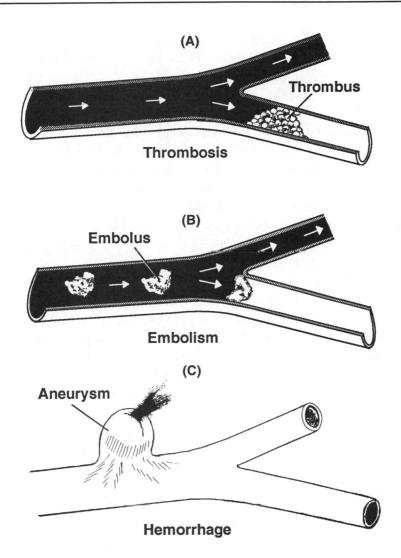

Figure 11–5. Types of injury to blood vessels that may result in a brain attack.

Sometimes the embolus may only *partially block* the flow of blood, or *may dissolve* or break down on its own accord. When stroke symptoms suddenly disappear after hours of apparent dysfunction, a condition known as a "small stroke," or a ***transient ischemic attack*** or ***TIA*** is apt to be diagnosed. The first consideration medically when TIAs are occurring is to locate and counteract the source of the emboli. The most common source is excessive clotting of the blood around an injured site within the circulatory system. For example, a heart valve may be slightly damaged and attempting to repair itself. As the body attempts to heal itself, clots of blood around the injury are sucked into the flow of blood passing in and out of the heart. As a result, some form of blood thinning agent is apt to be the treatment of choice (see Chapter 13).

A *ruptured blood vessel* is the third type of CVA. Much like an unprotected area of a garden hose where the walls have become weakened over the years and the inner rubber lining starts to extend out, blood vessels in one's head or body can do the same thing. A weakened region in a blood vessel that balloons outward from its original wall is called an *aneurysm*. Such areas represent the most vulnerable spots for breakage or rupture. When this occurs in the head, a pooling of blood, or *hemorrhage*, results (see Figure 11–5 [C]). When this occurs in the brain, the initial condition is often life-threatening, especially in the beginning hours and days after onset. If bleeding is deep in the brain, there is often little that can be done medically except to wait and see if the body naturally "plugs" the punctured vessel. Over 50% of the individuals with this type of internal injury die in the beginning hours and days. However, for those who do survive, there is often a more positive course of recovery than for those with an occlusive blood-related injury. People with hemorrhagic injuries can typically continue their recovery over a longer period of time than can people with occlusive injuries.

A growth in the head

Growths or tumors of the brain are a second physical cause of aphasia. Unlike an interrupted blood supply which cuts off needed nutrients to brain tissue, tumors either directly or indirectly interfere with normal brain activity. Directly, a tumor may actually invade and consume healthy brain regions. Indirectly, a tumor may push healthy brain tissue aside as it grows, increasing the internal pressure within the skull and in doing so make normal functions inoperative. A tumor may also cause a disruption of the blood supply, resulting in still another form of CVA. Any of these ways, whether direct or indirect, can produce aphasia.

There are two basic forms of brain tumors: (1) *benign*, and (2) *malignant*. A benign growth does not spread to other parts of the brain or body. In fact, it may remain dormant or unchanged over long periods of time. However, should such a tumor begin to grow, it typically does so within a self-contained sac or membrane. It is the added mass within the skull that poses the real threat to normal function. If the increased pressure against normal brain tissue is allowed to continue unchecked, permanent injury may result. If near the surface of the brain, this type of tumor may be treatable through surgery. A *meningioma* is a type of benign brain tumor. The other type of brain tumor, a malignant tumor, is far more serious and life-threatening. Once in the brain, these tumors spread readily and invade and consume living, normal brain tissue. Generally speaking, most are incurable. Because they cannot be eliminated, the treatment of choice is to retard their spread or growth. Malignant tumors of the brain include *gliomas* and *astrocytomas*.

A blow to the head

A third means of incurring aphasia is from a blow to the head. When such a blow induces changes in language, it typically comes from some form of *head trauma*. What is different about head trauma, when compared with either an interruption of blood or a tumor, is that entire brain functions, not just language, are typically compromised. Reasoning and memory are usually affected as well. Whereas these latter functions can be impaired with an interruption of blood or a tumor, they generally are spared when injury is confined to the left side of the brain. With head trauma, the entire brain is almost always involved, and the damage occurs in one of two forms: (1) *open head injury*, and (2) *closed head injury.*

Open head trauma refers to a penetrating wound that passes through the skull and directly into the brain. For example, a gunshot wound to the head is a form of open head trauma. Resulting language deficits depend largely on what parts of the brain were injured. If language areas were destroyed, a permanent aphasia is likely. However, the person's age is an important factor. If the victim is quite young, that is, adolescent or young adult, compensation of function in undamaged portions of the brain is often favorable. Even when open head trauma doesn't impinge directly on language areas, communication skills may suffer initially but then return to functional levels over time. However, underlying cognitive skills, especially abstract reasoning, usually do not. The extent of cognitive impairment depends on the extent and specific sites of injury.

Closed head trauma refers to a sudden blow to the head that is not penetrating. Either a fast moving object strikes an immobilized head (a baseball hitting a batter) or a fast moving head strikes an immobile object (a motorcycle rider striking his or her head on pavement). Today, it is this latter type of injury, from automobile and motorcycle accidents, that comprises the highest percentage of head trauma cases. Because the skull is not penetrated, the blow often results in a violent "jarring" of the entire structure within its bony encasement. This violent reverberation of brain tissue often renders the person unconscious or comatose.

You need to know that the type of change to language systems from either open or closed injury to the head is often quite different in form from damage caused by blood flow interruption or tumor. Besides the fact that trauma often involves a much younger age group, treatment is directed more toward compensating for thinking and memory dysfunctions in real-life realms, rather than confronting impaired communication skills. Because of the marked difference in dysfunction and treatment, this population of individuals is not addressed in this text. There is a separate and extensive body of literature dedicated to the needs of these individuals. You need to seek out a review of material addressing acquired head trauma or head injury on the Internet or at your public library.

Causes of injury to the brain

Most likely, your loved one's physical injury is known by now. Most likely, it involves some disruption to his or her blood flow. Remember that this is only the outward manifestation. Quite likely, the true cause of injury lies elsewhere in a mix of general health and aging issues. These issues are still important to discern, especially if you wish to minimize the risk of further injury (see Chapter 13).

The consequences of your loved one's head injury are apt to extend well beyond the inability to effectively use language and communication. The next chapter overviews other associated disabilities that may accompany your loved one's aphasia. Again, though, there is no rush to acquaint yourselves with more than is needed at the moment. You may wish, instead, to return to portions of the journey chapters and devote time and energy to these concerns. On the other hand, if you are confronting a number of related problems that are not communicatively based, then continuing on to Chapter 12 may assist your understanding considerably.

What may accompany aphasia

Besides impairments to language or communication, other differences may accompany your loved one's injury. A droopy or weakened right side of the face, the inability to move the right hand or leg, and loss of bowel or bladder control are some of the more *apparent* differences. There may be *less noticeable* changes too, ones that although hidden at first, are every bit as challenging. For instance, your loved one may not be able to eat food without having it silently seep into his or her lungs, see objects or people on the far right side, or endure physical or mental activity.

Whether apparent or camouflaged, these differences are apt to impact daily living and your loved one's sense of self. Sometimes the impact of these differences is minimal but at other times it is apt to be as profound as any changes in speech, language, or communication. This chapter overviews common impairments co-occuring with aphasia. Our aim here is simply to introduce you to these changes and to explain their basic nature. All of these changes are addressed more directly within the journey chapters under the headings of Recovery, Emotions, Daily life, and Relationship.

Co-occurring impairments can be categorized into two broad groups, (1) *physical differences,* and (2) *psychological or emotional differences*. Such a distinction is somewhat artificial, that is, physical change can prompt psychological change, and psychological change can influence physical attainment and function, but it is *the dominant feature* of the impairment that determines its classification here.

Physical changes found with aphasia

When injury to your loved one's brain interferes with language and communication abilities, it simultaneously may alter a number of other areas that affect his or her physical well-being. The degree to which these changes occur and the degree to which they impact daily life varies considerably from person to person and injury to injury. For this reason, some sections may be more pertinent to your loved one's condition than others: ignore those that are not.

Know, too, that substantial impairment in the early days after injury does not mean that substantial impairment will remain . . . although it might. Even when that impairment is substantial and lasting, however, its effects can usually be *lessened* or *accommodated in daily life*. Through exercise and adaptive aids, your loved one should be able to participate in chosen pursuits to some degree, and to reconstruct a destiny that rests more in his or her hands than in the hands of others. Many practical suggestions are contained within the journey chapters for achieving these specific ends.

Your challenge in coping with your loved one's physical impairments may be *no less* than his or hers! In fact, in many ways, it is much harder! It requires you to tolerate, accept, and permit a new use of altered physical status. As emphasized in the journey chapters, you may have some doubt or concern whether certain activities of daily life are even possible! Coming to allow your loved one to *try* to redefine life in his or her own terms, may not seem to be too difficult in theory. However, being able to truly stand back and allow her or him to try, especially if you have questions of your own, may not feel comfortable or easy. In Chapter 8 there is a detailed discussion of restoring the operatives of daily life to be fun and to accommodate expanding levels of function even when certain physical skills no longer exist.

Differences in movement

Total loss of movement of a body limb is called a **plegia** while partial loss of movement is a **paresis**. Since aphasia results from injury to the left side of the brain, it may seem strange that it is the right side of the body that is impaired. However, nerve tracts to the arms and legs cross over to the opposite side of the body just before leaving the brain. Thus, the left side of brain controls the movement of the right side of the body. When aphasia occurs, especially if the lesion is more frontal in the brain, your loved one may exhibit a right *hemiplegia* (total loss of movement of half of the body) or a right *hemiparesis* (partial loss of movement of half of the body).

In the beginning days of aphasia, a hemiplegic state is not uncommon. Due to swelling or **edema** around the site of injury, the degree of impairment often appears worse than it really is. Accordingly, if your loved one is unable to move his or her arm or leg at first, try not to panic. Improvement in these functions is apt to follow shortly as the brain adjusts to the insult. You should not be surprised either if impairment differs between limbs. It would not be strange to find movement of your loved one's leg, but not the arm or hand. Typically, if speech is totally absent, then movement of the right hand or arm is apt to be affected also. If speech is highly fluent, there is a greater likelihood of less impairment of both arm or leg, although in the early going some weakness or restricted range of movement may exist.

Whether the entire right arm or leg is immobilized or only partially affected, such a change is apt to affect a variety of common daily activities. Turning over in bed, sitting upright, getting dressed, standing, walking, or writing are all apt to suffer. As mentioned earlier, the picture you see now is not the picture that will likely exist months from now. Through the assistance of the rehab staff, particularly physical and occupational therapists, usually much can be done to restore or alleviate the impact of these physical impairments. Like aphasia, they will not simply disappear. But, also like aphasia, they need not preclude your loved one's living a life of personal choice.

Differences in physical and mental endurance

The existence of a plegia or paresis is one reason that your loved one is apt to struggle initially to participate in life. His or her overall level of physical and mental endurance is apt to suffer, too. This limitation may come, in part, from the increased effort to understand and cope with all that has happened. But *reduced participation in life* is more than adjusting to the physical and communicative changes. It is due to a processing difference within the brain itself; an altered mechanism and metabolism simply does not permit the same efficiency of thought or action as once existed. As a result, any sustained participation requires much more effort and time than ever before. Because of this, a generalized state of fatigue is apt to persist for weeks and months following injury.

This reduced state of function is likely to occur whether hemiplegia or hemiparesis is present or not. As a result, everyday tasks may need to be spaced apart. Eating, dressing, or visiting with friends may not be possible in the manner they customarily were in the past. Your loved one may appear interested and willing to participate, only to succumb to a state of near exhaustion midway through a task or activity. In the beginning days, his or her performance is apt to be far better in the early morning than later in the day. Not surprisingly, brief naps or rests during the daylight hours may be essential. After several weeks, you should get a better sense of how your loved one's physical and mental endurance has been affected.

Differences in bowel and bladder continence

An initial worry may be your loved one's loss of bowel and bladder control. Sudden insults to the brain often disrupt such functions. However, when this is the case, the disruption is usually of short duration—days or weeks. Sometimes it can linger on, and sometimes it lingers on because of communication difficulties. That is, your loved one may well know when he or she needs to use the toilet, but may be unable to let others know. Trained medical staff are usually familiar with, and sensitive to, this possibility. They routinely keep a urinal or bedpan visible and close at hand so the person with aphasia might initiate their use or gesture the need. In more severe cases, a toileting schedule may need to be adopted in the early going. Should this be necessary, then helping the person to the toilet for brief periods after meals in order to assure some uniformity in bowel care is a common practice. Be reassured, though, that even if this is necessary in the early going, incontinence is typically not an enduring problem. People with aphasia come to resume control over and responsibility for their toileting functions within several weeks or months after injury. It is possible, though, depending on the extent of paresis, that your loved one may need some ongoing assistance in carrying out certain parts of this process for a longer period of time.

Differences in eating and drinking

Immediately following onset, your loved one's ability to swallow is apt to diminish. Changes in strength, timing, and coordination of the muscles of the mouth or throat increase the likelihood that portions of swallowed food and liquid may seep into his or her airway or lungs. Normally when this happens, the body quickly reacts with a strong and forceful cough. But head injury often dulls this reflex and seepage may go undetected. When food or liquid has an open passage to the lungs, the person is at risk of contracting an *aspirant pneumonia*, an acute infectious state that, if not attended to quickly, may threaten your loved one's physical health and possibly his or her survival. As a result, oral intake of food and liquid is likely to be carefully monitored following injury. It may mean that your loved one needs to be fed through a narrow plastic tube extending from the nose to the stomach. Such a solution is typically short lived, giving him or her sufficient time to recoordinate disrupted functions so swallowing might occur without risk of aspiration. Should a feeding tube be necessary, oral intake of food and liquid should gradually resume over the next several days. The types of food and liquid introduced at first are likely to differ from a normal diet. Changes in food and liquid consistency, quantity, and rate of consumption are all likely to be carefully monitored until a more normal diet is possible.

Differences in seeing

Aphasia's onset may bring with it complaints of differences in vision. Your loved one may try to indicate that his or her eyeglass prescription does not seem right. He or she may indicate a need to schedule an eye examination. The difficulty in vision often involves changes in the person's focus, and objects or print may now appear somewhat blurred. This abrupt change in sight, though, most likely is not due to a difference in your loved one's eyes, but is a direct consequence of the brain injury. It is possible that some correction in his or her eyeglass prescription might help, although seldom is this outcome fully satisfying. Instead, it is common that such complaints about vision may spontaneously subside after a period of several months to a half-year postinjury.

Differences in seeing to the far right

Another common consequence of brain injury associated with aphasia is an inability to see objects in one's right field of peripheral vision— .far to the right side. In fact, your loved one may completely miss objects, events, or people when they are positioned to this side of his or her visual field. When this occurs, it often includes everything right of center, and since such a limitation entails half of one's visual field, it is known medically as a *right hemianopsia.* When severe, the injured person will eat food only from the left side of the plate or tray and totally ignore food on the right. When questioned about what was missed, this person is apt to look confused since the omissions are not apparent to him or her. Only when you redirect this person's gaze to the far right is he or she able to see the missing parts. It is not strange to hear a response like: "Oh, there's my coffee . . . I thought they had forgotten to give me some!"

A hemianopsia may or may not persist over time. However, if it does so for over a year's duration, it is likely to remain throughout one's life. When permanent, your loved one will need to learn to compensate. By that, we mean that he or she will need to learn to turn his or her head regularly to the far right to assure nothing is omitted. Such adjustments often become an automatic accommodation in daily life.

Differences in hearing

Just as visual changes are seldom a problem with the eyes, so too, a perceived decline in hearing is usually not a problem with your loved one's ears. Once again, the main disruption is likely traceable to the injury in the brain. On certain occasion, though, it may be due to a combination of hearing and brain injury. Possibly your loved one had a mild or moderate hearing loss before this injury. Language abilities were normal then and he or she could easily determine missed or mis-understood words in a conversational exchange. Now, though, due to the comprehension constraints from his or her aphasia, understanding everyday conversation is no longer possible. Similar to the eyeglass scenario earlier, it is possible that a hearing aid may help now, but only *partially*. To some degree, your loved one's difficulty understanding speech is due to the way speech is now received and deciphered in the brain. It is likely that he or she will need to acquire other strategies, like asking people to slow down their speech, avoiding conversation with more than one person at a time, or asking for occasional repetitions.

Differences in sensation

Your loved one may complain that portions of his or her face, mouth, or right side of the body may feel numb or tingly. When running his or her fingers across both sides of the face, there may be a distinct differ-ence in sensation. The left side is apt to feel normal while the right side feels partially "deadened," much like one's mouth after a visit to the dentist's office. Loss of sensation or *anesthesia,* like loss of movement, may be partial or complete, although it is seldom that *all* feeling is absent. Usually a diminished sensitivity to light touch and temperature differences may occur on the right side of the body. Deep pressure and pain usually remain largely intact.

Differences in thinking

We've stated that aphasia typically spares thinking. Also, we have reviewed how the integrity of thought may suffer in the beginning days of injury. However, your loved one, and even you, may wonder wheth-er his or her thinking is *completely* what it once was. It may seem as if complex topics or ideas are no longer as accessible as before. Your loved one may start to think that without ways of exchanging such con-tent, their underlying thoughts are gone, too. Perhaps at the very high-est levels of reasoning, this may be somewhat true. But to decide that *it is*, is a challenging and potentially error-prone process. Thought and language are highly interdependent. That is, for most of us without brain injury, we rely heavily on our language to define how and what we think. If language is disordered, as in the case of your loved one, it becomes difficult, if not impossible, to accurately determine how much of the difficulty in expression is one of language-based thinking and how much is simply language output. To some degree, it is likely both, but non-language-based thought is unquestionably far better preserved than language-based abilities. As a basic rule of thumb, constantly give your loved one the benefit of the doubt. Whether thinking precisely mirrors what it once was is not the point; he or she likely *approximates* past levels of thought when the effects of not having access and use of language can be minimized, excused, or circumvented.

Differences involving pain

Your loved one may experience periods of pain on the involved side of the body and seemingly specific to the arm, shoulder, or leg. Often such pain originates from misuse or disuse of involved limbs over an extend-ed period of time. To counteract this type of pain, regular exercise as prescribed by physical and occupational therapists is essential, espe-cially movements that strengthen and broaden the range of motion for the involved hand, arm, shoulder, or leg. Sometimes, though, this pain may originate from areas deep in the brain where the injury occurred rather than at the perceived site in the arm or leg itself. When this occurs, it is referred to as a ***phantom pain***, and its severity may vary considerably. Some people report a sharp pain as if stuck with a knife; others speak of an aching pain as if muscles are overworked; others describe it as a "hot" pain as if the hand or leg is on fire; and still oth-ers describe it as a radiating pain as if receiving a jolt of electricity. Whatever its form, phantom pain remains vividly real to the injured per-son, and is often unbearable. Should your loved one experience such pain, you will need to seek out a medical doctor who specializes in treating neurologically induced pain of a central nervous system origin.

Differences in brain wave activity . . . controlling seizures

Another common complication of head injury is that your loved one may have seizures. *Seizures* come from sudden and uncontrolled bursts of abnormal neurochemical activity within the brain. When someone incurs brain damage, there is an immediate, increased risk that seizures may follow. You should know that one's first exposure to a seizure, as either patient or caregiver, is often a *frightening experience*. Generally speaking, seizures disrupt the ability of the injured person to attend to purposeful movement or activity. In mild cases, the person may appear only momentarily dazed or preoccupied. But in more severe cases, he or she is apt to lose consciousness, fall, or experience twitching or jerking of one or more limbs. Whether the episode is mild or severe, the person suffering a seizure often feels different afterward. Symptoms following such an event include exhaustion, grogginess, and mental confusion.

The good news about seizures is that they usually do not cause additional brain injury. For this reason, there may be no need to seek emergency medical attention unless a doctor has so indicated. However, it is advisable to contact medical personnel shortly after your loved one's mental and physical condition stabilizes. Left untreated, seizures tend to recur. Repeated, untreated events might prove detrimental to one's health. A variety of effective medications is available to reduce that likelihood.

Usually, if your loved one is going to experience seizures associated with his or her head injury, they will occur within the first 12 months after onset. It is for this reason that many state governments forbid brain attack victims from driving an automobile during this period.

Psychological or emotional changes found with aphasia

There are other psychological or emotional changes that follow in the wake of aphasia and may be related to changes in communication as well as some of the other physical impairments just reviewed. They are often referred to collectively as *psychosocial features*. As a group of related problems bound to aphasia and its related disabilities, they represent some of the most challenging and enduring obstacles to recovery. Their management is a constant focus through the earlier journey chapters.

Differences in controlling one's emotions

Brain injury involving aphasia typically compromises whole brain functions at first. Because of this, your loved one is apt to experience changes in his or her "emotional thermostat." As a result, episodes of *appropriate* crying may occur far more readily than prior to injury, for example, upon seeing a close friend for the first time, or suddenly hearing a sentimental song or lyric on the radio. At other times, though, your loved one's tears may arise abruptly *without* apparent cause or reason. You may be discussing the weather with him or her when, without warning, he or she begins sobbing uncontrollably. This tendency to burst into tears at the "drop of a hat" is known to as **emotional lability.**

Many people assume that such apparent sorrow is a reflection of one's inner sadness or hopelessness over the present predicament. Friends and family may feel disheartened that they unknowingly worsened matters by saying whatever they did. It is usually not the topic, however, that caused the injured person to start crying, nor is it necessarily an overwhelming inner sadness. Instead, it is that this person's emotional regulation center in the brain is simply "ajar." In fact, he or she probably does not even know why he or she is crying either. It is simply that the brain-injured person cannot control these behaviors as he or she once did. Quite often, this emotional imbalance is only temporary, that is, it subsides in a matter of weeks or months.

If such a state of affairs exists with your loved one, it is important to recognize that its origin is not with you and your actions. Simply staying positive and moving to a new topic is often the best way of helping him or her out of these moments. If this doesn't work, then drawing his or her attention in an entirely different direction, as by squeezing her or his hand tightly, often helps.

Differences in mood . . . coping with depression

Few adults with aphasia escape feeling "down," especially as they become more aware of their changed status. But different from lability, which is more of an erratic and uncontrolled emotional "roller coaster," depression is suggestive of protracted periods of withdrawal or sadness in life. In the beginning of one's aphasia, it may be particularly hard for you to know whether your loved one's reduced participation is secondary to the injury itself or to depression. Communication may be so difficult that silence and withdrawal from talking may be natural reactions. When such withdrawal influences other common behaviors, like the person's sleep or eating habits, or the willingness to interact with loved ones, then depression becomes a more likely indication.

Depression can arise in response to physical and behavioral changes that have occurred. If this is the case, then it is referred to as *situational depression*. However, there is growing evidence to support the idea that depression is often linked to changes in the brain's chemistry following injury. That is, neurochemical activity that is essential to maintaining one's emotional stability may be permanently and adversely altered with left-sided infarctions. When this is the case, your loved one's negative feelings may not be simply situational adjustments but *physiologically induced depression*. His or her feelings of inadequacy may be more than simply *trying to adjust* to aphasia, they may be tied to distinct and discrete changes in neurochemical mood-determiners within the brain.

As highlighted in Chapter 6 and 7, when depression, regardless of its origin, persists, you need to consult with your loved one's physician or a trained specialist in this realm of dysfunction. Often, this condition can be aided by a combination of behavioral and drug modifications.

Differences in mood . . . feeling angry

Like depression, anger commonly accompanies aphasia and its related disabilities. It typically surfaces at some time in the recovery process, usually months after injury. When it does surface, it often emerges from a sense of "unfairness." Chapter 5, Person with Aphasia—Emotions describes these feelings and provides suggestions for coping with them.

Differences in one's perception of self

With aphasia and its other accompanying impairments, there comes an inner struggle to redefine and accept one's new and altered self. Chapter 2 defined such struggles as a prominent part of precisely what aphasia is! In fact, these aspects of aphasia are as much a part of the chronic disorder as on-going language and communication breakdowns. As well, the journey chapters (especially Chapters 6 and 7, Person with Aphasia—Emotions) highlighted how diminished self-worth and self-esteem impact reinvolvement in daily life. Getting better is as much a part of repairing these realms of life as it is repairing disordered communication.

Differences in "looking beyond" one's self

When one is stripped of key components of one's identity, it is not surprising that looking beyond one's self becomes a difficult, if not impossible, task. People with aphasia can become intensely preoccupied with who they are! Such a focus comes primarily from not seeing how their present form can, or will, fit comfortably within daily life, society, or their life-long view of themselves. Even though this preoccupation is more of a defensive or survival posture, a common consequence is that people with aphasia may seem to ignore others, their perspectives, and much of daily life—outside of themselves. Chapter 7, Person with Aphasia—Emotions—Feelings About Self—Daily Life, detailed a phenomenon known as "flow." Basically, this concept means subconsciously eliminating one's focus on self through pursuing chosen activities in life *that dominate* all other motives or thoughts. Finding flow again is not beyond those who have aphasia; even though they may think so initially. It will take time and effort, but it is possible. Chapters 7 and 8 are filled with suggestions for accomplishing these ends.

Differences in sexuality

Remaining physically attractive to a spouse or companion is commonly a desired and integral part of daily life. Given the multitude of physical and communicative changes, your loved one is apt to wonder whether he or she can still garner this type of response and respect from you. Chapter 6, Person with Aphasia—Relationship, directly addresses these issues and how you might better cope with them.

In this earlier section, coming to share intimately with one another in life was addressed within a metaphor of learning *to dance* again. Whether or not the act of "dancing" was even a preferred activity before injury, the message here is that there are ways of slowly reclaiming whatever you once had in feeling and action. Sitting next to one another, joking, touching, holding hands, and hugging are all preludes to stepping out on that "dance floor" again. In light of all that has happened it is not strange that you would give each other some time to recalibrate your response. Differences in your loved one's physical abilities or appearance may inhibit your ease and comfort to "dance." There should be no dishonor or stigma in feeling temporarily ajar, disoriented, or removed. It is perfectly normal and to be expected! What is not healthy is to let such feelings go unattended over an extended period of time. In Chapter 6 we offer ways of avoiding this latter situation.

Coping with more than aphasia

Adjusting to the injury causing aphasia brings more than impairment to language and communication and their consequences. It often ushers in other physical and psychological differences and consequences. For some people, the difficulties that are additional to aphasia may be minimal. But for others, they may change daily life as much, if not more, than faulty communication. **Just remember that no matter how many or how severe the impairments, there are always existing skills and resources, that if realigned from an inner desire to do more, can place meaning, purpose, and flow back in life.**

CHAPTER 13

What can be done to minimize further injury

Having endured the physical and emotional trauma of brain injury once, you and your loved one likely will want to do everything within your power to minimize its recurrence. Such a focus often is not simply a precaution or afterthought, but a passion. It is not strange to find victims and their caregivers totally overhauling their lifestyles in a manner that dramatically alters what they once were. Any factors which are perceived to be "related," regardless of the level of influence, are prime targets. Earlier in Chapter 10, we discussed the complexities involved in isolating the true cause(s) of your loved one's head injury. Maybe his or her head injury was known to be related to high blood pressure. Was this causal factor due to strain and stress at work, being overweight and not prone to exercising, a diet too concentrated with fatty, sweet, or salty foods, or more likely, some combination of all these? And if it was the latter, what was most contributory or in need of change? Another possibility is that your loved one was in *good shape* but a family history of vascular injury early in life predisposed him or her to this event. Regardless of which of these scenarios may apply, you and your loved one are likely trying to fashion a safer and more life-sustaining course now. This chapter is intended to overview how to minimize further injury. It is laid out in two main sections: (a) initial concerns—common treatments to minimize the prime cause of injury, and (b) subsequent concerns—common treatments that speak to the secondary, or tertiary causes of injury—often lifestyle changes. Before reviewing potential risk factors and ways of keeping the recurrence of head injury to a minimum, though, it is important to establish a basic plan of action.

Setting up a plan

Before proceeding, it is crucial to review any plan of action with your loved one's doctor and other specialists, that is, dietitian, physical therapist, occupational therapist, or speech-language pathologist. You may hear differing preferences among these professionals, and you may subsequently elect not to follow *all* of their recommendations. In addition, give careful thought and consideration to the pros and cons of each phase of any potential treatment plan before setting it into motion, especially if that plan involves radical changes to diet, exercise, or medications. Should your preferences for acting seem either incongruous, incomplete, or unclear when compared with the recommendations of others, consider obtaining a second or third opinion. Above all, you do not want to unknowingly compromise your loved one's health by introducing some aspect of change that is either too much or aversive. Once you know the range in which he or she might operate safely, you are far better able to determine which course of action might be best.

An example will serve to illustrate a number of these principles. I once knew a gentleman who wanted to run a marathon but was advised by his attending doctor that he might suffer another stroke if he did. He carefully weighed this professional's advice before choosing *his own* course. He began by walking to his street corner and back. Slowly he expanded this routine: down one side of the block and back, a full lap around the block, then a lap and a half, 2 laps, and finally 4 laps—a full mile. Next, he tried jogging slowly a half-lap and walking a half-lap. Over a couple of weeks, he increased his jogging distance until he was doing full laps. Months later, he was jogging the full mile. Over the next year and a half, he added to the miles until it became a minimum of 5 miles daily. More important than the end product, was the focus of this pursuit. It was his running that symbolized a changed style of life; it was this facet of daily life that got him out of bed in the morning and made his existence worthwhile.

Toward the end of his training, this gentleman had run 20 miles in a single outing! By race day, he knew that he was physically and mentally ready to do the 26 miles of a marathon. Even so, family members traded off and ran at his side throughout the race, just in case something unforeseen might happen. Nothing did! He has since run many, many more marathons. Running this first race came to represent more to him and his life than *not* running it ever had. He discovered along the way that running was a safe option and a wonderful conduit for charging his remade self and lifestyle. Had he not been able to run a short distance safely early on, he *likely* would have reconsidered his long-term goal. Undoubtedly, however, given this man's nature, drive, and desire, he would have redirected his energies to another similar pursuit that *was safer!*

You and your loved one will need to determine your *own* course for keeping the risk of reinjury to a minimum while permitting life's meaning and purpose to emerge and grow. What follows are some guidelines for initiating this pursuit.

Initial concerns

Immediately following onset, the first concern is to minimize the effects of injury as well as any risk of recurrence. You will recall from Chapter 10 that there are three prime causes of aphasia: (a) blood interruption to the brain, (b) a tumor or growth in the brain, and (c) a blow to the head.

Interruption of blood flow

When a **brain attack** is the precipitating cause of injury, treatment may vary according to when in the process it occurs. Very recently, there have been hopeful signs that if one's injury is due to an occlusion or blockage of a blood vessel within the brain, its effects may be reversed either through exposure to high concentrations of oxygen in the blood system or from the use of certain "blood-thinning" agents. Although such methods are only experimental at the moment, they appear promising enough to think that quick medical attention for any cerebral vascular accident may be more crucial than ever. Getting your loved one to a medical facility may not only improve his or her chances of survival, in certain instances, it may mean reversing many of the effects of permanent injury.

More likely, though, your loved one's impairment is too long postonset to reverse its symptoms or effects. When this more common scenario prevails, minimizing the existing damage and preventing further injury falls in one of three medical or health treatment realms: (a) medication, (b) surgery, and (c) changes in lifestyle.

Medication

Depending on what led to the interruption of blood to your loved one's brain, medication may aid in preventing further injury. If the existing brain attack resulted from an embolus, that is, a blood clot moving from elsewhere in the body to the head (see Figure 11–5 [**B**]), the doctor may prescribe an aspirin daily. This common, over-the-counter drug not only aids with pain, but it actively thins the blood without interfering significantly with normal clotting. However, if such migrating clots in the blood are frequent, due to ongoing injury within the circulatory system, like a damaged heart valve, a more aggressive blood-thinning agent may be necessary. Warfarin, Coumadin, or Heparin are common medications that serve this purpose. These medications aid in breaking down the size of the clot before it is released into the blood stream. These drugs, though, come with another, less desirable, side effect. Because they repress normal clotting functions, any internal or open bleeding may prove life-threatening. Should your loved one require such blood thinners, it is likely that compensations may be necessary in his or her living environment and lifestyle to minimize any risk of physical injury.

If blood flow was interrupted instead from a ruptured blood vessel, drug management is apt to be entirely different. Now the clotting of blood at the ruptured site is absolutely necessary for survival. The last thing the injured person needs is a blood thinner! Instead, it is more likely that rupturing of a blood vessel may be linked to excessive blood pressure. There are a number of effective medications that a doctor might rely on to accomplish a lowering of blood pressure.

Surgery

At times, surgery to restore a sufficient supply of blood to the brain may be necessary. When sustained flow is marginal due to the blockage of blood in both front and back passageways (see Chapter 11, the Circle of Willis), surgical deblocking or cleansing of a route may be recommended. The route of choice is often a carotid artery due to accessibility, and the professional of choice to perform this operation is a *vascular surgeon*. Such an operation involves entering the side of the neck with the greatest degree of occlusion and removing all debris causing the blockage. The surgery is called a *carotid endarterectomy*. This surgical procedure usually carries a low percentage of morbidity at the time of the operation but may need to be repeated at a later date, especially if other risk factors for the initial blockage have not been significantly reduced or eliminated.

Changes in lifestyle

Adoption of a healthier lifestyle is often the single best *preventative* measure toward reducing the risk of further brain injury. A later section of this chapter entitled *Subsequent concerns* overviews causative factors of lifestyle in more depth.

Growths or tumors

There are three ways that growths or tumors are treated. Again, these therapies may occur either alone or in combination. They are: (a) surgery, (b) radiation, and (c) medications.

Surgery

The treatment of choice for most benign tumors is surgical removal, assuming that access to the tumor is feasible. Benign tumors on the surface of the brain are readily excised. Often removal of these growths is possible without severe impairment to language, cognition, or memory, although some enduring impairment in one or more of these functions postsurgically is common. What is more concerning with benign growths is their tendency to recur. The likelihood of recurrence depends on the type and location of the growth.

Surgery may be indicated for certain types of malignant or cancerous growths as well. In such cases, though, the purpose of such operations is palliative, to reduce the size and negative impact of the tumor, not to cure the diseased state.

Radiation

High beam or locally intense radiation is often the choice of treatment for brain tumors that are surgically inaccessible. This technique involves directing a high beam x-ray signal directly on the tumor itself, thus destroying diseased tissue. With today's advances in brain imaging and x-ray delivery techniques, radiation treatment is far more precise and effective than in earlier years. Such treatment is often effective in reducing the size of the tumor, and for certain benign forms hidden deep in the brain, it is the treatment of choice. Malignant tumors are not typically arrested by such a procedure and, once again, are only treated as part of a palliative process.

Medications

Malignant tumors may also be actively treated with certain medications. If a malignancy is diagnosed, the doctor may recommend steroids to reduce liquid accumulation around the tumor site. In some instances, tumor size and its effects can be significantly reduced through such medications. Notable improvements in physical, mental, and speech/language functions may follow. However, as the tumor continues to grow and spread within the brain, increased levels of dysfunction in these realms will likely follow.

Blow to the head

As indicated in Chapter 11, there is an extensive body of literature pertaining to acquired head trauma later in life. Since the types of language and communication impairment are so different from those caused by an isolated insult to the left side of the brain, traumatic injuries are not covered here. Under National Organizations in Appendix C you will find an address and telephone number for the Brain Injury Association in America. Also, your loved one's speech-language pathologist should be able to help you in locating such sources.

Initial concerns about other differences that accompany aphasia

Chapter 12 overviewed common physical or psychological differences besides aphasia that may result from your loved one's brain injury. Like aphasia, other symptoms are most prominent and troublesome in the beginning weeks and months. Some, though, like movement of the right arm or leg, vision, pain, seizures, depression, reduced self-esteem associated with these impairments, and sexual dysfunction may endure over longer periods of time. Their management has been addressed throughout the journey chapters, particularly Chapters 5 through 7, Person with Aphasia/ Caregiver—Recovery. As a quick overview, though, we present a couple of clusters of nonaphasic concerns that commonly arise in the early weeks after injury, and suggestions of whom to turn to for their management.

Sitting, standing, and walking

Being able to move freely about in one's environment is a prime concern in daily life. Weakness throughout the entire right side of the body may interfere with your loved one's ability to sit up, transfer from a bed to a wheelchair, and walk. The professional who oversees these aspects of rehabilitation is a certified physical therapist (PT). If movement is restricted on your loved one's right side, a physical therapist's services will likely be needed.

Eating, dressing, and toileting

Impairments to these functions of daily living involve another rehabilitative specialist, a certified occupational therapist (OT). The first of these functions, eating, often involves a speech-language pathologist. The speech-language pathologist often oversees the evaluation and establishment of an eating treatment plan. Once oral intake of food and liquid is possible, treatment transfers to the OT and a dietitian who make sure that the plan is implemented properly. Being able to function independently in dressing and toileting skills are also OT treatment domains.

Subsequent concerns

The true cause of your loved one's aphasia likely began long before the injury occurred. Besides the natural aging process which, as of yet is irreversible, the most likely contributor was inattention to realms of basic health care. Even when other factors, such as one's genetic heritage, negatively impact this equation, attending to a healthy lifestyle is apt to be your loved one's best line of defense. As they pertain to minimizing further injury from brain attacks, the most important of these health care factors worth attending to are: blood pressure, diet, stress, physical exercise, substance abuse, and other physical ailments.

Monitoring blood pressure

Keeping your loved one's blood pressure within an acceptable range is a key component in lessening his or her risks of further injury. It is important that blood pressure be neither too low nor too high. The first of these conditions, too low blood pressure, is known as *hypotension*. The second type, too high a blood pressure, is *hypertension*.

Your loved one's doctor can tell you whether either of these conditions is of present concern. You need to know that *abnormal* blood pressure levels often are not felt or otherwise symptomatic. In fact, blood pressure levels may be quite "awry" without any interference in other daily activities or mental functions. For this reason, your loved one's blood pressure may need to be monitored closely until it is within an acceptable range. Obviously, trained medical personnel can do this, but there are devices commercially available that permit you to take these measurements in the home.

Depending on the modification desired, there are multiple ways of addressing blood pressure problems. Medications, elastic support sockings, diet, and exercise represent a partial list. Your loved one's physician is the best source for explaining and prescribing these options.

Establishing a healthy diet

Most of us likely could improve in this realm. For your loved one, though, it may be more important than ever to eat nutritious foods in primary food groups, that is, grains, vegetables, fruits, meat, and dairy products. Eating regular meals and supplementing one's diet with vitamins is often appropriate. Foods that are low in cholesterol and saturated fat are preferable in that they lessen the fatty deposits or plaques that accumulate in the blood system. Also, reducing one's consumption of salt and caffeine is helpful in reducing blood pressure.

Reducing daily strain and stress

People react differently to self-imposed, environmental, and work-related stress. Some people seem to do well or even excel, while others obviously sacrifice their personal comfort and well-being. Whether outwardly apparent or not, chronic exposure to stress is apt not to be healthy, especially when it elicits strong and lasting feelings of anger or hostility. Under such conditions, its presence is felt in ways besides one's emotions, that is, muscles may tighten and hands may sweat. As well, there are other bodily changes that may not be felt: cholesterol or adrenaline levels increase and these can adversely impact one's physical health. Whether patient or caregiver, you are not exempt from a host of challenging and stressful encounters in the initial months and years following injury. The journey chapters contain timely recommendations. In general, though, peer support groups, professional counseling, and directing one's energics more toward chosen pursuits are ways to counteract the effects of stress.

Building in safe and regular exercise

Besides diet, the most effective way of minimizing recurrence of brain injury is usually through a safe and regular exercise program. Regular exercise tends to strengthen the heart, promote relaxation, reduce stress, and improve blood pressure and cholesterol levels. Even though your loved one's head injury may affect his or her physical skills, these disabilities should not preclude exercise. Your loved one's physician should be able to advise you on the appropriateness and constraints of such a program. Most likely, it needs to begin slowly and be monitored carefully at first. Remember the marathon runner earlier in this chapter who progressed from walking around the block, to running a portion of the block, to running the block, to running a half-mile, to running a mile. Any new program needs to be undertaken gradually.

Physical and occupational therapists are excellent resources to consult for suggestions about the types of activities to consider and how they might be initiated and carried out. In addition, there are a number of exercise videos that demonstrate "low-impact" exercises performed in a sitting position, in warm water where heat and buoyancy may help facilitate involved arm or leg movement, and on stationary bicycles.

Eliminating substance abuse

If your loved one was a heavy user of tobacco or alcohol, he or she was likely advised earlier in life to modify these habits. Now there is even greater reason and urgency to revisit this advice. Both of these substances, when taken in large quantities, adversely affect long-term health. Smoking interferes with the optimal exchange of oxygen between respiratory and circulatory systems, and is known to be a prime factor in many forms of cancer. Consumption of large quantities of alcohol adversely affects higher thinking and memory functions. In addition, it may heighten the risk of seizure activity if such a possibility exists, as it does in people with brain injury. Simply put, threats to your loved one's health and general well-being from smoking or drinking are typically greater now than they were prior to injury. Remember that they were *not favorable* even then!

Attending closely to "other" physical ailments

Your loved one's injury may have been prompted somewhat from other pre-existing physical ailments, like heart disease or diabetes. When this is the case, attending to any special recommendations from his or her physician on how to minimize the negative effects of these conditions is important. For instance, physical exercise is still apt to be a preferred and beneficial activity, *but* under a far less rigorous and more carefully monitored format. Knowing how to exercise, how to check the degree of exertion, and when to stop are crucial factors. Your loved one's doctor needs to provide a specific prescription on how each of these steps should be carried out.

If diabetes was present before your loved one's aphasia, you likely know something about its nature and its influence on your loved one's health. Keeping his or her blood sugar level well monitored and within a tolerable range becomes even more important now. Depending on the severity of diabetes, a treatment plan is apt to involve diet, exercise, medications, or a combination of these.

Avoiding further injury

Much of the information in this chapter falls under the heading of just "good common sense." Society has become more knowledgeable of the frailties of the human body when it is not attended to properly, especially over the extended duration of one's life. **People are living longer today, and with that promise and hope there is greater emphasis, concern, and responsibility about health. Taking care of ourselves in many of the realms overviewed here provides the greatest assurance and insurance that later life will remain as productive and free of disability as possible.**

Continuing the journey

You have just completed the final "side trip" on this journey. Maybe you chose to read all the information chapters (Chapters 9–13) at one time, or more likely, you have selectively attended to them as you made your way through Chapters 4–8. If the latter is the case, you likely need to return to somewhere of importance along the current road. However, down the road you will eventually return to this juncture to complete the final chapter of the journey. In Chapter 14, we glance into the future . . . beyond the "two year juncture" described in Chapter 8. We bring you selected stories of others who have made, or are still making, this journey successfully. Regardless of where you and your loved one are in this process, we invite you to share in the experiences of some of your fellow travelers!

Living life productively in spite of aphasia

The impact of aphasia on daily life is usually profound and everlasting. Whatever your life once was is now dramatically different, but more significant than this, is the impact of aphasia on what life might be, now and in the future. As you read this, it may be weeks, months, or years after the injury actually occurred. No matter where you are in the progression of your journey toward recovery, there is nothing more important or fundamental to coping with aphasia's consequences than realizing and internalizing that **aphasia need not dominate your actions or the living of daily life hereafter**! Whether you, yourself, incurred this injury, or you are the caregiver or friend to someone who did, you separately and jointly have choices that can free you from its apparent domination over what you do, who you are, and how you go about conducting daily life.

Quite often the choices before you don't feel like "true" choices. That is, they either feel like things you would never have chosen, or things that offers no real choice at all. Instead of whether to take a high-paying position in the city and commute daily long distances to work or take a low-paying position and live in a quiet rural setting, the choices now feel more like what to do once you've lost your home to fire without adequate insurance: seeking a loan to rebuild or moving into an apartment. As such, these options don't bear any semblance of choice; in fact, they may only evoke anger and dread, and feel more like an "imposed sentence" than something offering direction or purpose. Each day you cannot help wondering what life would have been like had this "fire" not occurred.

Reflecting back on incurring aphasia and suffering its consequences is an understandable part of moving forward with life. When directed toward making better choices at the moment, this process is not only valuable, but essential. However, when it becomes a point of "fixation" that interferes with making other informed choices, it becomes *more* of the problem than the injury itself. The simple truth is, your house of old *did* burn down, either partially or in full. Also, its precise form and contents as you knew them before are not retrievable! No matter how hard you work or how much you wish, this reality stands squarely before you! Coming to terms with this fact does not mean you need forget the occurrence of the injury; it will never be forgotten. What it does mean is that every moment from here until death need not be predicated on this happening. You and your loved one have all the requisites to rebuild a comfortable home today; you have each other and whatever your current resources include.

Much has already been written about helping you realize and accept your current position in daily life. Many suggestions, especially in Chapters 11 and 12, addressed ways for optimizing the choices before you: where and how to begin, who should be responsible for what, where and how to add to your plans over time, and how to keep their outcomes secure, progressing, and positive in the years ahead. If you have already read these chapters, and had time to mold them into your own form and direction, you may feel comfortable with your progress and direction. However, if you are struggling with this process or just beginning, you may welcome a better glimpse of where these choices might eventually lead. That is what this final chapter is about, providing a collection of three case scenarios, or stories, of people with aphasia and their caregivers who have faced and rebuilt their partially destroyed pasts. For many, their new "domiciles" probably are not totally of choice on the normative scale of old, but are "of choice" when compared with letting aphasia stand in the way of a productive and self-determined daily existence.

Tim and Nan

It has now been 11 years since Tim had a stroke; he was a mere 35 years of age at the time it occurred. His wife, Nan, had known him since their youth; they had remained closely bonded as people and as a couple since their high school days. Tim was an optometrist and a recognized leader in his state professional association, while Nan was a well-respected elementary school teacher. They did not have children, and had blossoming, middle-aged careers when the blood to Tim's brain unexpectedly stopped flowing one day. During the first weeks after injury, there was a near total loss of speech and movement on the right side of his body. In a matter of moments, a "fire" had taken a significant portion of a home they had mutually put together over two decades. It left both of them emotionally and physically immobilized.

Within 6 months, Tim was talking, walking, and understanding most aspects of everyday conversation. Over the next couple of years, he continued to make slow, steady progress in all of the realms of communication and physical function. Although his current talking, walking, reading, and writing still stand in the way of a normal lifestyle, the basics of everyday life are well within Tim's skills. What has proven the most challenging adjustment, though, for both Tim and Nan, has been Tim's feelings of total despair about life and himself. He not only was unable to return to his job as an optometrist, but he devalued most of what he could do now in life as trivial and unimportant. In the beginning years of recovery, he spent much of his time idly at home with little purpose or direction. Nan did her best to prompt areas of interest both within and outside the home, but she was curtailed by Tim's minimal receptivity and her limited free time. Given their young ages and the financial constraints of maintaining a household, she had no choice but to continue her work as a school teacher.

Changing the emptiness of Tim's days did not begin until several years after his injury. It is likely that Tim needed much of that time, *3 years*, to finally come to grips with the reality of who he was! Matters began to move in a preferred direction once he decided to start attending to a small backyard garden, an old hobby of his. Although reluctant at first, he finally agreed to do so with Nan's ongoing encouragement and support. From doing a few gardening projects of "his own" the first year, he steadily enlarged these functions and responsibilities. Several summers later, he had assumed responsibility for much of the flower and vegetable beds in the yard. As well, he had begun growing flowers and plants from seed in an attached greenhouse and he was now mowing and maintaining the yard.

One summer day, approximately 6 years after Tim's injury, he and Nan were hosting a backyard barbecue when a friend noticed the quality of care he had afforded his flowers and vegetables. Somewhere out of the blue, he asked Tim if he might consider overseeing some flower beds outside a restaurant he was managing. After some thought, Tim agreed, and so began a long, slow progression of again living life through some chosen pastimes outside the home.

He carefully attended the flower beds of this restaurant for a couple of summers and then his friend took a different position, managing the dining facility and grounds at a private country club. But before accepting this new position, he ensured that he could bring his own gardener with him. Now, instead of the few flower beds at the restaurant, Tim oversees multiple flower gardens surrounding the main lodge of this private club. It is much to his delight and pleasure that these gardens provide a constant bouquet of floral beauty and color throughout the summer months.

The momentum and the personally derived pleasure from being a part of this process has prompted Tim to begin undertaking lawn and gardening projects elsewhere in the community. This past summer Tim expanded his business as he began mowing and caring for a neighbor's yard. Add to this the care of his own yard and the responsibilities at the country club, and Tim's summer months are becoming filled with activities of his own choice. Besides slowly establishing a routine outside the home that benefits himself as well as others, Tim is also building a number of supportive "communities" where he is viewed as an "insider" rather than an "outsider."

It is important to know, too, that Tim's journey remains ongoing. Although the summer months have come to assume some character of his liking, the winter months have been far more challenging. Until 5 or 6 years ago, it was not uncommon that as the last outdoor gardening activities waned, so did Tim's emotional well-being. To offset his blues, he tried to busy himself with snow removal and housecleaning chores at home and a regular schedule of physical exercises in the basement. Yet, these were not enough, and with Nan's urging and support, he began volunteering at a nearby nursing home, socializing with someone in need of a friend. He was paired initially with an elderly gentleman who had no immediate family and who had suffered a stroke like Tim's. This gentleman could still talk but, like Tim, not as well as he had before the stroke. Over the next couple of years, they came to know one another quite well. Tim visited him quite regularly during the winter months, and even when he returned to his summer lawn and gardening activities, he still would drop by occasionally to just chat. Then, the inevitable happened; his friend died mid-winter of the third year. For the duration of that winter, Tim stayed home; it just didn't seem "right" going back to that facility without his friend present.

The following fall, though, Tim returned to the nursing home to be paired with another person who might benefit from his company. The staff then assisted in locating another gentleman for Tim to visit. Although being back and helping someone else also helped Tim, it simply wasn't enough to offset his winter blues. It was about this time that another friend of Tim's, one who had several hours a week to devote to finding something else to fill Tim's time, began taking him bowling. It was an activity of Tim's choice, that is, Tim had requested that they give it a try. He had not thrown a bowling ball since his stroke. Like the process described in Chapter 11, going bowling eventually turned out to be an opportunity to merge skill with challenge to produce a state of flow in Tim, but not at first!

Tim's first attempts at bowling were anything but perfect. He started toward the lane with his old bowling ball in his right hand only to realize mid-way that he lacked the necessary strength in that hand to grip it. On the second step, the ball came loose and it bounced thunderously off the floor. Tim's first instinct was to think, "Hey, I can't do this!" However, his second thought was: "No, that's not right . . . I just can't do it that way . . . but maybe there's any another way!" Through some joint problem-solving with his friend, he switched the ball to his left hand. Although that remedied his problem, his former way of approaching the lane no longer worked.

Bowling left-handed required that Tim reach the point of release on his right foot, just the opposite of what he had done when using his right hand. He tried several times to coordinate ball, forward momentum, and release so that all of them might mesh, but alas, it was simply too much to do at this point! So, together, he and his partner devised a way that he could walk to the foul line, position his body properly toward the pins, rock the ball several times back and forth with his left hand, and then release it. Even then, it took numerous visits to the bowling alley to refine his skills to a point where he could keep the ball consistently in the lane and out of the gutters. Throughout this period, there were various "ups and downs" in his demeanor and willingness to persevere. But as frustrating as some parts were, they were less objectionable to him than sitting at home doing nothing. In fact, there were distinct periods in these bowling outings where he totally forgot that he was aphasic or hemiparetic. He became so involved in the process of trying to get his ball down the alley and to hit the pins, that nothing else mattered—including his injury or himself—it was the task that was his sole focus.

Unquestionably, bowling helped to keep Tim more engaged in life that winter. But in the greater scope of wishing to add to his self-esteem and worth, his involvement still fell short in his mind. Tim had long judged the worth of actions in terms of their societal merit and how much they actually added to life beyond the person involved. One prime measure of that worth to Tim was whether they were reimbursable, and whether people would pay money for the service rendered. If so, it signaled to him that the activity was something of value. As a result, he and the same friend set about looking for other activities or tasks in the winter that might satisfy this end.

Another winter has passed since then, and in that interim, Tim has begun shoveling snow at a home besides his own. It happens that the neighbor who hired him to tend her lawn has now hired him to remove snow from her driveway and walks. Since Tim and his client know one another from that earlier contact, it made this winter addition another "protected" setting where he might begin working. This activity, along with his visitation to the nursing home, his participation in a community aphasia group, and an occasional visit to the bowling alley, have begun to put his winter emotions on a more tolerable scale.

That all aspects of their daily lives are as they would like to have them is neither accurate nor fair to imply. Tim and Nan continue to work toward a more harmonious balance to life, 11 years after Tim's injury. Today, however, matters are more of personal choice than they were several years ago, and certainly they are much better than they were 5 or 6 years prior. What is most striking about Tim and Nan's story is not all that they've accomplished, which is significant, but its *evolution*. For them, overcoming aphasia and its consequences has not been a process collapsible into weeks or months; rather it has been a continuing growing and learning experience of years, and now more than a decade. In their own chosen ways, they continue to make living life a high priority.

Betty and Billie

There were 2 ½ years between Betty's first stroke, and her second, fatal stroke. She had been a high-spirited, energetic lady, who in her late 70s had never experienced more than "minutes" of what one might call "down time." She had spunk, a broad smile, a bright wit, and the charisma of a lady of the theater, although she had never been in a formal theatrical production. She lived alone in a small home outside San Antonio, Texas, on 10 acres of land where she could cater to her second love in life—animals. Betty's outbuildings were homes for her other family: her chickens, cats, goats, and horses. Of these, it was the horses that captured her heart the most. By the time of her first stroke, she had outlived two husbands and had spent much of the preceding 2 years attending to the second husband's struggle with lung cancer. She had just returned to her first love—oil painting, when her first stroke occurred.

Betty's initial injury to the left side of her brain was extensive. It involved much of the entire region dedicated to expressive communication and movement on the right side of her body. During the first 3 months, she received extensive rehabilitative services at a rehab center in San Antonio. During that interim, communication and mobility improved, although not remarkably. At the time of discharge, her speech was largely broken and unclear with only occasional words to help one decipher her message. Self-care activities, such as dressing, eating, and using the toilet, were now possible, but a severe right-sided weakness and diminished overall endurance made standing and walking a limited and difficult process. Despite these setbacks, though, Betty's mind, memory, and spunk remained largely intact.

With rehab ending and Betty's severe communicative and physical impairments remaining, a discharge decision was rather predetermined; she would need to be placed in a long-term nursing care facility or in a protected setting where constant ongoing supervision was possible. It was the rehabilitative team's recommendation that her current needs were simply too much for any one person to manage alone; they urged nursing home placement. However, it was apparent that this option was not Betty's first choice nor her daughter, Billie's. Given the choices available, Billie elected to return to Wisconsin with her mother and see if she couldn't live with her. If after a trial period she could not manage Betty's needs alone, then placing her in a nursing home near her would at least allow frequent access and visitation.

Billie lived in a small rented home with her significant other. Neither of them had expected Betty's arrival, nor did they have the financial means to enlarge their living quarters. To make room for Betty, an upstairs bedroom was set up for her use. Although this was not the best arrangement because of Betty's physical limitations, she and Billie negotiated the stairs each morning and evening. The clear advantage for everyone was it provided all parties with some personal privacy. Since Billie and her significant other were not available during the work week, Billie placed her mother in an adult daycare center, Monday through Friday. Although this configuration was not perfect for either Betty or Billie, everyone favored it over placing Betty permanently in a nursing home.

By one year following the stroke, Betty's communication was slowly improving. She was talking more, more words were making sense, and more of her messages were understandable. However, she frequently encountered situations in which parts of her messages were either unclear or irretrievable, and depending on the importance of the intended message, Betty's level of frustration varied also. There was little functional change in her right arm, hand, or leg, although her overall physical endurance was slightly better and she was walking longer distances. There was nothing in daily life, however, that mattered much to her. Betty's contact with others at the adult daycare center was minimal and none of that contact seemed to offer her an improved feeling of self-satisfaction. Her daughter, Billie, worked long hours in an administrative and bookkeeping position for a nonprofit agency. She did all she could within her free time, however, to keep life at home harmonious between herself, her mother, and her significant other—all in a dwelling only slightly larger than 1,000 square feet.

In the second year of recovery, Betty was linked with a volunteer in the community who was willing to devote 2–4 hours weekly to help get her become engaged in some activities away from the daycare center and home. Initially, they began by visiting art supply stores and galleries. Betty longed to continue her past involvement with oil painting, but she was unsure whether she could do so without the use of her dominant right hand. In the spring of her second year with her aphasia, she and this volunteer enrolled in an adult noncredit oil painting class in the community, and from the moment of entry, Betty's demeanor and attitude about daily life changed.

What was most noteworthy about these changes was that they extended well beyond the painting course; they were equally apparent at home. From almost the first 10 minutes of the first session, she became engaged again as an active participant in the living of daily life. Although, like Tim's bowling, not all aspects of Betty's painting worked as she might have hoped, it was unquestionably welcomed as a focus and a goal.

Because she could not make brush strokes with her right hand, Betty relied on the use of ther left hand. These strokes were not as fluid or as precise as they had been, especially in the beginning, and she anguished over these differences. To Betty, they made her paintings appear "messy" or "unkempt," qualities not present in her prior efforts. Also, she could not readily mix colors as she once had. This particular skill had been automatic, something she never had to think about. She had never written down any notes about *how* to mix colors; creating the varied reds or blues of a Texas sunset were simply something that *she did*! Now, though, she would stare at her subject, stare at her box paints, and finally fidget unsuccessfully with several color combinations on her palette.

After considerable time had elapsed, she would come to place something on that canvas. Usually when it was done, the overall composition delighted her immensely. It was like Tim finally getting that ball to hit the pins. But the process, like Tim learning to bowl with his opposite hand, was unmistakably different and, at times, tremendously challenging. To some observing it from afar, it may have appeared more like an unsatisfying than a satisfying experience. It *was* Betty's choice, however, and that alone created its value. Painting in an alternative form compared with not having the opportunity to try was the difference between living life and not participating at all. After months of redefining her painting style, Betty's pleasure became even greater. Once she was able to internalize that the product of old was not going to return, she settled into finding pleasure with what was possible.

Changes at home appeared at the same time as Betty's resumption of painting. Instead of falling asleep in her chair after supper, she began retiring to her room early either to work on a canvas or to begin sketching something new. In some ways, the sketching was more appealing to Betty; it didn't involve mixing or adding colors. She came to painting class each week, always with more done and with more in mind to do, either with that painting or another one. Never in this struggle to match skill with challenge did she give any indication of not wanting to continue or that the frustrations of the moment were enough to stifle or stop her desire to try.

In the fall, during her third year with aphasia, Betty suffered a second stroke, now on the opposite side of the brain, and never regained consciousness. Her death cut short a journey that inspired many she met along the way. Warm and witty, Betty learned to create pleasure again—in a medium that had always inspired her. Her story is not about the length of her journey or its completion as it was too short to really complete. Instead, the story is about her process and what it took for her to reengage in living life. When Betty was painting, even in the modified manner she used following her first stroke, she was beyond permitting her aphasia and hemiparesis to interfere with her chosen participation in everyday life. Had Betty's journey continued, I have no doubt that she would be painting weekly now, and in a manner more *acceptable* to her, albeit unlike what it once was.

John and Elizabeth

Fourteen years had passed since John's stroke at age 62. It had come just years before his retirement from IBM as a personnel manager. His wife, Elizabeth, a long-time accomplished elementary school teacher, was likewise looking forward to their days of travel and relaxation. Both had lived active, productive lives, raising a son who was exceptional as a student and athlete, and contributing their time and talents to community, youth, and church organizations and events. John, for instance, had coached Little League baseball when his son played and later umpired in the league. He was admired for the quality and fairness of his work as a personnel manager, but he was adored for the person he was. John was a people person; he loved to interact with others, and especially with children.

At the time of John's stroke, speaking ceased and there was no movement on the right side of his body. Elizabeth retired from work and basically set out to find everything that might help John regain his former self. He received extensive speech-language, occupational, and physical therapy in a variety of hospital and rehabilitative settings over the next 3 years. After each ended, Elizabeth searched out and pushed for more of anything that might help. By 3 years into his recovery, he was walking short distances regularly although there was no functional use of his right hand. He could attend to most self-care activities around the house if given adequate time, something Elizabeth fostered and rewarded from early on. The real loss, though, was his speech; he had no recognizable words. He could make vocal sounds with ease, but these utterances consisted of a repetitious linking of vowels, none of which approximated a true word. However, his excellent use of vocal tone and facial expressions often were enough to compensate. People who really knew John and his topic of conversation often could understand his spoken message even though there were no decipherable words.

Over the next 5 years, John intermittently went to a Veteran's Hospital where he continued to receive varied forms of communication therapy. The emphasis during this period was more on finding other ways that John might communicate with others than on remediating his speech. Pointing to lists of printed words, writing, and gesturing were explored. Although there were steady gains within clinical settings, little of this improvement transferred to real life. John and Elizabeth's communication remained largely unchanged at home throughout this period. John, though, saw these opportunities at the VA Hospital as ways to press his potential further. Often, it afforded him one of the few opportunities to interact regularly with others who understood and could compensate for his communication difficulties.

After 8 years with aphasia, he started on a different course in life. With the support of a speech-language pathologist and a series of community volunteers, he began exploring activities of his own choice outside the home. Over the next 6 years, that list grew substantially. From attending an occasional afternoon matinee with a volunteer, to shopping for Elizabeth, to becoming a weekly participant in child-care settings outside the home, John began to expand his life to take on more meaning, purpose, and value. It was activities within protected environments outside the home that permitted John, with his limited communication, to begin to experience a part of life he may have thought was behind him.

Some of these changes came to be because of the insight of a community volunteer. This volunteer had accompanied John on a shopping outing for Elizabeth and had noticed that any child within 50 feet of him was an instant magnet. John typically carried pieces of hard candy with him for himself, but in these settings they immediately served as a bridge to young children he got to know and over time, it didn't really matter whether he could talk or not. Noticing these encounters, John's volunteer began looking into settings where John might interact with children. Of those explored, he elected to attend a daycare for disadvantaged children in an economically deprived neighborhood. With the aid of the volunteer, they set about developing a mutual routine that would benefit John, the children, and the entire staff. He used talking books to read to them; he interacted through a variety of supported and unsupported individual and group tasks. Weekly, over the next several years, "Grandpa John" visited this location, his children, and the staff. From the cook in the kitchen who usually had a donut and a carton of milk awaiting his arrival, to the janitor in the hallways who often engaged John as he made his way to or from the preschool classroom, he was *accepted* and *valued* as an integral member of that community.

There were other settings and stories of John's continued personal growth and reinvolvement in daily life after this one. Most recently, he had begun filming students in a first grade physical education class at an elementary school near his home so they and their teacher might share and work on mutual points of interest. Had he not passed away in his sleep last year for reasons unrelated to his stroke 14 years earlier, he likely would have become a valued and integral member of that community as well. The children not only loved seeing themselves on a large television monitor, but they loved how John consistently positioned himself as their ally. He laughed with them and championed their efforts, no matter how fantastic or lacking; he was there with them and they with him.

The value of John's reinvolvement in life outside his home did more than increase his own quality of life. It demonstrated to Elizabeth that there were aspects of John's life outside their home that could be relied on, and this temporarily freed her of the responsibility of trying to make life work for her husband. She never questioned the value of these pursuits, only supported them. She could see their value in John's overall demeanor, pleasure, and enthusiasm for living life. Never, in the first 5 years with aphasia, had she been able to get him out of bed before 9 o'clock in the morning. He was a chronic, late-night television watcher. But on the mornings he visited *his* children, he was up early and anxious to be at the front door well ahead of his departure time. Typically, even in stormy or cold wintry conditions, John never considered canceling or *not attending*. For Elizabeth, this devotion and constancy was confirmation enough of the importance of these additions to daily life.

Putting aphasia's presence behind you

In different ways, for different reasons, and with different support systems, Tim and Nan, Betty and Billie, and John and Elizabeth all determined and maintained their own pace and direction in making life work again. Although their circumstances and solutions differed, they shared common features with one another. For the most part, the commonalties among them related back to the very keys we offered you in the opening chapter of this book. In each scenario, there were common threads of:

1. coming to understand and manage aphasia's nature *in their own ways.*

2. not having to confront or resolve aphasia's dilemmas *alone.*

3. building a better life gradually from the bottom up, and not *racing ahead aimlessly.*

4. using time as their *ally,* not their enemy.

5. not depending on any *one person* to make all the parts work.

6. finding *harmony and balance* in life even with aphasia present.

Each year, approximately 80,000 Americans join the Tim, Betty, and John on a journey of their own. For many, the greatest asset outside of themselves are their own Nan's, Billie's, or Elizabeth's. At any one time, there are over a million people with aphasia in America attempting to live a better life in spite of aphasia. If your loved one is one of them, you obviously are *not* alone, and, more importantly, you are not obligated to live a lesser form of life because of this injury. The choices before you are real ones, not simply whether to rebuild a "fire-ravaged home," but whether to pursue pleasure in living life now, something totally apart from that "house" of old. Once you know it, understand it, and adequately attend to it, you need to allot aphasia and its associated disabilities the significance they deserve—*to put them behind you*! So, it is up to you to look to activities in life that permit you to experience and enjoy life now and to enhance that enjoyment in the years ahead.

We have savored the opportunity to drive along with you to this point in time. If you have successfully negotiated the terrain to here . . . you are ready to manage what lies ahead alone! We wish you well; have a safe and productive trip . . . that new home and way of life are straight ahead . . . keep moving forward!

Glossary of terms

Acalculia: An inability to perform simple mathematical calculations.

Activities of Daily Living (ADLs): Common term used by rehabilitation specialists to refer to primary cares of daily life such as: personal hygiene, dressing, grooming, eating, drinking, walking, and sitting.

Acute: The initial symptoms and consequences of impairment, injury, or disease; certain diseases may be severe but span a short duration and as such they are called "acute illnesses."

Adaptive Device: A device that permits participation in an activity that otherwise would not be possible.

Alzheimer's Disease: A progressive and irreversible form of dementia. Often begins with intermittent states of mental confusion, disorientation, and loss of recent memory loss. Subsequently leads to severe impairment in all realms of thinking, memory, language, and communication.

Ambulation: The act of walking with or without assistance or adaptive devices.

Anesthesia: Loss of sensation to a portion of the body or a limb (*see* Chapter 12).

Aneurysm: A region in the wall of a blood vessel that has become weakened due to injury or aging and visibly "pooches" out; often a potential site for a hemorrhage (*see* Chapter 11).

Angiogram: An x-ray test that permits doctors to see the course and condition of a person's blood vessels by injecting a radio-sensitive dye directly into the bloodstream.

Anomia: An inability to retrieve common, well-known words from one's mental dictionary. Also, a form of aphasia where the substantive or meaningful words are disproportionally omitted (*see* Chapter 10).

Aphasia: An acquired impairment of language that typically disrupts communication and speech by robbing its victim of ease and accessibility to one's inner words (language symbols) whether spoken, written, or gestured (*see* Chapter 2).

Apoplexy: A common "older" medical term for a vascular stroke or "brain attack."

Apraxia: An inability to perform volitional or purposeful motor movements, not because of muscular weakness but because of an inability to plan and execute those movements; apraxia of speech is a commonly co-occurring impairment with aphasia (*see* Chapter 10).

Arteriogram: An x-ray test of a damaged artery to determine its status, that is, whether it is open, blocked, weakened, or hemorrhaging.

Arteriosclerosis: A hardening of the artery walls due to atherosclerosis.

Assisted Exercise: An exercise requiring the assistance of another person or an adaptive device.

Ataxia: An impairment of the brain resulting in lack of coordination, unsteady gait, and poor balance; often tied to injury to the brain stem.

Atherosclerosis: An impairment of the blood vessels due to a gradual accumulation of fatty deposits within their inner lining, especially arteries; if severe, normal blood flow may be permanently obstructed.

Audiologist: A health care specialist with expertise in the assessment and treatment of hearing impairments.

Beta Blocker: A medication that decreases the strain and work on the heart by decreasing its rate.

Blood Pressure: The force or pressure exerted by the heart in pumping blood through the vascular system.

Brain Attack: More recent term of the American Heart Association to refer to cerebral stroke; used to differentiate the term "stroke" from "heart attack" by referring to the location of injury.

Brain Stem: A lower portion of the brain that connects the spinal cord to the mid-brain and cerebral hemispheres; involved in the regulation of primary vegetative functions of life, such as breathing, blood pressure, and consciousness.

Broca's Aphasia: A type of aphasia named after the French neurologist who first described its features; characterized by restricted speech accompanied by retaining a functional understanding of spoken words (*see* Chapter 10).

Cardiovascular: Referring to the heart and its outgoing (arteries) and incoming (veins) blood vessels.

Carotid Artery: A main frontal corridor of blood from the heart to the brain (*see* Chapter 11).

Catheter: A rubber tube inserted into the body; often referring to tubing placed directly into a person's urinary tract to help alleviate urinary dysfunction (incontinence) in the beginning days or weeks after injury.

Cerebellum: The lower brain appendage behind the brain stem that is instrumental in the coordination of body movements.

Cerebral Dominance: The concept that certain higher level brain functions, such as language, music, art, or logical thought are more localized in one hemisphere of the brain than the other (*see* Chapter 9).

Cerebral Hemispheres: The two large, paired spherical bodies of the human brain that are integral to thought, language, and speech (*see* Figure 9–1 in Chapter 9).

Cerebral Vascular Accident (CVA): Any sudden disruption to the flow of blood to the brain that results in permanent injury or dysfunction.

Chronic: The symptoms or consequences of impairment, injury, or disease that endure over a long period of time; typically aphasia is a "chronic" disorder.

Circumlocution: The use of many words to express a concept that might have been captured with a few.

Communication: The sharing of feelings, ideas, and information through many means, one of which is language. music, art, dance, or pantomime are others (*see* Chapter 9).

Computer Tomography (CT) Scan: A computerized X ray of a portion of the body that helps differentiate abnormal or damaged structures from normal structures.

Contracture: The shortening or tightening of tissue around a joint; a common consequence following a "brain attack" and often requiring active "range of motion" exercises to counteract.

Cortex: The outer lining of the cerebral hemispheres; comprised largely of nerve cell bodies; integral to functions of thought, language, and communication (*see* Chapter 10).

Decubitus Ulcer: A bedsore or pressure sore; usually preventable by regular repositioning of the person in bed so undue pressure against a prominent area of contact is lessened.

Dementia: An impairment of thinking and reasoning; may be progressive or not; Alzheimer's disease is a progressive, irreversible dementia.

Depression: An acute or chronic condition characterized by hopelessness, emotional despair, lethargy, and an inability to "act" or initiate daily functions; may be physically or psychologically triggered in people with aphasia (*see* Chapter 12).

Diabetes: A chronic disorder in which the body is unable to metabolize carbohydrates, thus leading to excessively high levels of blood sugar; unless carefully controlled through medication, exercise, or diet, this disorder can threaten other body functions and organs; a potential factor to a brain attack.

Diagnosis: The identification of cause or reason for injury, impairment, or disease.

Disability: The inability to perform a function or activity within a "normal" range when compared with noninjured persons.

Diuretic: A type of medication that eliminates salt (sodium) from the body and helps to reduce high blood pressure and edema.

Dysarthria: A speech impairment due to injury to nerve tracts leading to muscles (mouth, tongue, jaw, voice box, and lungs) directly involved in the production of spoken words (*see* Chapter 10).

Dyslexia: An inability to read while thought and reasoning remain largely intact; may be developmental or acquired.

Dysphagia: An inability to swallow; a common occurrence in the early stages of injury after a brain attack (*see* Chapter 12).

Dysphasia: Term used instead of aphasia to mean a partial loss of language as opposed to a complete loss; a more accurate descriptor of injury in most cases of aphasia.

Edema: Swelling of body parts around a site of injury; due primarily to the accumulation of excessive fluid.

Embolism: The sudden blockage of blood flow from free-floating debris becoming wedged in a smaller vessel (*see* Figure 11–5b in Chapter 11).

Embolus: Free-floating debris in a blood vessel.

Endarterectomy: A surgical procedure for deblocking blood flow to the brain; typically performed on the carotid artery in the neck.

Expressive Aphasia: A common descriptor for people with aphasia who struggle to talk yet understand most of what is said to them; Broca's Aphasia (*see* Chapter 10).

Flaccidity: An absence of muscle tone typically resulting in a "floppy," nonfunctional limb or extremity.

Flexion: Movement of a joint which brings the operative parts closer together; opposite of extension.

Fluent Aphasia: A category of aphasias characterized by a near normal "flow" of spoken words although such utterances may not be clear or understandable (*see* Chapter 10).

Functional: A common term and treatment objective that typically refers to one's ability or capacity to act independently in a realm of impairment; may also refer to a category of skills that pertain to purposeful activities in daily life such as eating, dressing, walking, or speaking.

Gait: Referring to one's ability to walk.

Global Aphasia: The most severe of aphasias; suggestive of severe impairment in comprehension and use of language; a common occurrence in the beginning hours and days of injury but not necessarily indicative of long-term impairment (*see* Chapter 10).

Handicap: Personal or social ramifications felt or experienced from having suffered a chronic injury or disability; it entails the "perceived" disadvantages of being permanently injured, either by self or others, whether they may be fully accurate or not.

Hemianopsia: The loss of half of one's visual field due to an injury to the opposite side of the brain; often possible to train injured person to compensate (*see* Chapter 12).

Hemiparesis: A partial loss of movement on one side of the body due to muscle weakness from a brain injury; loss involves face, body, arm, and leg (*see* Chapter 12).

Hemiplegia: A total loss of movement on one side of the body (*see* Chapter 12).

Hemi-Walker: A broad-based walker-cane combination designed to stabilize the gait of people with a marked hemiparesis.

Hemorrhage: The rupturing of a blood vessel (*see* Figure 11–5c in Chapter 11).

Hypertension: A condition of perpetual high blood pressure; often without visible symptoms and a common factor in the cause of a brain attack or heart disease.

Impairment: The physical or psychological result of injury or disease to an organ or body function.

Incontinence: The inability to control one's discharge of urine or feces; usually due to a loss of sphincter control when secondary to a brain attack.

Infarction: The area of brain tissue damaged in injury.

Intermediate Care: A rehab center other than the hospital where intensive treatment might be provided over a brief period of weeks or months or a long-term setting where minimal health care and daily life assistance are necessary.

Ischemia: The result of lack of oxygen to a vital area in the body, such as the brain.

Jargon: A type of speech common to people with certain types of fluent aphasia; spoken words may or may not contain "real" words; even when parts of speech are recognizable, they may still be totally incomprehensible (*see* Chapter 10, Wernicke's Aphasia).

Lability: An inability to control one's emotions (either crying or laughing) that is not due to situational reaction to injury or function; physiologically based (*see* Chapter 12).

Language: An agreed-on system of spoken, written, or gestured symbols for expressing thoughts, feelings, or ideas in one's culture or society.

Lesion: The area of damage to the brain from stroke, tumor, or trauma.

Long-term Care: Ongoing care for people with prolonged personal and medical care needs that cannot be provided independently; may be provided in a residential care setting or at home.

Magnetic Resonance Imagery (MRI) Scan: A highly sophisticated type of computerized x-ray imagery that provides vivid pictorial details of internal hard and soft body tissues; a procedure used when attempting to specify the precise region, nature, and extent of injury to the brain after a brain attack.

Motor: Any portion of either nerve or muscle function involved with movement of body parts.

Muscle Tone: Degree of tension in a muscle at rest; *see* **Flaccidity** and **Spasticity**.

Myocardial Infarction: An injury in the heart due to blockage of blood to that region; a type of heart attack.

Necrosis: The death of living tissue; the loss of nervous tissue due to the blockage of blood to a specific region in the brain.

Neglect: An inability to "recognize" or "sense" an injured side of the body; unconscious perceptual omission.

Neologism: Speech utterances that have no recognizable form or meaning, such as: "nehrst furbis farctis."

Neoplasm: A tumor.

Neurologist: A medical doctor who specializes in disorders, injury, or diseases of the nervous system; a primary health care provider for people with aphasia.

Nonfluent Aphasia: A category of aphasias characterized by halting, broken, or absent speech (*see* Chapter 10).

Nystagmus: Rapid, involuntary movements of the eyeballs when tracking an object horizontally across one's visual field; often indicative of brain injury.

Occupational Therapy (OT): A rehab specialty that targets the restoration of optimal function in Activities of Daily Life (ADLs) and hand movement on the involved side of the body (*see* Table 4–1 in Chapter 4).

Paralysis: Total or near total loss of motor function to a body part or limb.

Paresis: Partial loss of motor function to a body part or limb.

Perception: The ability to receive and distinguish information through the prime senses of vision, touch, taste, hearing, smell, and position in space.

Perseveration: The continued use of a gesture, spoken word, or vocal utterance that is not appropriate but cannot be inhibited or stopped; a common consequence of brain injury following stroke (*see* Chapter 12).

Physiatrist: A medical doctor who specializes in physical medicine or the rehabilitation of body parts or functions compromised through physical impairment or disease.

Physical Therapy (PT): A rehab specialty that targets the restoration of optimal movement of involved extremities (arm and leg) following stroke; especially prominent in rehabilitating daily functions of standing, transferring, and walking (*see* Table 4–1 in Chapter 4).

Prognosis: The projected outcome of injury or disease; may pertain to the projected outcome of recovery with or without treatment.

Quad-Cane: Broad-based cane with four legs that provides increased stability when standing or walking.

Range of Motion: The extent of movement possible in a particular joint from passive manipulation; also, a set of physical exercises designed to keep such movement as viable as possible.

Receptive Aphasia: A common descriptor of people with aphasia who struggle to understand spoken language; Wernicke's Aphasia (*see* Chapter 10).

Recreational Therapy (RT): A rehab specialty that targets the use of leisure or recreational activities as part of the therapeutic process (*see* Table 4–1 in Chapter 4).

Rehabilitation: The restoration of physical, mental, communicative, social, or vocational skills following a disabling injury or disease.

Skilled Nursing Facility/Care: Long-term institutionalized care that requires continuous nursing and medical personnel; often provided for people with chronic injury or disability who need moderate to maximal assistance

Social Services: A rehab specialty that targets resolution of personal, social, or familial problems associated with a brain attack (*see* Table 4–1 in Chapter 4).

Spasm: A sudden, involuntary contraction of a muscle or a muscle group; often associated with pain and dysfunction.

Spasticity: Increased muscle tone often resulting in contractures and pain; a common consequence of stroke that requires continuous stretching and range of motion exercises to counterbalance.

Speech: The verbal expression of one's language (*see* Chapter 9).

Speech-Language Pathology (SLP): A rehab specialty that targets the restoration of speech, language, and communication following injury (*see* Table 4–1 in Chapter 4).

Spontaneous Recovery: Refers to the early tendency of most stroke survivors to improve to some degree whether provided rehabilitative therapies or not; likely related to reduced edema around the site of injury.

Stroke: Synonymous with a "brain attack"; injury to the brain secondary to some form of interruption in the blood supply (*see* Chapter 11).

Stroke/Aphasia Group: A community group of stroke/aphasia survivors and/or caregivers who provide emotional and social support.

Subluxation: A condition of separation or dislocation of a body part; commonly in the shoulder joint on the involved side of the body.

Supine: Horizontal positioning of the body with head facing up.

Tachycardia: Rapid heart rate.

Thrombosis: An interruption in the flow of blood through a vessel due to a gradual accumulation of debris at the site of blockage.

Thrombus: The debris at the site of a thrombosis (*see* Figure 11–5a in Chapter 11).

Transfer: The physical act of moving a person with moderate to severe hemiparesis from bed to chair or chair to chair.

Transient Ischemic Attack (TIA): A small or mini-stroke; a brief, usually reversible episode of brain attack symptoms that may last over a period of minutes or hours; often an indicator of a person being at risk for a subsequent stroke (*see* Chapter 11).

Triglyceride: A common form of fat found in the blood.

Vasospasm: A brief abnormal constriction of a blood vessel.

Vital Signs: The prime indicators of life; that is, measures of blood pressure, body temperature, and breathing; these signs must stabilize before any regular rehabilitation can commence.

Wernicke's Aphasia: A type of aphasia named after the German neurologist who first described its features; characterized by fluent flow of jargon but with little or no comprehension of the spoken word; a severe fluent aphasia (*see* Chapter 10).

Printed resources

Newsletters

Be Stroke Smart
National Stroke Association
8480 Orchard Road, Suite 1000
Englewood, CO 80111-5015
(800) 787-6537

Let's Rap
Communicative Disorders Clinic
University of Michigan
1111 E. Catherine Street
Ann Arbor, MI 48109-2054

Newsletter: National Aphasia Association
National Aphasia Association
P.O. Box 1887, Murray Hill Station
New York, NY 10156
(800) 922-4622

Speaking Up
Action for Dysphasic Adults
1 Royal Street
London, England SE1 7LL

Stroke Connection and A Stroke of Luck
American Heart Association
7272 Greenville Avenue
Dallas, TX 75231
(214) 373-6300

Books and booklets pertaining to stroke/aphasia for families and caregivers

Ahn, Jung, & Ferguson, Gary. (1992). *Recovering From a Stroke.* New York: HarperPaperbacks.

Ancowitz, Arthur. (1993). *The Stroke Book: One-on-One Advice About Stroke Prevention, Management, and Rehabilitation.* Thorndike, ME: Thorndike Press.

Bell, Lorna, & Seyfer, Eudora. (1987). *Gentle Yoga* (2nd ed.). Berkeley, CA: Celestial Arts.

Boone, Daniel. (1984). *An Adult Has Aphasia* (5th ed.). Austin, TX: Pro-Ed Publishers, Inc.

Caring for a Person With Aphasia. (1994). Dallas, TX: American Heart Association.

Castleman, Michael. (1993). *An Aspirin A Day.* New York: Hyperion.

Eisenson, Jon. (1990). *Understanding Stroke and Aphasia.* Austin, TX: Pro-Ed Publisher, Inc..

Ewing, Sue, & Pfalzgraf, Beth. (1990). *Moving Beyond Stroke and Aphasia.* Detroit, MI: Wayne State University Press.

Foley, Conn, & Pizer, H. F. (1990). *The Stroke Fact Book.* Golden Valley, MN: Courage Press.

Gordon, Neil F. (1993). *Stroke: Your Complete Exercise Guide.* Champaign, IL: Human Kinetics Publishers.

Hay, Jennifer. (1995). *Stroke: Questions You Have, Answers You Need.* Allentown, PA: People's Medical Society.

Horne, Jo. (1991). *A Survival Guide for Family Caregivers.* Minneapolis, MN: CompuCare Publishers, Inc.

Lisle, Rebecca. (1996). *When Granny Couldn't Speak.* London, UK: Action for Dysphasic Adults.

Marshall, Jane, & Carlson, Eva. (1993). London, UK: Action for Dysphasic Adults.

Book 1: *How To Help the Dysphasic Person in the Early Stages.*

Book 2: *How To Help the Dysphasic Person With Comprehension and Speech.*

Book 3: *How To Help the Dysphasic Person With Reading and Writing.*

Book 4: *How To Help With Total Communication.*

Book 5: *Complicating Factors With Dysphasia.*

The Road Ahead: A Stroke Recovery Guide. (1989). Englewood, CO: National Stroke Association.

Sarno, Martha Taylor. (1986). *Understanding Aphasia: A Guide for Family and Friends.* New York: New York University Medical Center, Education Center.

Shimberg, Elaine Fantle. (1990). *Strokes: What Families Should Know.* New York: Random House Inc., Ballantine Books.

Singleton, Lafayette, & Johnson, Kirk. (1993). *The Black Health Library Guide to Stroke.* New York: Henry Holt and Company.

Weiner, Florence, Matthew, Lee, & Bell, Harriet. (1994). *Recovering at Home After a Stroke.* New York: The Berkeley Publishing Group.

Where Do I Go From Here? (1993). Ann Arbor, MI: Communicative Disorders Clinic, University of Michigan.

Youngson, R. M. (1987). *Stroke! A Self-Help Manual for Stroke Sufferers and Their Relatives.* Oxford, England: David and Charles Publishers.

Personal accounts of stroke/aphasia

Bergquist, W. H., McLean, R., & Kobylinski, B. A. (1994). *Stroke Survivors.* San Francisco: Jossey-Bass, Inc.

Collins, E. (1992). *Unprepared!* Minneapolis: Deaconess Press.

Josephs, A. (1992). *The Invaluable Guide to Life After Stroke.* Long Beach, CA: Amadeus Press.

Kasell, P. (1990). *The Best of the Stroke Connection.* Golden Valley, MN: Courage Center.

Knox, David. (1971). *Portrait of Aphasia.* Detroit, MI: Wayne State University Press.

Lavin, John. (1985). *Stroke: From Crisis to Victory.* New York: Franklin Watts.

Newborn, Barbara. (1997). *Return to Ithaca.* Rockport, MA: Element Books, Inc.

Paullin, Ellen. (1988). *Ted's Stroke: The Caregiver's Story.* Cabin John, MD: Seven Locks Press.

Sarton, May. (1988). *After the Stroke: A Journal.* New York: W. W. Norton & Co.

Shirk, Evelyn. (1991). *After the Stroke: Coping With America's Third Leading Cause of Death.* Buffalo, NY: Prometheus Books.

West, Paul. (1995). *A Stroke of Genius: Illness and Self-Discovery.* New York: Viking Press.

Wulf, Helen. (1986, revised). *Aphasia, My World Alone.* Detroit: Wayne State Press.

Young, J. (1997). *Up From the Ashes.* Sarasota, FL: Inner Path Publishing.

❖ APPENDIX C

National, state, and international agencies associated with stroke/aphasia

National Agencies

American Heart Association
7272 Greenville Avenue
Dallas, TX 75231
(800) 553-6321

American Speech-Language-Hearing Association
10801 Rockville Pike
Rockville, MD 20852
(800) 638-8255

The Brain Injury Association
1776 Massachusetts Avenue, N.W.,
  Suite 100
Washington, DC 20036
(202) 296-6443

National Aphasia Association
P.O. Box 1887
Murray Hill Station
New York, NY 10156
(800) 922-4622

National Easter Seal Society
230 W. Monroe, Suite 1800
Chicago, IL 60606
(800) 221-6827

National Family Caregivers Association
9621 E. Bexhill Drive
Kensington, MD 20895-3104
(301) 949-6430

**National Institute of Neurological
  Disorders and Stroke**
Public Health Service Bldg. 31 Room 8A-06
31 Center Drive
Bethesda, MD 20892-2540
(800) 352-9424

National Stroke Association
96 Inverness Drive, Suite I
Englewood, CO
(800) 787-6537

Visiting Nurse Association of America
3801 E. Florida Avenue, Suite 900
Denver, CO
(303) 753-0218

The Well Spouse Foundation
P.O. Box 801
New York, NY 10023
(212) 724-7209

State Agencies

All entries below are alphabetized by state. We begin each state's listings with its department or commission on aging. This agency should be helpful in locating a support group near you. If not, we recommend contacting the National Aphasia or Stroke Associations; their addresses and phone numbers are listed above. In addition, you will find a list of "known" or "established" support groups by cities within states. The name of the group, the address to write for further information, the type of membership, the contact person, and that person's phone number follow. This listing is not inclusive, nor is the information necessarily current, although we have made a concerted effort to ensure these qualities at the time of publication. We urge you to contact the National Aphasia Association for additional entries and information.

ALABAMA

Commission on Aging
502 Washington Avenue
Montgomery, AL 36130
(205) 261-5743

ALASKA

Older Alaskans Commission
Department of Administration
Pouch C-Mail Station 0209
Juneau, AL 99811
(907) 465-3250

ARIZONA

Aging and Adult Administration
1400 West Washington Street
Phoenix, AZ 85007
(602) 542-4446

Phoenix

St. Joseph's Hospital
Stroke/Caregiver/Aphasia Discussion Groups
Easter Seals Society
903 N. 2nd Street
Phoenix, AZ 85004

Stroke/Aphasia
Mary Ellen Mussman
(602) 406-6686

Scottsdale

HealthSouth Meridian Point Rehab Hospital
11250 N. 92nd Street
Scottsdale, AZ 85258

Stroke/Aphasia
Barbara Hendrickson
(602) 860-0671, ext. 169

Scottsdale Memorial Hospitals–North
10450 N. 92nd Street
Scottsdale, AZ 85258

Stroke/Aphasia
Sue Okun
(602) 860-3636

The Senior Citizen Center
10440 East Via Linda
Scottsdale, AZ 85258

Stroke/Aphasia
Roger Ross
(602) 922-9389

Sun City

Sun City's Aphasia Group
Community Education Center
Thunderbird & 103rd Avenue, #10
Sun City, AZ 85351

Aphasia
Eileen Wolpert
(602) 933-4176

Tucson

University of Arizona Aphasia Groups
Dept of Speech and Hearing Sciences
P.O. Box 210071
Tucson, AZ 85721-0071

Aphasia
Pagie Beeson
(520) 621-7070

ARKANSAS

Division of Aging & Adult Services
Dept of Social and Rehabilitative Services
Donaghey Bldg., Suite 1428
7th & Main Streets
Little Rock, AR 72201
(501) 371-2441

Fayetteville

Stroke Support Group of Northwest Arkansas
University of Arkansas
Speech and Hearing Clinic
410 Arkansas
Fayetteville, AR 72701

Stroke/Aphasia
Barbara Shadden
(501) 575-4509

CALIFORNIA

Department of Aging
1600 K Street
Sacramento, CA 95814
(916) 322-5290

Concord

Pat Martin Stroke Support Group of
    Contra Costa County
1865 Granada Drive
Concord, CA 94519-1326

Stroke/Aphasia
Marge Boyer
(510) 685-4217

Inglewood

Stroke Support Group
Daniel Freeman Hospitals, Inc.
333 N. Prairie Avenue
Inglewood, CA 90301

Stroke/Aphasia/TBI/Dementia
Tammie Bean
(310) 823-8911, ext. 4136

Long Beach

Stroke/Aphasia Support Groups
5901 E. 7th Street
Long Beach, CA 90822

Stroke/Aphasia
Irene Hennessy
(310) 494-5415

Stroke Association of Southern California
Long Beach Chapter
P.O. Box 8340
Long Beach, CA 90808

Stroke/Aphasia
Marianne Simpson
(562) 985-9971

Los Angeles

Aphasia Community Group
Cedars Sinai Medical Center
8700 Beverly Blvd, Rm 7418
Los Angeles, CA 90048

Aphasia
Sherri Washington
(310) 855-3136

Stroke/Aphasia Support Groups
Stroke Association of Southern California
2001 S. Barrington Avenue, Suite 308
Los Angeles, CA 90025

Stroke/Aphasia
Susan Blatt
(310) 575-1699

Martinez

Veterans Stroke Support Group
VA Outpatient Clinic, Speech Pathology (126)
150 Muir Road
Martinez, CA 94553

Stroke/Aphasia
Cami Bebarta
(510) 372-2641

Mission Viejo

Aphasia/Stroke Support Groups
Newport Language, Speech & Audiology
   Center, Inc.
26137 La Paz Road; Suite 104
Mission Viejo, CA 92691

Stroke/Aphasia
Nan Weaver
(714) 581-5206, ext. 117

Oakland

Aphasia Center of California
3996 Lyman Road
Oakland, CA 94602

Aphasia
Roberta Elman, Ph.D.
(510) 336-0112

Palos Verdes Estates

Keyhole Unit
Southern California Aphasia Network
721 Paseo del Mar
Palos Verdes Estates, CA 90274

Aphasia
S. Tres Mennis
(310) 378-8026

Pinole

West Contra Costa County Stroke
   and Aphasia Support Group
Doctor's Hospital
2151 Appian Way
Pinole, CA 94564

Stroke/Aphasia
Flo Leverenz
(510) 235-7999

San Francisco

Stroke Club; Stonestown YMCA
333 Eucalyptus Street
San Francisco, CA 94132

Stroke/Aphasia
Kathy Orsi
(415) 759-9632, ext. 217

Santa Monica

The Pathfinders Speech Group
Santa Monica College
1900 Pico Boulevard
Santa Monica, CA 90405

Stroke/Aphasia
Sandy Burnett
(310) 450-5150, ext. 9442

COLORADO

Aging and Adult Services Division
Department of Social Services
717 17th Street; P.O. Box 181000
Denver, CO 80218
(303) 866-5122

Akron

Determinaires Stroke Club
Senior Community Center
166 Cedar Avenue
Akron, CO 80720

Stroke/Aphasia
Willis and Rosalie Allen
(970) 345-2390

Aurora

Aurora Stroke Club
Aurora Senior Center
30 Del Mar Circle
Aurora, CO 80012

Stroke/Aphasia
Zita Walker
(303) 371-0406

Boulder

Conversations Groups
Dept of Speech Language Hearing Sciences
Speech Language Hearing Clinic
University of Colorado-Boulder
Campus Box 409
Boulder, CO 80309

Stroke/Aphasia
Gail Ramsberger
(303) 492-3043

Boulder Stroke Club
Boulder Meridan
801 Gillespie Drive
Boulder, CO 80303

Stroke/Aphasia
Roberta Martine
(303) 538-3534

Broomfield

Broomfield Stroke Support Group
Broomfield Senior Center
280 Lemar Street
Broomfield, CO 80038

Stroke/Aphasia
Alice Finnegan
(303) 469-0536, ext. 28

Castle Rock

Sky Cliff Stroke Center
Plum Creek Plaza
960 S I-25, Unit E
Castle Rock, CO 80104

Stroke/Aphasia
Karolynn Clint
(303) 688-3925

Ft. Collins

Ft. Collins Community Stroke Group   Stroke/Aphasia
Trinity Lutheran Church   Angie Steele
301 E. Stuart Street   (970) 482-5712, ext. 157
Ft. Collins, CO 80525

Ft. Morgan

Northeast Colorado Stroke Support Group   Stroke/Aphasia
Methodist Church   Ham Jackson, M.D.
117 East Bijou   (970) 867-6555
Ft. Morgan, CO 80701

Grand Junction

Western Slope Stroke Support Group   Stroke/Aphasia
St. Mary's Rehab Center   Jo Sullivan
1100 Paterson Road   (970) 244-6164
Grand Junction, CO 81506

Greeley

North Colorado Young Stroke Survivors Group   Stroke/Aphasia
N. Colorado Medical Center   Naomi Rider
1801 16th Street   (970) 350-6279
Greeley, CO 80631

Weld County Stroke Support Club   Stroke/Aphasia
600 37th Avenue Court   Wanda Potter
Greeley, CO 80634   (970) 352-5785

Gypsum

Eagle County Stroke Club   Stroke/Aphasia
P.O. Box 152   Nettie Reynolds
Gypsum, CO 81637   (970) 534-9325

Lakewood

Young Stroke Survivors Group   Stroke/Aphasia
5755 West Alameda   Nancy Walters
Lakewood, CO 80226   (303) 466-4830

Montrose

Montrose Memorial Stroke Group   Stroke/Aphasia
Montrose Memorial Hospital Rehab Center   Laurie Deltondo
800 S. 3rd Street   (970) 240-7369
Montrose, CO 81401

Pueblo

Stroke Survivors Support Group of Pueblo
McLelland Library/Joseph H. Edwards
   Senior Center
710 1/2 E. Mesa Avenue
Pueblo, CO 81006

Stroke/Aphasia
Charles Couchman
(719) 583-8498

Trinidad

Spanish Peaks Stroke Support Group
Medbrook Rehab
916 Arizona
Trinidad, CO 81082

Stroke/Aphasia
Karen Malone, SLP
(719) 846-4473

CONNECTICUT

Department of Aging
175 Main Street
Hartford, CT 06106
(203) 566-3238

Bridgeport

Stroke Support Group
Ahlbins Centers for Rehab Medicine
226 Mill Hill Avenue
Bridgeport, CT 06610

Stroke/Aphasia
Beth Geoghegan
(203) 366-7345

New Britain

Hospital for Special Care Stroke Support Group
Hospital for Special Care
2150 Corbin Avenue
New Britain, CT 06053

Stroke/Aphasia
Jennifer Tanger
(860) 827-1958, ext. 5091

Stamford

ABI/TBI/Stroke Support Groups
Easter Seals Rehab Center
26 Palmers Hill Road
Stamford, CT 06902

Dementia/Head Trauma/Stroke/
   Aphasia
Larry Segall
(203) 325-1544, ext. 27

Windsor

Indepedence Unlimited, Inc.
2138 Silas Deane Highway, Suite 100
Rocky Hill, CT 06067

Aphasia
Marcia Britting
(860) 257-3221

DELAWARE

Division on Aging
Dept of Health and Social Service
1901 N. DuPont Highway
New Castle, DE 19720
(302) 421-6791

DISTRICT OF COLUMBIA

Office on Aging
1424 K Street N.W., 2nd floor
Washington, DC 20005
(202) 724-5622

FLORIDA

Program Office of Aging and Adult Services
Dept of Health and Rehab Services
1317 Winewood Boulevard
Tallahassee, FL 32301
(904) 488-8922

De Land

The Aphasia Interactive Support Group	Aphasia
Memorial Hospital West Volusia	David Wall
701 W. Plymouth Avenue	(904) 943-4692
De Land, FL 32720	

Jupiter

Stroke of Hope Aphasia Group at Jupiter	Aphasia
Jupiter Medical Center	Liz Blake
1210 S. Old Dixie	(561) 745-0400
Jupiter, FL 33458	

Palm Gardens

Stroke of Hope Club, Inc.	Stroke/Aphasia
Palm Beach Gardens Aphasia Group	Liz Blake
Palm Beach Gardens Medical Center	(561) 745-0400
3360 Burns Road	
Palm Beach Gardens, FL 33410	

Sarasota

Community Stroke Network
Senior Friendship Center, Inc.
1888 Brother Geenen Way
Sarasota, FL 34236

Stroke/Aphasia
Mary Twitchell
(941) 917-7626

Tampa

Tampa Aphasia Support Group
David Barksdale Center
214 N. Boulevard
Tampa, FL 33606

Aphasia
Marie McMahon
(813) 839-2373

Royal Palm Beach

The Aphasia Group of Golden Rule Stroke Club
Beverly Health Care and Rehab
600 Business Parkway
Royal Palm Beach, FL 33411

Stroke/Aphasia
Sandy White
(561) 798-4182

GEORGIA

Office of Aging
878 Peachtree St, N.E., Rm 632
Atlanta, GA 30309
(404) 894-5333

Lawrenceville

Stroke Support Group
Gwinnett Medical Center
1000 Medical Center Blvd
Lawrenceville, GA 30045

Stroke/Aphasia
Elizabeth Osterholz
(770) 995-4322

HAWAII

Executive Office on Aging
Office of the Governor
335 Merchant Street, Room 241
Honolulu, HI 96813
(808) 548-2593

Kahului

Maui Stroke Club
Rehab at Maui
140 Hoohana Street, Suite 201
Kahului, HI 96732

Stroke/Aphasia
Donna Tamashiro
(808) 877-0606

IDAHO

Office on Aging
Rm 114-Statehouse
Boise, ID 83720
(208) 334-3833

ILLINOIS

Dept of Aging
421 E. Capitol Avenue
Springfield, IL 62701
(217) 785-3356

Chicago

Stroke Awareness Group
University of Chicago Hospitals
5841 S. Maryland Avenue, Room RT644S
Chicago, IL 60637

Stroke/Aphasia
Margaret O'Hara
(773) 702-7450

Evanston

Young Adults Stroke Survivors Support Group
Northwestern University Speech & Language
  Clinic
2299 N. Campus Drive
Evanston, IL 60208

Stroke/Aphasia
Ann Oehring
(847) 491-5012

La Grange

Aphasia Community Group
Columbia-LaGrange Memorial
  Hospital/Rehab Dept
5101 S. Willow Springs Road
LaGrange, IL 60525

Stroke/Aphasia
Kara Torri
(708)352-1200, ext. 4769

Wheaton

Aphasia Support Group
Marionjoy Rehab Hospital
26 West 171 Roosevelt Road
P.O. Box 795
Wheaton, IL 60189

Stroke/Aphasia
Michele Wesling
(630) 462-4226

INDIANA

Dept of Aging and Community Services
251 N. Illinois St.
P.O. Box 7083
Indianapolis, IN 46207
(317) 232-7006

Bloomington

Indiana University Aphasia Support Group   Aphasia
Indiana Univeristy Speech and Hearing Center   Laura Murray, Ph.D.
200 S. Jordan Avenue   (812) 855-6251
Bloomington, IN 47405

Elkhart

Elkhart Area Aphasia Support Group   Aphasia
Elkhart Hospital   Judy Loutzenhiser
600 East Boulevard   (219) 295-7628
Elkhart, IN 46516

Goshen

Goshen Community Aphasia Group   Aphasia
P.O. Box 723   Susan Woodhull
Goshen, IN 46526   (219) 262-1471

Richmond

Oakridge Stroke Club   Stroke/Aphasia
Oakridge Rehab Center   Mary Felty
1042 Oak Drive   (765) 966-7788, ext. 47
Richmond, IN 47374

South Bend

St. Joseph's Aphasia Community Group   Aphasia
St. Joseph's Medical Center   Judy Loutzenhiser
801 E. LaSalle   (219) 295-7628
South Bend, IN 46634

IOWA

Department of Elder Affairs
Suite 236, Jewett Bldg.
914 Grand Avenue
Des Moines, IA 50319
(515) 281-5187

Des Moines

The Aphasia Group
Mercy Hospital Center/Laurel Center
300 Laurel Street
Des Moines, IA 50314

Aphasia
Susan Fagg
(515)247-4434

The Stroke Club
Easter Seals Society of Iowa
2920 30th Street
Des Moines, IA 50310

Stroke/Aphasia
Julie Patten
(515) 274-1529, ext. 2

KANSAS

Department of Aging
610 W. Tenth
Topeka, KS 66612
(913) 296-4986

Hays

Northwest Kansas Stroke Support Group
Senior Citizens Center
201 E. 7th Street
Hays, KS 67601

Stroke/Aphasia
Gerry Heil
(913) 623-5695

Overland Park

MARH Motivators/Young Stroke Support Group
Mid America Rehab Hospital
5701 W. 110th Street
Overland Park, KS 66211

Stroke/Aphasia
Susan Ramsey
(913) 491-2400

KENTUCKY

Department for Aging Services
Department of Human Resources
DHR Bldg., 6th floor
275 E. Main Street
Frankfort, KY 40601
(502) 564-6930

LOUISIANA

Office of Elderly Affairs
P.O. Box 80374
Baton Rouge, LA 70898
(504) 925-1700

MAINE

Bureau of Maine's Elderly
Dept of Human Servies
State House-Station #11
Augusta, ME 04333
(207) 289-2561

MARYLAND

Office on Aging
State Office Bldg.
301 W. Preston Street, Room #1004
Baltimore, MD 21201
(301) 225-1102

Annapolis

Annapolis Stroke Club
701 Glenwood Avenue
Annapolis, MD 21401

Stroke/Aphasia
Nancy Tietge
(410) 263-6982

Bethesda

Young Stroke Group/Speech Therapy Group
10100 Old Georgetown Road
Bethesda, MD 20814

Stroke/Aphasia
Joan Lipman Green
(301) 664-4490

Columbia

Speakeasy
Florence Baines Senior Center
5470 BeAvenuerkill Road
Columbia, MD 21044

Stroke/Aphasia
Barbara Miller
(410) 313-7213

Glen Burnie

The Stroke Club
Comprehensive Rehab Care
200 Hospital Drive, Suite LL-10
Glen Burnie, MD 21061

Stroke/Aphasia
Linda Thompson
(410) 553-9714

Silver Spring

Speech Language Therapy Group
Montgomery County Stroke Club
P.O. Box 2052
Silver Spring, MD 20915

Stroke/Aphasia
Janet Gritz
(301) 622-2282

MASSACHUSETTS

Executive Office of Elder Affairs
38 Chauncy Street
Boston, MA 02111
(617) 727-7751

Boston

Aneurysm Group
Massachusetts General Hospital
Brain Injury & AVM Center
Vincent Burnham Bldg., BBK710
Fruit Street Boston, MA 02114

TBI/Stroke/Aphasia
Deidra Buckley
(617) 726-5531

Braintree

Aphasia Community Group
Braintree Hospital
250 Pond Street
Braintree, MA 02185

Aphasia
Meredith Hilditch
(617) 848-5353 ext-2196

Canton

Boston Aphasia Community Group
30 Pleasant Gardens Road
Canton, MA 02021

Aphasia
Barbara Wymer
(617) 828-0411

Framingham

Aphasia Support Group
Healthsouth Sports Medicine & Rehab
463 Worcester Road
Framingham, MA 01701

Aphasia
Sharon Wade
(508) 820-1208

Holyoke

Holyoke Hospital Aphasia Therapy Group
Holyoke Hospital
575 Beech Street
Holyoke, MA 01040

Aphasia
Esmat Ezzat
(413) 534-2508

Springfield

Aphasia Support Group
Weldon Center for Rehab/Mercy Hospital
233 Carew Street
Springfield, MA 01102-9012

Aphasia
Angela Mansolillo
(413) 748-6800

MICHIGAN

Office of Services to the Aging
P.O. Box 30026
Lansing, MI 48909
(517) 373-8230

Ann Arbor

Ann Arbor Aphasia Support Group
1111 East Catherine St
Ann Arbor, MI 48109

Aphasia
Sue Cowles
(313) 764-8440

Bay City

Bay Area Support Group
Bay Medical Center for Rehab
West Campus/3190 E. Midland Road
Bay City, MI 48708

Stroke/Aphasia
Michael Adamczyk
(517) 677-6736

Birmingham

Communication Loss Support Group
William Beaumont Hospital
Beaumont Rehab and Health Center
746 Purdy
Birmingham, MI 48009

Stroke/Aphasia
Group Leader
(248) 258-1090

Garden City

Stroke Support Group
Garden City Osteopathic Hospital
Nursing Rehab Unit
6245 N. Inkster Road
Garden City, MI 48135

Stroke/Aphasia
Stacy Suida, CTRS
(313) 458-4392

Kalamazoo

Aphasia/Language Maintenance Group
Van Riper Speech/Language & Hearing Clinic
Western Michigan University
1000 Oakland Drive
Kalamazoo, MI 49008

Aphasia
Clinic Secretary
(616) 387-8047

Kalamazoo Stroke Club
Coover Center
918 Jasper
Kalamazoo, MI 49001

Stroke/Aphasia
Dick Heinzelman
(616) 382-0515

Travenuerse City

Grand Travenuerse Area Stroke Club
Bethlehem Lutheran Church
1050 Peninsula Drive
Traverse City, MI 49684

Stroke/Aphasia
Jim Batsakis or April Ritner
(616) 935-6380

Troy

Cane & Able: Stroke Recovery Group
William Beaumont Hospital
44201 Dequindre Road
Troy, MI 48098

Stroke/Aphasia
Bob Dale or Polly McIlrath
(248) 828-6003

Wyandotte

Down River Aphasia Support Group
Wyandotte Hospital Rehab & Orthopedic Center
2300 Biddle Avenue
Wyandotte, MI 48192

Aphasia
Kathy Zych
(313) 284-4233, ext. 3290

MINNESOTA

Board on Aging
Metro Square Bldg., Room 204
Seventh & Robert Streets
St. Paul, MN 55101
(612) 296-2770

Crosby

Cuyuna Regional Medical Center
Crosby, MN 56441

Stroke/Aphasia
Elli Brennan
(218) 546-6861

Park Rapids

Headwaters Stroke Support Group
Park Rapids City Library
Highway 34
Park Rapids, MN 56470

Stroke/Aphasia
Roger Giddes
(218) 732-7135

MISSISSIPPI

Council on Aging
301 W. Pearl Street
Jackson, MI 39203
(601) 949-2013

MISSOURI

Division on Aging
Dept of Social Services
P.O. Box 1337; 505 Missouri Boulevard
Jefferson City, MO 65102
(314) 751-3082

NEBRASKA

Department of Aging
P.O. Box 95044-301; Centennial Mall-South
Lincoln, NB 68509
(402) 471-2307

LINCOLN

Madonna Outpatient Aphasia Group
Madonna Rehab Hospital
5401 South Street
Lincoln, NB 68506

Aphasia
Teresa Cloet
(402) 483-9873

NEVADA

Division on Aging
Department. of Human Resources
505 E. King Street
Kinkead Bldg., Room 101
Carson City, NV 89710
(702) 885-4210

NEW HAMPSHIRE

Council on Aging
105 London Road-Bldg. #3
Concord, NH 03301
(603) 271-2751

Manchester

Aphasia Support Group
Catholic Medical Center
100 McGregor Street
Manchester, NH 03102

Aphasia
Joyce A. Santostefano
(603) 641-6700

NEW JERSEY

Division on Aging
Department of Community Affairs
P.O. Box 2768; 363 W. State Street
Trenton, NJ 08625
(609) 292-4833

Camden

Stroke Club
Our Lady of Lourdes Medical Center
1600 Haddon Avenue
Camden, NJ 08103

Stroke/Aphasia
Jack Fujiki
(609) 757-3864

Madison

North Jersey Stroke Discussion Group
Grace Episcopal Church
4 Madison Avenue
Madison, NJ 07940

Stroke/Aphasia
Stanley Levine
(908) 754-6482

Newton

Newton Memorial Stroke Club
175 High Street
Newton, NJ 07860

Stroke/Aphasia
Mrs. Richard Maglin
(201) 729-7424

Rutherford

NJ Aphasia Community Support Group
55 Kip Avenue
Rutherford, NJ 07070

Aphasia
Nicholas Mikula, Jr.
(973) 523-3896

NEW MEXICO

State Agency on Aging
224 E. Palace Avenue, 4th Floor
La Villa Rivera Bldg.
Santa Fe, NM 87501
(505) 827-7640

NEW YORK

Office for the Aging
New York State Plaza
Agency Bldg. #2
Albany, NY 12223
(518) 474-4425

Bayside

Selfhelp Clearview Senior Center Stroke Club
208-11 26th Avenue
Bayside, NY 11360

Stroke/Aphasia
Audrey Barzideh, CSW
(718) 224-7888

Bronx

Aphasia Support Group (Veterans Only)
Bronx Veterans Affairs Medical Center (126)
130 W. Kingsbridge Road
Bronx, NY 10468

Aphasia
Natalie Sutcliffe
(718) 584-9000, ext. 6500

Lehman College Aphasia Community Group
Lehman College-Speech and Hearing Center
250 Bedfort Park Boulevard West
Bronx, NY 10468

Aphasia
Robert Goldfarb
(718) 960-6085

Stern Stroke Center Club NW-1
Montefoire Medical Center
111 E. 210th Street
Bronx, NY 10467

Stroke/Aphasia
Dan Rosenbaum
(718) 920-6402

Brooklyn

Communication Therapy Group
Brooklyn College-Speech and Hearing Center
2900 Bedford Avenue; Room 4400B
Brooklyn, NY 11210-2889

Stroke/Aphasia
Jerry Koller
(718) 951-5186

FOCUS (Families Organized for Community
    Understanding of Stroke)
Brooklyn College
Speech and Hearing Center
Brooklyn, NY 11210

Stroke/Aphasia
Sam Chwat
(212) 242-8435

Buffalo

The Aphasia Group
State University of New York at Buffalo
127 Park Hill
Buffalo, NY 14260

Aphasia
Carol Ann Sellers
(716) 645-3400, ext. 127

Buffalo Hearing and Speech Center
50 E. North Street
Buffalo, NY 14203

Stroke/Aphasia
Stephanie Grosshans
(716) 837-9541

Flushing

Stroke Club; Flushing Hospital   Stroke/Aphasia
45th Avenue & Parsons Boulevard   Lynn Antonelli
Flushing, NY 11355   (718) 670-5515

New York City

Aphasia Community Groups   Aphasia
Rusk Institute of Rehab Medicine   Karen Riedel
400 E. 34th Street   (212) 263-6027
New York, NY 10016

STAS (Surviving and Thriving After Stroke)   Stroke/Aphasia
Dept of Rehab Medicine; Mt. Sinai Hospital   Helene Goldstein
1 Gust Avenue L. Levy Place   (212) 241-9188
New York, NY 10029-6574

Manhattan Stroke Survivors Club   Aphasia
400 Central Park West; Apt. 8R   Samuel Freedman
New York, NY 10026   (212) 666-3269

Port Jefferson

St. Charles Hospital Aphasia Group   Aphasia
Rehab Center; 200 Belle Terre Road   Michelle Zlotnick
Port Jefferson, NY 11777   (516) 474-6330

St. Albans

Communication Group (for Veterans)   Stroke/Aphasia
Veterans Administration Hospital   Milena Ippilito-Micek
1262 Linden Blvd and 179th Street   (718) 526-1000, ext. 3744
St. Albans, NY 11425

Staten Island

Staten Island University Hospital   Stroke/Aphasia
Stroke Self-Help Group   Josephine Greico
475 Seaview Avenue   (718) 226-9173
Staten Island, NY 10305

Syracuse

Survivors of Stroke Luncheon Group   Stroke/Aphasia
Arise, Inc.   Joseph Lincoln
501 E. Sayette Street   (315) 472-3171
Syracuse, NY 13202

White Plains

Aphasia Group
Burke Rehab Center of White Plains
72 Chase Road
Scarsdale, NY 10583

Aphasia
Barbara Martin
(914) 723-7006

Stroke Support Groups
White Plains Hospital
Davis Avenue & E. Post Road
White Plains, NY 10601

Stroke/Aphasia
Ilana Kafkafi
(914) 681-1114

NORTH CAROLINA

Division on Aging
1985 Umpstead Drive; Kirby Bldg.
Raleigh, NC 27603
(919) 733-3983

Burlington

Alamance County Stroke Club
Alamance Regional Medical, Rehab Services
1240 Huffman Mill Road
Burlington, NC 27215

Stroke/Aphasia
Lisa Pennington
(910) 538-7500

Charlotte

Charlotte Mecklenburg Stroke Club
Charlotte Institute of Rehab
1100 Blythe Boulevard
Charlotte, NC 28203

Stroke/Aphasia
Marla Porter
(704) 355-4395

Concord

Cebarrus Stroke Club
42 Hillcrest Avenue S.E.
Concord, NC 28025

Stroke/Aphasia
Gene MacRae
(704) 782-4023

Durham

Durham VA Medical Center Stroke Support Group
Audiology & Speech Pathology Service (126)
508 Fulton Street
Durham, NC 27705

Stroke/Aphasia
Candice Scharver
(919) 286-0411, ext. 6328

Fayetteville

Fayetteville Stroke Club
Southeastern Regional Rehab Center
1638 Owen Drive
Fayetteville, NC 28302

Stroke/Aphasia
Betsy Robbins
(910) 609-6520

Greensboro

Guilford County Stroke Club
Moses H. Cone Hospital
1200 Elm Street
Greensboro, NC 27401

Stroke/Aphasia
Elizabeth Hildreth P.T.
(910) 574-8120

Henderson

Vance/Granville Stroke Club
Med Visit
1924 Ruin Creek Road
Henderson, NC 27536

Stroke/Aphasia
Emily Moss
(919) 438-8461

Hickory

Frye Stroke and Head Injury Group
Frye Regional Rehab Center
420 N. Center
Hickory, NC 28601

Stroke/Aphasia
Marsha Sigmon
(704) 324-3603

Mooresville

Mooresville Stroke Club
Lake Norman Regional Medical Center
610 E. Center Avenue
Mooresville, NC 28115

Stroke/Aphasia
Juanita Davis
(704) 664-5554

Pinehurst

Moore County Stroke Club
Moore Regional Hospital Auditorium
P.O. Box 3000; Page Road
Pinehurst, NC 28374

Stroke/Aphasia
Leslie Gentry/Sandy Black
(910) 215-1658

Wilmington

New Hanover Stroke Club
New Hanover Regional Medical Center
P.O. Box 9000
2131 S. 17th Street
Wilmington, NC 28403

Stroke/Aphasia
Sharon Roberts
(910) 815-5615

NORTH DAKOTA

Aging Services
Department of Human Services
State Capitol Bldg.
Bismarck, ND 58505
(701) 224-2577

Fargo

Together Group
Merit Care Hospital
720 4th Street N
Fargo, ND 58122

Stroke/Aphasia
Marion Sansted
(701) 235-2583

OHIO

Department on Aging
50 W. Broad St-9th floor
Columbus, OH 43215
(614) 466-5500

Akron

Stroke Support Group
Edwin Shaw Rehab Hospital
1621 Flickinger
Akron, OH 44312

Stroke/Aphasia
Denise Simcox
(216) 784-2174, ext. 502

Dayton

Miami Valley Hospital Aphasia Support Group
Speech Pathology Department
1 Wyoming Street
Dayton, OH 45409

Aphasia
Gail Waddell
(513) 208-6277

Oxford

Miami Speech and Hearing Stroke Support Group
Dept. of Communications
Miami University
162 Bachelor Hall
Oxford, OH 45056

Stroke/Aphasia
Louise Van Vliet
(513) 529-2500

OKLAHOMA

Special Unit on Aging
Department on Human Services
P.O. Box 25352
Oklahoma City, OK 73125
(405) 521-2281

Edmond

The Northside Stroke Club
Horizon Specialty Hospital
1100 E. 9th Street
Edmond, OK 73034

Stroke/Aphasia
Case Manager
(405) 341-8150

Oklahoma City

Aphasia Support Group
Integris Jim Thorpe Rehab Hospital
   at South West Medical Center
4219 S. Western
Oklahoma City, OK 73109

Aphasia
Gary Brotherton
(405) 644-5281

OREGON

Senior Services Division
313 Public Service Bldg.
Salem, OR 97310
(503) 378-4728

Corvallis

Corvallis Stroke Club
ORI/Easter Seals Society of Oregon
999 N.W. Circle Boulevard
Corvallis, OR 97330-1408

Stroke/Aphasia
Angela Latta
(541) 753-2273

PENNSYLVANIA

Department of Aging
231 State Street
Harrisburg, PA 17101
(717) 783-1550

Clarks Summit

Stroke Support Group of Allied Rehab Services
220 Barry Drive
Clarks Summit, PA 18411

Stroke/Aphasia
Jean Preston
(717) 587-1035

Darby

The One-Step-at-a-Time Stroke Club
Mercy Fitzgerald Hospital
1500 Lansdowne Avenue
Darby, PA 19023

Stroke/Aphasia
John Brown
(610) 237-4289

Erie

Stroke Support Group
HealthSouth Great Lakes Rehab Hospital
143 E. 2nd Street
Erie, PA 16507

Stroke/Aphasia
Lorri MacIssac, MS., CCC-SLP/L
(814) 878-1385

Lancaster

Stroke Survivors Club
Homestead Village
1800 Village Circle
Lancanster, PA 17604

Stroke/Aphasia
Nancy Cavanaugh
(717) 291-8383

Philadelphia

Magee Rehab Aphasia Community Support Group
Six Franklin Plaza
Philadelphia, PA 19102

Aphasia
Debora DiRaddo
(215) 587-3204

Friends of Moss Rehab Aphasia Center
Moss Rehab Hospital
1200 W. Tabor Road
Philadelphia, PA 19141

Aphasia
Fran Gross
(215) 456-9025

Pittsburgh

Aphasia Support Group of Western Pennsylvania
Passavant Hospital
9100 Babcock Boulevard
Pittsburgh, PA 15237

Aphasia
Jack Simon
(412) 487-3320

Conversation/Stroke Survivors Groups (Vets only)
VA Pittsburgh Healthcare System
7180 Highland Drive
Pittsburgh, PA 15206

Stroke/Aphasia
Kristie Spencer
(412) 365-5112

Reading

Aphasia Support Group
Reading Rehab Hospital
1623 Morgantown Road
Reading, PA 19607

Aphasia
Kathy Longenecker
(610) 796-6423

Scranton

Marywood University Adult Aphasia Group
2300 Adams Avenue
Scranton, PA 18509

Aphasia
Janet Bisset, Ph.D.
(717) 348-6299

Wilkes Barre

Stroke Support Group
John Heinz Institute
150 Mundy Street
Wilkes Barre, PA 18702

Stroke/Aphasia
Jane Novinger
(717) 826-3890

RHODE ISLAND

Department of Elderly Affairs
79 Washington Street
Providence, RI 02903

PROVIDENCE

The Aphasia Support Group
Roger Williams Medical Center
Speech Pathology Dept.
825 Chalkstone Avenue
Providence, RI 02908

Aphasia
Gloria Gemma
(401) 456-2228

SOUTH CAROLINA

Commission on Aging
915 Main Street
Columbia, SC 29201
(803) 758-2576

SOUTH DAKOTA

Office of Adult Services and Aging
700 N. Illinois Street
Kneip Bldg.
Pierre, SD 57501
(605) 773-3656

TENNESSEE

Commission on Aging
706 Church Street, Suite 201
Nashville, TN 37219
(615) 741-2056

Memphis

Stroke and Aphasia Clubs of Memphis
Raymond F. Skinner Center
712 Tanglewood
Memphis, TN 38104

Stroke/Aphasia
Joan and Jim Cunningham
(901) 937-7545

Stroke Club East Central Church
6655 Winchester
Memphis, TN 38115

Stroke/Aphasia
Jean Miller
(901) 375-8140

Nashville

Aphasia Community Group
Vanderbilt Stallworth Rehab Hospital
2201 Capers Avenue
Nashville, TN 37212

Aphasia
Patty Hammond
(615) 963-4057

TEXAS

Department on Aging
P.O. Box 12786 Capitol Station
1949 IH 35, South
Austin, TX 78741
(512) 444-6890

Amarillo

People with Aphasia & Language Difficulties
　　of the Golden Spread (PALDOGS)
Sports & Occupational Medicine Center
5111 Canyon Drive
Amarillo, TX 79110

Stroke/Aphasia
Maggie Stear
(806) 467-7071

Arlington

Aphasia Support Group
3301 Matlock Road
Arlington, TX 76015

Aphasia
Karen Burnette
(817) 472-4849

Dallas

Dallas Community Aphasia Support Group
Vickery Towers at Belmont Retirement Center
Belmont & Greenville Streets
Dallas, TX 75206

Aphasia
Jan Murphy Babler
(214) 826-2325

North Texas Stroke Survivors
8543 Stillwater Drive
Dallas, TX 75243

Stroke/Aphasia
Pat Boland
(800) 553-6321

Denton

Denton Area Stroke Club
1008 University Drive (Wyatt's Cafateria)
Denton, TX 76201

Stroke/Aphasia
Lucy Trail
(817) 458-7786

VERMONT

Office on Aging
103 S. Main Street
Waterbury, VT 05676
(802) 241-2400

VIRGINIA

Department on Aging
101 N. 14th Street;18th floor
James Monroe Bldg
Richmond, VA 23219
(804) 225-2271

Falls Church

The Northern Virginia Brain Injury Association   TBI/Stroke/Aphasia
Falls Church High School   Kay Kehoe
7521 Jaguar Trail   (703) 978-7975
Falls Church, VA 22042

Fisherville

Shenandoah Valley Stroke Club   Stroke/Aphasia
P.O. Box 1000   Karen Cook
Fisherville, VA 22939   (540) 932-4030

WASHINGTON

Aging and Adult Services Administration
Department of Social & Health Services
OB-44A
Olympia, WA 98504
(206) 753-2502

Bremerton

Green Mountain Rehab   Stroke/Aphasia
900 Pacific Avenue   Sharon Feeney
Bremerton, WA 98337   (360) 373-9119

Everett

Everett Stroke Support Group   Stroke/Aphasia
Providence Center for Outpatient Rehab   Mary Ann Varnum
2940 W. Marine View Drive   (206) 258-7984
Everett, WA 98201

Mt. Vernon

Skajit Valley Stroke Support Group
Labor and Industries Meeting Room
525 College Way, Suite H
Mt. Vernon, WA 98273

Stroke/Aphasia
Barbara Bond-Howard, MA, CTRS
(360) 757-0476

Seattle

North West Hospital
Center for Medical Rehab
1550 North 115th Street
Seattle, WA 98133

Stroke/Aphasia
Joan Jaeger
(206) 368-1769

Tacoma

Tacoma Area Stroke Support Group
6315 S. 19th Street
Tacoma, WA 98465

Stroke/Aphasia
Mary Kelly
(206) 752-2675

Vancouver

Vancouver Stroke Club
Southwest Washington Medical Center
400 Mother Joseph Place
Vancouver, WA 98668

Stroke/Aphasia
Belva Watson
(360) 892-6947

WEST VIRGINIA

Commission on Aging
Holly Grove-State Capitol
Charleston, WV 25305
(304) 348-3317

Morgantown

HealthSouth MountainView Stroke
   Support Group
HealthSouth MountainView Regional
   Rehab Hospital
1160 Van Voorhis Road
Morgantown, WV 26505

Stroke/Aphasia
Gina Mazure
(304) 598-1100, ext. 2430

WISCONSIN

Bureau of Aging
Division of Community Services
One West Wilson St, Room 480
Madison, WI 53702

(608) 266-2536

Madison

Madison Area Stroke Club
Meritor Hospital
202 S. Park Street
Madison , WI 53705

Stroke/Aphasia
Debbie Brey
(608) 267-6173

Mazomanie

Living with Aphasia, Inc.
6344 Hillsandwood Road
Mazomanie, WI 53560

Aphasia
Jon G. Lyon
(608) 767-3838

Milwaukee

St. Luke's Aphasia Support Group
St. Luke's Hospital
2900 Oklahoma Avenue
P.O. Box 2901
Milwaukee, WI 53215-2901

Stroke/Aphasia
Janice Secreto-Pfaffl
(414) 649-7772

WYOMING

Commission on Aging
Hathaway Bldg.-Room 139
Cheyenne, WY 82002
(307) 777-6111

International Agencies

The Association Internationale Aphasie in Brussels offers a guide for people seeking information about individual and group treatment services throughout the world. Their address is:

> Association Internationale Aphasie
> Avenue des Héros, 50
> B 1160 BRUXELLES
> Phone: 32.2.672.40.51
> Fax: 32.2.675.12.45

Countries listed in this resource guide are: Austria, Australia, Argentina, Bahamas, Belgium, Canada, Czechoslovakia, Denmark, Finland, France, Great Britain, Greece, Iceland, India, Ireland, Italy, Luxembourg, Malaysia, Netherlands, New Zealand, Norway, Poland, Portugal, Senegal, Spain, Sweden, Switzerland, and United States

CANADA

Alberta (English speaking)

Neighborhood Chat
Capital Health, Suite 300
10216 124th Street
Edmonton, Alberta T5N 4A3

Stroke/Aphasia
Coordinator, Neighborhood CHAT
(403) 413-7982

Montreal (French speaking)

Association Québecoise des Personnes Aphasiques
Centre de recherche due Centre hospitalier
   Côte-des-Neiges
4565 Chemin Reine-Marie
Montréal, Québec H3W 1W5

Aphasia
Claire Charest
(514) 340-3540

Quebec (French speaking)

Association des Personnes Intéressées a L'aphasie
525 Boulevard Hamel Est
CDN Quebec G1M 2S8

Aphasia
Marie-Marc Coté
(418) 647-3684

Ottawa (English and French speaking)

Aphasia Centre of Ottawa-Carleton
211 Bronson Avenue
Ottawa, Ontario KIR 6J5

Aphasia
Gillian Gailey
(613) 567-1119

Metro Toronto (English speaking)

The Pat Arato Aphasia Centre
53 The Links Road
North York, Ontario M2P 1T7

Aphasia
Aura Kagan
(416) 226-3636

St John's (English speaking)

Stroke/Aphasia
L.A. Miller Centre
100 Forest Road
St. John's, NF A1B 3V6

Stroke Survivors Support Group
Judy Wells
(709) 737-6560

York and Durham Regions (English speaking groups, although consultation given in other languages)

York-Durham Aphasia Centre
12184 Ninth Line
Stouffville, Ontario L4A 3N6

Aphasia
Ruth Patterson
(905) 642-2053

GREAT BRITAIN

There are numerous support and self-help groups for people confronting aphasia throughout England. The best way to sort out which might serve your needs is to contact:

Action for Dysphasic Adults
1 Royal Street
London SE1 7LL
Phone: 0171-261-9572
Fax: 0171-928-9542

Agencies or businesses providing technical or treatment-related assistance, materials, or aids

Communication aids

CAUTION: Visual communication aids to supplement spoken language have been available for decades. Of late, the computer age has resulted in a number of new products with varied claims and functions. Such communicative supplements have proven particularly valuable for children and for adults with poor or minimal speech but intact language and cognition. Aphasia, though, is a disorder of language. Therefore, selection of symbols (regardless of their form) for people with aphasia is **not** as "simple" or "assured" as it may be claimed! Prior to purchasing any supplemental device, be sure that its benefits complement your loved one's needs and linguistic skills. A certified speech-language pathologist should be able to assist you in making informed choices.

Attainment Company, Inc.
P.O. Box 930160
Verona, WI 53593-0160
(800) 327-4269
Supplier of many augmentative options for communication. Free catalog available.

Crestwood Company
6625 N. Sidney Place
Milwaukee, WI 53209
(414) 352-5678
Manufacturer of supplemental communication devices and boards. Free catalog available.

IBM Special Needs Systems
1000 N.W. 51st Street
Boca Raton, FL 33432
(800) 426-4832
Information on computers that may help people with communication difficulties. See note above. Free literature available.

Imaginart
307 Arizona St
Bisbee, AZ 85603
(800) 828-1326
Manufacturer of visual communication alternatives, also producer of treatment materials. Free catalog available.

Innocomp
26210 Emery Road, Suite 302
Warrensville Heights, OH 44125
(800) 382-8622
Manufacturer of supplemental communication products. Free catalog available.

Interactive Therapeutics, Inc.
P.O. Box 1805
Stow, OH 44224-0805
(800) 253-5111
Manufacturer of visual communication alternatives. Catalog available.

Lifeline Systems, Inc.
640 Memorial Drive
Cambridge, MA 02139-4851
(800) 543-3546
Manufacturer a telephone-based alerting system that permits nonspeaking individuals to access emergency services. Free brochures available.

Prentke Romich Co.
1022 Heyl Road
Wooster, OH 44691
(800) 262-1984
Manufacturer of augmentative communication devices. Free catalog available.

Trace Research and Development Center
Waisman Center
University of Wisconsin
1500 Highland Avenue
Madison, WI 53707-2280
(608) 262-6966
Center for research and development of technical devices to help augment the needs of nonspeakers.

Communication materials

CAUTION: As with visual or computer-based aids, so too, treatment or language stimulation materials require careful selection and monitoring. It is essential that they be properly geared to needs and skill levels. Randomly selecting from such materials can be more detrimental than beneficial. Consult with a trained professional before proceeding.

Communication Skill Builders
3830 E. Bellevue
P.O. Box 42050
Tucson, AZ 85733
(602) 323-7500
Offers a variety of stimulus materials and augmentative communication aids.

Creative Learning
206 Sacramento Street, Suite 305
Nevada City, CA 95959
(916) 265-0584
Offers specialized software for people attempting to recovery from stroke and aphasia.

Imaginart
307 Arizona Street
Bisbee, AZ 85603
(800) 828-1376
Manufactures picture stimuli, treatment workbooks, and interactive exercises.

Interactive Therapeutics, Inc
P.O. Box 1850
Stow, OH 44224-0805
(800) 253-5111
Produces communication boards and booklets for verbally restricted adults.

Parrot Software
P.O. Box 250755
West Bloomfield, MI 48325-0755
(800) PARROT-1
Offers a variety of software programs for speech and language stimulation.

Recreational materials

Access Tours
P.O. Box 2985
Jackson, WY 83001
(800) 929-4811
Travel-related materials for the Western United States for people with restricted mobility.

Access Living
310 S. Peoria Street, Suite 201
Chicago, IL 60607
(312) 226-5900
Provides information and assistance geared toward maintaining optimal independence in daily life, especially for individuals with physical disabilities.

Access to Recreation
2509 E. Thousand Oaks Boulevard, Suite 430
Thousand Oaks, CA 91360
(800) 634-4351
Provides a catalog of adaptive devices that may help individuals with a hemiparesis increase their ease with activities such as bowling, fishing, or hunting.

Independent Living Aids, Inc.
27 East Mall
Plainview, NY 11803-44-4
(516) 752-8080
Personal and recreational aids to improve
independence. Catalog available.

Outdoors Forever
P.O. Box 4832
East Lansing, MI 48823
(517) 337-0018
Plans and organizes outdoor activities for
persons with disabilities.

Wilderness Inquiry
1313 Fifth Street SE, Suite 327
Minneapolis, MN 55414
(612) 379-3858
Plans and guides wilderness outings for
people with or without physical impairments.

Resource information

AbleData
8455 Colesville Rd, Suite 935
Silver Spring, MD 20910
(800) 227-0216
A database company that provides information on assistive technology for people with
physical, sensory, or cognitive limitations.

Adaptability
Dept 2228
Colchester, CT 06415
(800) 288-9941
Products for independent living, mobility
aids. Free Catalog

Communicative Disorders Clinic
1111 E. Catherine
University of Michigan
Ann Arbor, MI 48109-2054
Publishes a resource guide for consumers,
also hosts an annual gathering for adults
with aphasia and their caregivers.

National Stroke Association
8480 E. Orchard Rd, Suite 1000
Englewood, CO 80111-5015
(800) 787-6537
Publishes an extensive consumer's guide
entitled, *Adaptive Resources*.

Index